T0226421

Cerebellar Diseases

Editors

ALIREZA MINAGAR
ALEJANDRO A. RABINSTEIN

NEUROLOGIC CLINICS

www.neurologic.theclinics.com

Consulting Editor
RANDOLPH W. EVANS

November 2014 • Volume 32 • Number 4

ELSEVIER

1600 John F. Kennedy Boulevard • Suite 1800 • Philadelphia, Pennsylvania, 19103-2899

http://www.theclinics.com

NEUROLOGIC CLINICS Volume 32, Number 4
November 2014 ISSN 0733-8619, ISBN-13: 978-0-323-32660-5

Editor: Joanne Husovski
Developmental editor: Donald Mumford

Neurologic Clinics (ISSN 0733-8619) is published quarterly by Elsevier Inc., 360 Park Avenue South, New York, NY 10010–1710. Months of issue are February, May, August, and November. Periodicals postage paid at New York, NY, and additional mailing offices. Subscription prices are $300.00 per year for US individuals, $517.00 per year for US institutions, $145.00 per year for US students, $375.00 per year for Canadian individuals, $627.00 per year for Canadian institutions, $415.00 per year for international individuals, $627.00 per year for international institutions, and $210.00 for Canadian and foreign students/residents. To receive student/resident rate, orders must be accompanied by name of affiliated institution, date of term, and the *signature* of program/residency coordinator on institution letterhead. Orders will be billed at individual rate until proof of status is received. Foreign air speed delivery is included in all *Clinics* subscription prices. All prices are subject to change without notice. **POSTMASTER:** Send address changes to *Neurologic Clinics*, Elsevier Health Sciences Division, Subscription Customer Service, 3251 Riverport Lane, Maryland Heights, MO 63043. **Customer Service: Telephone: 1-800-654-2452 (U.S. and Canada); 314-447-8871 (outside U.S. and Canada). Fax: 314-447-8029. E-mail: journalscustomerservice-usa@elsevier.com (for print support); journalsonlinesupport-usa@elsevier.com (for online support).**

Reprints. For copies of 100 or more of articles in this publication, please contact the Commercial Reprints Department, Elsevier Inc., 360 Park Avenue South, New York, New York, 10010-1710; Tel.: +1-212-633-3874; Fax: +1-212-633-3820, and E-mail: reprints@elsevier.com.

Neurologic Clinics is also published in Spanish by Nueva Editorial Interamericana S.A., Mexico City, Mexico.

Neurologic Clinics is covered in *Current Contents/Clinical Medicine, MEDLINE/PubMed (Index Medicus), EMBASE/Excerpta Medica, and PsycINFO, and ISI/BIOMED.*

Contributors

CONSULTING EDITOR

RANDOLPH W. EVANS, MD
Clinical Professor of Neurology, Baylor College of Medicine, Houston, Texas

EDITORS

ALIREZA MINAGAR, MD, FAAN, FANA
Professor, Department of Neurology, LSU Health Sciences Center Shreveport;
Department of Psychiatry, Overton Brooks VA Medical Center, Shreveport, Louisiana

ALEJANDRO A. RABINSTEIN, MD, FAAN, FANA
Department of Neurology, Mayo Clinic, Rochester, Minnesota

AUTHORS

HESAM AKBARIAN-TEFAGHI, BS
Department of Neurosurgery, LSU Health Sciences Center Shreveport, Shreveport, Louisiana

NADEJDA ALEKSEEVA, MD
Department of Psychiatry, Overton Brooks VA Medical Center, Shreveport, Louisiana

SUDHEER AMBEKAR, MD
Department of Neurosurgery, LSU Health Sciences Center Shreveport, Shreveport, Louisiana

SHIN C. BEH, MD
Department of Neurology, University of Texas Southwestern Medical Center, Dallas, Texas

BRITTANI CONWAY, MD
Neurology Resident, Department of Neurology, Jackson Memorial Hospital, Miami, Florida

SUDHIR DATAR, MD
Department of Neurology, Mayo Clinic, Rochester, Minnesota

DEBRA E. DAVIS, MD
Associate Professor of Clinical Neurology, Department of Neurology, LSU Health Sciences Center Shreveport, Shreveport, Louisiana

LOURDES M. DᴇʟROSSO, MD, FAASM
Assistant Professor of Pediatrics, University of Pennsylvania School of Medicine, Sleep Physician, The Children's Hospital of Philadelphia, Philadelphia, Pennsylvania

ELLIOT M. FROHMAN, MD, PhD
Departments of Neurology and Ophthalmology, University of Texas Southwestern Medical Center, Dallas, Texas

TERESA C. FROHMAN, PA-C
Department of Neurology, University of Texas Southwestern Medical Center, Dallas, Texas

EDUARDO GONZALEZ-TOLEDO, MD, PhD
Department of Radiology, LSU Health Sciences Center Shreveport, Shreveport, Louisiana

BHARAT GUTHIKONDA, MD, FACS
Associate Professor, Department of Neurosurgery, LSU Health Sciences Center Shreveport, Shreveport, Louisiana

ROMY HOQUE, MD, FAASM
Assistant Professor of Neurology, LSU Health Sciences Center Shreveport, Shreveport, Louisiana

RONAK JANI, MD
Neuroimaging Fellow, DENT Neurologic Institute, Amherst, New York

VIJAYAKUMAR JAVALKAR, MD, MCh
Resident, Department of Neurology, LSU Health Sciences Center Shreveport, Shreveport, Louisiana

ROGER E. KELLEY, MD
Department of Neurology, Tulane University School of Medicine, New Orleans, Louisiana

MISBBA KHAN, MD
Former Resident, Department of Neurology, LSU Health Sciences Center Shreveport, Shreveport, Louisiana

AMIR HADI MAGHZI, MD
Department of Neurology, University of California, San Francisco, San Francisco, California

CORY MARKHAM, BS
Department of Neurosurgery, LSU Health Sciences Center Shreveport, Shreveport, Louisiana

JEANIE McGEE, DHEd, MSHS
Department of Neurology, LSU Health Sciences Center Shreveport, Shreveport, Louisiana

LASZLO MECHTLER, MD
Professor of Neurology and Oncology, DENT Neurologic Institute, Roswell Park Cancer Institute, Buffalo, New York

ALIREZA MINAGAR, MD, FAAN, FANA
Professor, Department of Neurology, LSU Health Sciences Center Shreveport; Department of Psychiatry, Overton Brooks VA Medical Center, Shreveport, Louisiana

KEVIN MORROW, BS
Department of Neurosurgery, LSU Health Sciences Center Shreveport, Shreveport, Louisiana

ANIL NANDA, MD, FACS
Chairman, Department of Neurosurgery, LSU Health Sciences Center Shreveport, Shreveport, Louisiana

ARASH NAZERI, MD
MS Research Center, Neuroscience Institute, Tehran University of Medical Sciences; Interdisciplinary Neuroscience Research Program, Tehran University of Medical Sciences, Tehran, Iran; Kimel Family Translational Imaging-Genetics Research Laboratory, Centre for Addiction and Mental Health, University of Toronto, Toronto, Canada

MENARVIA NIXON, MD
Department of Neurosurgery, LSU Health Sciences Center Shreveport, Shreveport, Louisiana

MARYAM NOROOZIAN, MD
Director, Associate Professor of Neurology, Memory and Behavioral Neurology Division, Department of Psychiatry, Tehran University of Medical Sciences, Tehran, Iran

THOMAS J. PFIFFNER, MD
Neuroimaging Fellow, DENT Neurologic Institute, Amherst, New York

AMY A. PRUITT, MD
Professor of Neurology, University of Pennsylvania, Philadelphia, Pennsylvania

ALEJANDRO A. RABINSTEIN, MD, FAAN, FANA
Department of Neurology, Mayo Clinic, Rochester, Minnesota

TINA ROOSTAEI, MD, MPH
MS Research Center, Neuroscience Institute, Tehran University of Medical Sciences; Interdisciplinary Neuroscience Research Program, Tehran University of Medical Sciences, Tehran, Iran

MOHAMMAD ALI SAHRAIAN, MD
Associate Professor, Department of Neurology, Sina Hospital, Tehran University of Medical Sciences; Head, MS Research Center, Neuroscience Institute, Tehran University of Medical Sciences, Tehran, Iran

ALIA SHAKIBA, MD
Psychiatrist, Department of Psychiatry, Tehran University of Medical Sciences, Tehran, Iran

WILLIAM SHEREMATA, MD, FRCP(C), FACP, FAAN
Professor Emeritus of Clinical Neurology, University of Miami, Multiple Sclerosis Center of Excellence; Department of Neurology, Multiple Sclerosis Center of Excellence, Miller School of Medicine, Miami, Florida

LETICIA TORNES, MD
Assistant Professor, Clinical Neurology, University of Miami, Multiple Sclerosis Center of Excellence; Department of Neurology, Multiple Sclerosis Center of Excellence, Miller School of Medicine, Miami, Florida

SHIHAO ZHANG, MD
Department of Neurosurgery, LSU Health Sciences Center Shreveport, Shreveport, Louisiana

Contents

have cerebellar manifestations once they enter the progressive stages of the disease. Of the cerebellar findings, tremor is by far the most common.

Cerebellar infarction presents with symptoms of nausea, vomiting, and dizziness and thus mimics benign conditions such as viral gastroenteritis or labyrinthitis, which constitutes a good proportion of patients seen in the emergency department. A physician is often faced with the task of identifying the few cases in which cerebellar stroke is the underlying cause instead. In-depth knowledge of the signs and symptoms of cerebellar infarction is therefore essential. Large infarctions or the ones with hemorrhagic conversion can lead to tissue swelling and complications such as obstructive hydrocephalus and brainstem compression. This article summarizes the current multidisciplinary approach to cerebellar stroke.

The clinical presentation of cerebellar hemorrhage can range from symptoms mimicking ischemic stroke to catastrophic neurologic decline. Symptomatology largely depends on the size of the hemorrhage and the degree of perilesional edema. The posterior fossa is a tight compartment with virtually no additional space to accommodate the mass effect. Thus, the hematoma and its associated swelling can cause obstructive hydrocephalus and brainstem compression, in severe cases contributing to early mortality, but outcome can be good if surgical intervention is appropriately timed. This article summarizes the current multidisciplinary approach to cerebellar hemorrhage, and addresses the controversies regarding its optimal management.

The cerebellum is responsible for refining ocular movements, thereby guaranteeing the best possible visual acuity and clarity despite changes in body or head positions or movement of the object of interest. The cerebellum is involved in the control of all eye movements, in their real-time, immediate modulation, and in their long-term adaptive calibration. The flocculus-paraflocculus complex and the caudal vermis (nodulus and uvula) together constitute the vestibulocerebellum. Lesions affecting these different regions give rise to 3 principal clinical cerebellar syndromes. This article discusses the various neuro-ophthalmic manifestations of various cerebellar disorders, as well as some therapeutic options for oscillopsia.

Our understanding of the contribution of the cerebellum to neurocognition is still in a nascent stage, essentially because of the historical neglect of the nonmotor role of the cerebellum. But it is also because the cerebellum acts primarily as a rather subtle modulator of neurocognitive processes. If this modulating function is impaired, deficits arise that are quantitatively and qualitatively different from the deficits produced by lesions of the supratentorial structures. This article reviews in further detail the current understanding of cognitive deficits associated with cerebellar impairments and unravels its modulating role in cognitive and behavioral processes.

For a long time, cerebellum was only known for its role in movement coordination and until recently, its role in non-motor brain function was largely ignored. Recent evidences has expanded the concept of coordination, from voluntary movements and orientation of the body to nearly every cerebral function including emotion regulation, social cognition, and time perception. This article aims to review the current evidences supporting the role of the cerebellum in the pathophysiology of psychiatric disorders, including studies using volumetric and/or functional imaging techniques, genetic and molecular studies, and clinical reports. The implication of these findings, their potential use, and future directions are also discussed.

Although the cerebellum can be affected by any infection that also involves other parts of the brain parenchyma, cerebrospinal fluid, or nerve roots, a limited range of infections targets cerebellar structures preferentially. Thus, a primarily cerebellar syndrome narrows infectious differential diagnostic considerations. The differential diagnosis of rapidly evolving cerebellar signs suggesting infection includes prescription or illicit drug intoxications or adverse reactions, inflammatory pseudotumor, paraneoplastic processes, and acute postinfectious cerebellitis. This article discusses the diagnosis and differential diagnosis of viral, bacterial, fungal, and prion pathogens affecting the cerebellum in patterns predictable by pace of illness and by involved neuroanatomic structures.

NEUROLOGIC CLINICS

RELATED INTEREST

Role of Neuroimaging in the Evaluation of Tremor,
February 2010 (Vol. 20, No. 1)
In Neuroimaging Clinics
Davina J. Hensman, and Peter G. Bain, *Editors*

NOW AVAILABLE FOR YOUR iPhone and iPad

Preface

Cerebellar Diseases

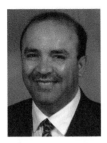 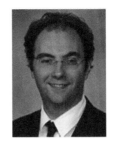

Alireza Minagar, MD, FAAN, FANA   Alejandro A. Rabinstein, MD, FAAN, FANA
Editors

For centuries, research and obtaining knowledge about the human cerebellum and its exact role in the regular function of the central nervous system have been eclipsed by numerous research efforts to unravel the mysteries within the rest of the human brain. Only recently, scientists have paid more attention to the cerebellum and its functions beyond a simple and smooth coordinator of human motor activities. Increasingly, knowledge and insight gained from molecular genetics, neuropathology, neuroimaging, and neuroanatomy have been applied to better understand the nature and pathophysiologic mechanisms of human cerebellar diseases. Now and more than ever in human history, we know and are still learning about the cerebellum and its physiology and pathophysiology. Gradually but persistently, the roles of this large and unique segment of the central nervous system, occupying the bulk of the posterior fossa, in activities beyond controlling the motor system are emerging. Presently, we are slowly understanding the complexities and delicacies of the cerebellar function and correlate them with the clinical features in our patients.

This interesting issue is entirely dedicated to the cerebellum and includes articles on its functional neuroanatomy and different cerebellar pathologies. Among the various excellent reviews contained in this issue, we find of particular interest two articles uniquely devoted to the role of the cerebellum in human cognition and psychiatric diseases. Clearly, the cerebellum is much more than a simple center for coordination of movements, and progressively its role in other aspects of human behavior is being uncovered.

We have been most fortunate to benefit from the expertise and collaboration of a number of world class neurologists, neurosurgeons, psychiatrists, neuroradiologists, and neuroscientists who eagerly and generously contributed their superb articles to this issue of *Neurologic Clinics*. We are eternally grateful to these wonderful individuals without whom this monograph would have never materialized. We also say thank you to the hardworking staff members at Elsevier and particularly Mr Donald Mumford and Ms Joanne Husovski, for their unwavering commitment during preparation of this

Neurol Clin 32 (2014) xiii–xiv
http://dx.doi.org/10.1016/j.ncl.2014.09.001
0733-8619/14/$ – see front matter © 2014 Elsevier Inc. All rights reserved.

neurologic.theclinics.com

issue. Finally, we appreciate our patients, who have taught us so much about the fascinating diseases of the cerebellum.

Alireza Minagar, MD, FAAN, FANA
Department of Neurology
LSU Health Sciences Center
Shreveport, LA 71130, USA

Alejandro A. Rabinstein, MD, FAAN, FANA
Department of Neurology
Mayo Clinic
200 First Street SW
Rochester, MN 55905, USA

E-mail addresses:
aminag@lsuhsc.edu (A. Minagar)
Rabinstein.alejandro@mayo.edu (A.A. Rabinstein)

The Human Cerebellum

A Review of Physiologic Neuroanatomy

Tina Roostaei, MD, MPH[a,b,1], Arash Nazeri, MD[a,b,c,1],
Mohammad Ali Sahraian, MD[a,d,*], Alireza Minagar, MD[e]

KEYWORDS

- Cerebellar lobules • Cerebellar circuitry • Compartmentalization • Plasticity
- Cerebellar connections

KEY POINTS

- Based on the afferent/efferent connections and functions, the cerebellum can be subdivided into the vestibulocerebellum, spinocerebellum, and cerebrocerebellum.
- Traditionally, the cerebellum is viewed as a brain region entirely devoted to motor control and learning; however, recent studies suggest that cerebellum is also engaged in cognitive and affective tasks.
- The cerebellar cortex is a 3-layered structure with stereotypical circuitry and distribution of cell types.
- The cerebellum consists of myriads of functional units (modules) that function independent of each of other.

The cerebellum (Latin for "little brain") is approximately one-tenth of the cerebrum in size and weight and is situated in the posterior cranial fossa. It is connected directly or indirectly to a variety of structures, including brainstem, spine, and diverse cerebral subcortical and cortical regions. The cerebellum contains almost 80% of the total brain neurons[1] and is composed of highly regular arrays of neuronal units, each sharing the same basic cerebellar microcircuitry. Its circuitry is classically viewed to be involved in motor control and motor learning. The cerebellum does not contribute

The authors have no conflict of interest to disclose.
[a] MS Research Center, Neuroscience Institute, Sina Hospital, Tehran University of Medical Sciences, Hassan Abad Square, Tehran 1136746911, Iran; [b] Interdisciplinary Neuroscience Research Program, Tehran University of Medical Sciences, Poursina Street, Tehran 1417863181, Iran; [c] Kimel Family Translational Imaging-Genetics Research Laboratory, Centre for Addiction and Mental Health, University of Toronto, 250 College Street, Toronto ON M5T 1R8, Canada; [d] Department of Neurology, Sina Hospital, Tehran University of Medical Sciences, Tehran 1136746911, Iran; [e] Department of Neurology, Louisiana State University-Health, 1501 Kings Highway, Shreveport, LA 71103, USA
[1] These authors contributed equally to this work.
* Corresponding author. MS Research Center, Neuroscience Institute, Sina Hospital, Hassan Abad Square, Tehran, Iran.
E-mail address: msahrai@tums.ac.ir

to movement initiation, and thus its damage is not associated with paralysis. However, coordinated, precise, and smooth execution of voluntary movements and their adaptive modification rely on an intact cerebellum. Moreover, there is an increasing recognition of the cerebellum's role in nonmotor cognitive and affective functions. In recent years, novel tools and resources have emerged that can spur new lines of research in cerebellar anatomy and physiology (**Box 1**).[2,3]

The first sections of this review describe neuroanatomy and major physiologic subdivisions and functions of the cerebellum. Next, histology and neural circuitry of the cerebellum along with cerebellar functional units are addressed. Lastly, relevance of cerebellar circuitry and firing patterns to motor learning are discussed.

LARGE-SCALE NEUROANATOMY OF THE CEREBELLUM

The cerebellum is located posterior to the brainstem and the fourth ventricle and is rostrally separated from the cerebrum by an extension of the dura matter called *tentorium cerebelli*. It consists of 2 lateral hemispheres and a narrow midline zone (ie, the cerebellar vermis, from the *Latin* for worm), and its surface has many parallel thin transverse folds called *folia* (**Fig. 1**). The cerebellum consists of an outer layer of highly convoluted gray matter (cerebellar cortex) surrounding a highly branched body of white matter known as the *arbor vitae* (Latin for "tree of life"), which in turn surrounds the 3 pairs of deep cerebellar nuclei embedded in the central cerebellar white matter (corpus medullare). From medial to lateral, the deep nuclei are the fastigial, interposed (consisting of globose and emboliform nuclei), and dentate nuclei. Anatomically, the cerebellum is divided into 3 lobes by 2 transverse fissures. The primary fissure separates the anterior from the posterior lobe, and the posterolateral fissure lies between the posterior and flocculonodular lobe. The cerebellum is further subdivided into 10 transverse lobules marked by Roman numerals (lobules I–X) (**Fig. 2**). Each lobe/lobule encompasses a central portion in the vermis along with the adjacent 2 lateral segments in the hemispheres.

The cerebellum is attached to the brainstem through its 3 pairs of peduncles (inferior, middle, and superior) (see **Fig. 1**A, B). All efferents and afferents of cerebellum

---

Box 1
Toolboxes and resources for studying the cerebellum

- Healthy aging, normal development, and various central nervous system disorders are associated with cerebellar atrophy and/or volume changes. Tools dedicated to investigating these cerebellar volume differences were recently developed (eg, spatially unbiased atlas template of the cerebellum and brainstem [SUIT],[15,16] multiple automatically generated templates of different brains [MAGeT-Brain][17,18]). These methods could be used to automatically generate volumetric measurements of the cerebellum and/or assess local cerebellar volume changes with voxel-wise approaches. Further, specific patterns of cerebellar volume changes/atrophy could be elucidated using these techniques.

- Human Connectome Project (http://www.humanconnectome.org/) seeks to explore structural and functional connectivity in the human brain. Advanced high-resolution functional, structural, and diffusion magnetic resonance images of cerebellum along with other structures are provided in this data set.[19]

- A useful resource for investigators who are interested in patterns of gene expression across cerebellum is transcriptomic databases. In the recent years, spatiotemporal transcriptomic maps of cerebellum have become publically available (cerebellar development transcriptome[20] and various datasets in the Allen brain atlas[21]).

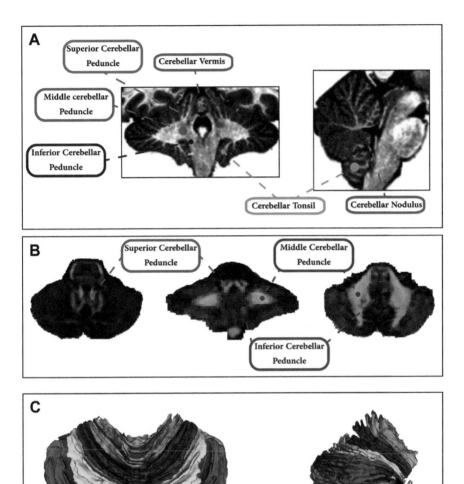

Fig. 1. Cerebellar gross anatomy. (*A*) Coronal (*left*) and sagittal (*right*) views of high-resolution magnetic resonance images of cerebellum with T1/T2 ratio contrast (to enhance white matter/gray matter contrast). (*B*) Axial (*left and right*) and coronal (*middle*) views of the cerebellar peduncles shown in color-coded directional maps (*red*: left–right, *green*: anterior–posterior, *blue*: inferior–superior) modulated by fractional anisotropy estimated from diffusion tensor imaging. (*C*) Superior (*left*) and lateral (*right*) views of 3-dimensional reconstruction of cerebellar surface (spatially unbiased infratentorial and cerebellar template [SUIT] atlas[15,16]). Lobules IV, V, VI, VIIA (crus I, crus II), VIIB, VIIIA, VIIIB, and IX are shown in different colors. ([*A*] *Adapted from* The Human Connectome Project public data. Available at: http://www.humanconnectome.org/. Accessed February 1, 2014.)

pass through these peduncles to reach their targets (**Table 1**). The middle cerebellar peduncle is the largest and is composed almost exclusively of pontocerebellar fibers that stem from the contralateral pontine nuclei and relay signals from the cerebral cortex. Lying medial to the middle cerebellar peduncle is the inferior peduncle, which consists of restiform (afferent) and juxtarestiform (mainly efferent) bodies. The superior

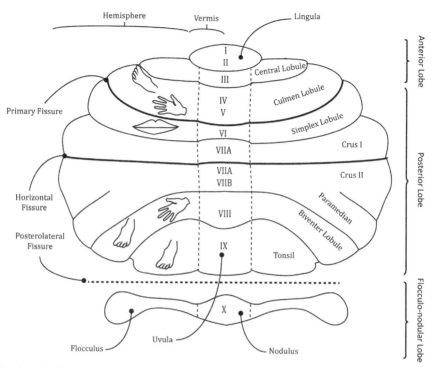

Fig. 2. Unfolded view of the cerebellar cortex showing lobes, fissures, lobules, along with cerebellar somatotopy (left cerebellum only).

peduncle is mainly composed of efferent fibers originating from the dentate and interposed nuclei and, to a smaller extent, the fastigial nucleus.

MEDIOLATERAL SUBDIVISIONS OF THE CEREBELLUM

Although from the anatomic viewpoint the cerebellum is divided into 3 major transverse lobes, this structure is functionally segregated longitudinally. Aside from the flocculonodular lobe (archicerebellum/vestibulocerebellum, a small and evolutionarily primitive part of the cerebellum), the medial (vermis) and intermediate (paravermis) lobes are most commonly called the *spinocerebellum*, with the lateral zone (hemispheres) regarded as the cerebrocerebellum.[4]

Vestibulocerebellum

The flocculonodular lobe receives vestibular inputs from the ipsilateral vestibular nerve (the only primary fibers reaching the cerebellum directly) and the vestibular nuclei (superior, medial, and inferior). It also receives visual inputs from the midbrain (pretectal area) and the visual cortex. A unique feature of this lobe is that it sends outputs directly to the vestibular nuclei, bypassing the deep nuclei.

The medial vestibulocerebellum primarily controls axial musculature by modulating activity of the vestibular nuclei, whereas the flocculi (lateral vestibulocerebellum) are involved in eye pursuit movement and coordination of eye and head movements by controlling medial vestibular nuclei activity. Vestibulo-ocular reflex (VOR) is the compensatory counterrotation of the eyes during head movement that functions to stabilize images on the retina. Motor adaptations and adjustments to the VOR are

Table 1
Major cerebellar afferents and efferents

Peduncle	Tracts	Distribution	Laterality	Location of Cell Bodies
Cerebellar Afferents				
Inferior	Olivocerebellar tract	Cerebellar cortex and deep cerebellar nuclei	Contralateral	Inferior olivary nucleus
	Vestibulocerebellar tract	Flocculonodular lobe, caudal uvula, and fastigial nucleus	Ipsilateral	Vestibular nuclei and vestibular ganglion
	Posterior spinocerebellar tract	Lower extremity regions of the cerebellar cortex and nuclei	Ipsilateral	Clarke column
	Cuneocerebellar tract	Upper extremity and trunk regions of the cerebellar cortex and nuclei	Ipsilateral	Cuneate and external cuneate nuclei
	Rostral spinocerebellar tract	Upper extremity and trunk regions of the cerebellar cortex and nuclei	Ipsilateral	Intermediate zone and horn of the cervical enlargement
	Reticulocerebellar tract[1]	Cerebellar hemispheres and vermis, along with fastigial and interposed nuclei	Bilateral	Lateral reticular nucleus of the medulla oblongata
	Trigeminocerebellar tract	Related somatotopic regions of the cerebellar cortex and nuclei	Ipsilateral	Trigeminal nucleus
Middle	Pontocerebellar tract	Neocerebellar cortex and dentate nucleus	Contralateral	Pontine nuclei
Superior	Anterior spinocerebellar tract[a]	Lower extremity regions of the cerebellar cortex and nuclei	Ipsilateral	Clarke column
Cerebellar Efferents				
Inferior	Cerebellovestibular tract	Vestibular nucleus	Ipsilateral	Fastigial nucleus, vermis, and vestibulocerebellar cortex
Superior	Cerebellorubral fibers	Red nucleus	Contralateral	Dentate and interposed nuclei
	Cerebellothalamic fibers	Ventrolateral thalamic nucleus	Contralateral	Dentate and interposed nuclei
	Uncinate fasciculus	Vestibular, pontomedullary reticular, and thalamic nuclei	Contralateral	Fastigial nucleus
	Nucleo-olivary tract[b]	Inferior olive	Contralateral	Deep cerebellar nuclei

[a] The tract crosses 2 times: once in the spinal cord, and once again in the cerebellar white matter.
[b] Inhibitory (GABAergic).
Adapted from Standring S. Gray's anatomy: the anatomic basis of clinical practice. 40th edition. London: Churchill Livingstone/Elsevier; 2008.

critical in various contexts (eg, tracking a slowly moving target) and rely on the integrity of flocculus. Hence, floccular lesions are associated with ipsilateral punctuated pursuit and impairments in tasks that require VOR adaptation or suppression (eg, suppression of the VOR during combined head and eye tracking). VOR adaptation has been used as a model system to probe neural underpinnings of cerebellar function.[5]

Spinocerebellum

Spinocerebellum receives extensive somatosensory information directly and indirectly from the trunk and limbs through its connections with the spinal cord, the head and face through its connections with trigeminal nuclei, and visual and auditory systems. Posterior spinothalamic and cuneocerebellar tracts transmit proprioceptive inputs from lower and upper extremities, respectively, whereas the anterior and rostral spinothalamic tracts convey efference copies of the spinal motor discharges from lower and upper extremities, respectively. The spinocerebellum contains somatotopic maps of body parts (see **Fig. 2**).[6] The vermis receives inputs from the trunk and proximal portions of limbs, whereas the intermediate parts (paravermis) of the hemispheres receive inputs from the distal portions of limbs. The Purkinje cells in the vermis modulate vestibulospinal and reticulospinal activity through the fastigial nucleus. The outputs of these pathways are important in motor outputs to axial and proximal musculature, and thereby contribute to postural control and balance. In contrast, the Purkinje neurons located in the paravermal cortex project to the interposed nucleus, which in turn projects to the magnocellular red nucleus and the ventrolateral thalamus to regulate distal limb movements through modulation of rubrospinal and corticospinal activity, respectively. It is believed that the cerebellum is constantly comparing between planned motor commands (efference copy) and the actual somatosensory feedbacks to adjust motor outputs if necessary.[4] Further, mounting evidence suggests that the spinocerebellum implements an internal dynamic model[7] of the limbs that could translate any given end point to a series of accurately timed sequences of muscle contractions and can anticipate the future position of a limb in the course of a movement based on sensory position inputs. The dorsal vermis and fastigial nuclei play an important role in the accuracy of saccadic and precise conjugate eye movements. Lesions of these regions could lead to saccadic dysmetria and/or vergence abnormalities.[8]

Neocerebellum

The lateral zone (cerebrocerebellum) encompasses by far the largest part of the cerebellum and is reciprocally connected with the cerebral cortex. Along with cerebral association areas, this part of the cerebellum has expanded tremendously in humans.[1] It receives inputs exclusively from the cerebral cortex (parietal lobe in particular) through the relay neurons within the pontine nuclei, forming the cortico-pontocerebellar pathway. Lateral cerebellar hemispheres project through the dentate nuclei to the contralateral ventrolateral thalamic and parvocellular red nuclei. Axons of these thalamic nuclei terminate in motor areas of the premotor cortex and primary motor area of the frontal lobe. The neurons in the parvocellular division of the red nucleus project to the inferior olivary nucleus, relaying feedbacks from the neocerebellum.

Lesions in the cerebellar hemispheres could lead to deficits in motor planning, delays in the onset of movements, and irregularities in timings of movement components.[4] In addition, the neocerebellum was recently implicated in various cognitive functions (discussed later).

THE CEREBELLUM AND COGNITION

Converging evidence from functional imaging, tracing, and clinical studies have supported a role for cerebellum in higher cognitive functions. Transneuronal tracing methods have delineated cerebellar connections with various nonmotor cortical regions (eg, prefrontal cortex) that could serve as neural substrates for contributions of the cerebellum to cognitive function.[3] In addition, functional imaging studies have consistently provided support for cerebellar activation during cognitive tasks involving working memory, language, time perception, executive functioning, and emotional processing.[3]

Acquired cerebellar damages could lead to development of a complex pattern of behavioral deficits, termed *cerebellar cognitive affective syndrome*.[2] This syndrome is characterized by cognitive impairments, such as executive dysfunction, impaired working memory, disturbances in visuospatial cognition, and language deficits, and personality and affective changes that may include blunting of affect and/or disinhibited behavior.

CEREBELLAR CORTEX

The cytoarchitecture and microcircuitry of the cerebellar cortex seem to be identical regardless of the cortical region, connections, and functions, and it is composed of 3 layers (**Fig. 3**A). The granular layer, the deepest of the 3, is densely packed with a large number of the granule cells, along with interneurons. These cells are mainly Golgi

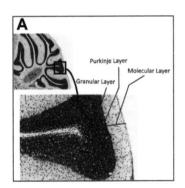
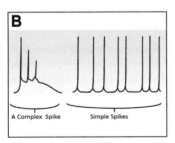
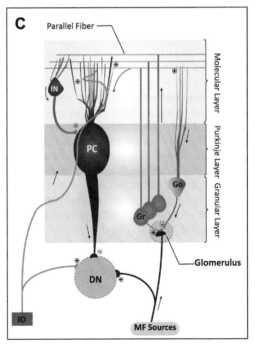

Fig. 3. (*A*) A sagittal histologic section of the mouse cerebellum stained with Nissl showing layers of cerebellar cortex. (*B*) Two spike patterns of Purkinje cell activity. (*C*) Schematic diagram of cerebellar cortex and basic cerebellar neural circuitry. DN, deep cerebellar nucleus; Go, Golgi cell; Gr, granule cell; IN, molecular layer inhibitory interneuron; IO, inferior olive; MF, mossy fibers; PC, Purkinje cell.

cells, but may also include Lugaro cells and unipolar brush cells in some cerebellar regions. This thick layer functions as the input layer for the cerebellar cortex, because the mossy fibers (1 of the 2 major cerebellar afferent pathways, discussed shortly) terminate in the granular layer, forming synaptic structures called cerebellar glomeruli. In the middle lies a narrow zone called the Purkinje layer, which serves as the output layer of the cerebellar cortex. This layer is mainly composed of cell bodies of Purkinje cells along with Bergmann glia cells. The most superficial layer (molecular layer) consists of flattened dendritic trees of Purkinje cells. In addition, the axons of the granule cells ascend to the molecular layer, where they split into 2 parallel fibers. Parallel fibers make synaptic contacts with the dendritic tress of the Purkinje cells as they move horizontally in the molecular layer. The molecular layer is also home to 2 types of inhibitory interneurons: stellate cells and basket cells (see **Fig. 3**C).

CEREBELLAR CIRCUITRY

The cerebellum receives its main excitatory inputs through 2 major pathways: mossy fibers and climbing fibers. The climbing fibers arise exclusively from the contralateral inferior olivary complex and directly form synapses with the Purkinje cells in the cerebellar cortex. In contrast, the mossy fibers deliver inputs indirectly to the Purkinje layer and originate from a variety of structures, including the pontine nuclei, spinal cord, vestibular nuclei, and the reticular formation mainly through inferior and middle cerebellar peduncles. Both mossy and climbing fibers send collaterals to the deep cerebellar nuclei (see **Fig. 3**C). Aside from these main pathways, aminergic and cholinergic inputs presumably function as global modulators of cerebellar activity.[9]

Mossy fibers form excitatory synapses with the neurons in the deep cerebellar nuclei and the granule cells. In the granular layer, a mossy fiber gives rise to a series of enlargements called *rosettes* that make contact with dendritic enlargement of the granule cells (dendritic claw) to form cerebellar glomeruli. Terminals from Golgi cells also infiltrate these structures and make inhibitory synaptic contacts with the granule cell dendrites. A sheath of glial cells encases the entire complex. Each mossy fiber diverges substantially as it reaches the granular layer by sending collateral branches to several cerebellar folia, with each collateral generating multiple rosettes. Granule cells are the excitatory neurons that emit the parallel fibers. These fibers also demonstrate considerable divergence as they pass through and make synaptic contacts with the dendritic trees of several Purkinje cells in the molecular layer. The activity of these fibers could generate simple spikes in the Purkinje cells (see **Fig. 3**B). Granule cells also target Golgi cells and other inhibitory interneurons: stellate cells and basket cells. Stellate and basket cells form inhibitory synapses (GABAergic) onto Purkinje cell dendrites and cell bodies, respectively.

Purkinje cells also receive inputs from the inferior olive via climbing fibers. In the cerebellar cortex, each climbing fiber innervates up to approximately 10 Purkinje cells. However, in sharp contrast to the parallel fibers, each Purkinje cell is exclusively innervated by the terminals of a single climbing fiber. Climbing fibers "climb" the dendritic tree of the Purkinje cells, making hundreds of synaptic connections. The input from the climbing fibers is so strong that a single action potential from a single fiber is capable of generating a protracted complex depolarization waveform in the Purkinje cell (see **Fig. 3**B).

Purkinje cells exert inhibitory effects on their targets by γ-aminobutyric acid (GABA) neurotransmission and their axons form the sole output of the cerebellar cortex. After projecting collaterals that innervate nearby parts of the cerebellar cortex, the axons travel into the deep cerebellar nuclei where they converge within small domains. In turn, the deep nuclei function as the outputs of the cerebellum. The cerebellar efferents (nucleofugal fibers) originating from the deep nuclei pass through superior and inferior peduncles and make excitatory synapses with their targets, except for the nucleo-olivary projections. The only exception to this general rule in the cerebellar circuitry (Purkinje-deep nuclei pathway) is the fibers projecting directly from the Purkinje cells to the vestibular nuclei.

An important hallmark of cerebellar circuitry is that inhibitory and excitatory inputs are compared in both the cerebellar cortex and the deep nuclei.[4] At the level of the deep nuclei, excitatory inputs from the mossy and climbing fiber collaterals converge with inhibitory inputs from the Purkinje cells. The inhibitory inputs from the latter shapes the excitatory signal from the former. In the cerebellar cortex, signals from the parallel fibers directly activate Purkinje cells, but also inhibit these cells through activation of inhibitory interneurons (stellate, basket, and Golgi interneurons). Stellate cells modulate activity of the same set of Purkinje cells activated by the parallel fibers, whereas axons from the basket cells run perpendicular to the parallel fibers and exert inhibitory effects on the flanking Purkinje cells (lateral inhibition). Another important feature of cerebellar circuitry is the occurrence of recurrent loops at different levels, such as the cerebral cortex via thalamic nuclei. Another recurrent loop could be found within the cerebellar cortex, where the Golgi interneurons are activated by parallel fibers and in turn provide inhibitory inputs back to the granule cells.

CEREBELLAR COMPARTMENTALIZATION AND MICROZONES

Histologic examination of the cerebellar cortex reveals a homogeneous sheet of tissue with a stereotypical internal structure.[10] However, this structure has been compartmentalized using anatomic, molecular, and physiologic approaches to longitudinal zones.[10] A longitudinal zone is a narrow, rostrocaudally extended sagittal region of the cerebellar cortex in which Purkinje cells receive climbing fiber inputs from specific subregions of inferior olive and project to specific cell groups of the deep cerebellar nuclei. Each of these nuclear subregions in turn projects to a specific set of targets in the central nervous system.

Vermis, paravermis, and cerebellar hemispheres are each divided into 3 to 5 longitudinal zones from midline to lateral. Each longitudinal zone could be further subdivided to even narrower compartments known as microzones.[10] The Purkinje cells of each microzone have a similar somatotopic receptive field (ie, activated by an essentially identical peripheral stimulus) and receive climbing fiber inputs from a cluster of inferior olivary neurons that are coupled together by gap junctions. These Purkinje cells project to particular clusters of neurons in the deep cerebellar/vestibular nuclei, and part of the nuclei output projects back to the same cluster of olivary neurons. Molecular layer interneurons and Golgi cells' inputs and outputs are also limited to the microzones they belong to. Given that the parallel fibers tend to span multiple sagittal zones, microzones are not unique in their mossy fiber inputs. The combination of microzones along with their associated clusters within inferior olivary and deep cerebellar nuclei could be regarded as functional units (modules) of the cerebellum. Thus, cerebellum is regarded as a computational machine consisting of a large number of almost independent modules, which are similar in terms of internal structure, and as such, perform the same computation on any kind of input (motor or nonmotor) that they receive. In addition, several spatially distinct microzones receiving inputs from the same olivary neurons form multizonal microcomplexes that may have a crucial role in parallel processing and integration of information from a multitude of mossy fiber sources.[10]

CEREBELLAR PLASTICITY AND LEARNING

Recordings from cerebellar neuronal activities in vitro and in vivo, under natural conditions and after pharmacologic and genetic manipulations, have greatly contributed to the current understanding of the physiologic basis underlying cerebellar motor performance, motor learning, and consolidation.[11] These studies suggest that, in addition to the rate of neuronal firing, the spatiotemporal firing pattern of Purkinje cells also play an important role in cerebellar coding (reviewed elsewhere).[11] The electrical activity of Purkinje cells is characterized by a combination of simple and complex spikes. Simple spikes are single action potentials and their firing pattern is determined by the intrinsic activity of Purkinje cells, together with their inputs from parallel fibers and molecular layer interneurons. Complex spikes are sequences of short-interval action potentials with diminishing amplitudes (see **Fig. 3**B) that are generated in response to olivary neuron inputs through climbing fibers. Olivary neurons innervating a given microzone show coherent and synchronous firing pattern and subthreshold membrane potential oscillations. Inputs from external stimuli can reset the phase of these subthreshold oscillations, which in turn may influence the temporal pattern of Purkinje complex spikes and lead to switching to a different motor program mode.[11] As with complex spikes, simple spike firing patterns are also best preserved within microzones.

Climbing fibers are believed to convey the error signals to the cerebellum.[12] These signals are crucial for motor learning because they could help cerebellum adapt the motor commands based on errors from prior movements. At the level of the cerebellar cortex, the timing of climbing and parallel fiber activation with respect to each other is critical for cerebellar plasticity and learning. Coincidence of inputs from these 2 fibers leads to a distributed and synergistic plasticity[13] within the cerebellar functional modules. Plasticity is distributed in the sense that it occurs along almost all types of synapses (both at the level of cerebellar cortex and deep nuclei) and intrinsic neuronal excitability within the cerebellar circuitry, and it is synergistic in the sense that long- or short-term depression at excitatory synapses occurs in coordination with long- or short-term potentiation at inhibitory interneuronal connections, and vice versa.

Abnormal expression of ion channels or defective channels in the cerebellar neurons lead to inappropriate excitability of the cells, alter their firing rates or spike patterns, and impede proper neuronal plasticity. Investigators have posited that such cerebellar channelopathies contribute to cerebellar deficits in ataxic disorders.[14]

REFERENCES

1. Herculano-Houzel S. Coordinated scaling of cortical and cerebellar numbers of neurons. Front Neuroanat 2010;4:12.
2. Schmahmann JD, Sherman JC. The cerebellar cognitive affective syndrome. Brain 1998;121(4):561–79.
3. Buckner RL. The cerebellum and cognitive function: 25 years of insight from anatomy and neuroimaging. Neuron 2013;80(3):807–15.
4. Kandel E, Schwartz J. Principles of neural science. 5th Edition. McGraw-Hill Education; 2013.
5. Broussard DM, Titley HK, Antflick J, et al. Motor learning in the VOR: the cerebellar component. Exp Brain Res 2011;210(3–4):451–63.
6. Manni E, Petrosini L. A century of cerebellar somatotopy: a debated representation. Nat Rev Neurosci 2004;5(3):241–9.
7. Imamizu H, Kawato M. Cerebellar internal models: implications for the dexterous use of tools. Cerebellum 2012;11(2):325–35.

8. Robinson FR, Fuchs AF. The role of the cerebellum in voluntary eye movements. Annu Rev Neurosci 2001;24(1):981–1004.

9. Schweighofer N, Doya K, Kuroda S. Cerebellar aminergic neuromodulation: towards a functional understanding. Brain Res Brain Res Rev 2004;44(2):103–16.

10. Apps R, Hawkes R. Cerebellar cortical organization: a one-map hypothesis. Nat Rev Neurosci 2009;10(9):670–81.

11. De Zeeuw CI, Hoebeek FE, Bosman LW, et al. Spatiotemporal firing patterns in the cerebellum. Nat Rev Neurosci 2011;12(6):327–44.

12. Apps R, Garwicz M. Anatomical and physiological foundations of cerebellar information processing. Nat Rev Neurosci 2005;6(4):297–311.

13. Gao Z, van Beugen BJ, De Zeeuw CI. Distributed synergistic plasticity and cerebellar learning. Nat Rev Neurosci 2012;13(9):619–35.

14. Shields SD, Cheng X, Gasser A, et al. A channelopathy contributes to cerebellar dysfunction in a model of multiple sclerosis. Ann Neurol 2012;71(2):186–94.

15. Diedrichsen J. A spatially unbiased atlas template of the human cerebellum. Neuroimage 2006;33(1):127–38.

16. Diedrichsen J, Balsters JH, Flavell J, et al. A probabilistic MR atlas of the human cerebellum. Neuroimage 2009;46(1):39–46.

17. Chakravarty MM, Steadman P, Eede MC, et al. Performing label-fusion-based segmentation using multiple automatically generated templates. Hum Brain Mapp 2013;34(10):2635–54.

18. Park MT, Pipitone J, Baer L, et al. Derivation of high-resolution MRI atlases of the human cerebellum at 3T and segmentation using multiple automatically generated templates. Neuroimage 2014;95:217–31.

19. Van Essen DC, Ugurbil K, Auerbach E, et al. The human connectome project: a data acquisition perspective. Neuroimage 2012;62(4):2222–31.

20. Sato A, Sekine Y, Saruta C, et al. Cerebellar development transcriptome database (CDT-DB): profiling of spatio-temporal gene expression during the postnatal development of mouse cerebellum. Neural Netw 2008;21(8):1056–69.

21. Jones AR, Overly CC, Sunkin SM. The Allen brain atlas: 5 years and beyond. Nat Rev Neurosci 2009;10(11):821–8.

Clinical Manifestations of Cerebellar Disease

Vijayakumar Javalkar, MD, MCh, Misbba Khan, MD, Debra E. Davis, MD*

KEYWORDS

- Gait ataxia • Limb ataxia • Nystagmus • Dysdiadochokinesia • Dysmetria
- Kinetic tremor • Action tremor • Cerebellar mutism

KEY POINTS

- Clinical manifestations of cerebellar disease include ataxia and tremor as being the most prominent clinical signs, as well as nystagmus, dysarthria, and cognitive dysfunction.
- Recognition of the cerebellar pattern of disease can aid in the prompt and correct diagnosis, and lead to appropriate treatment and rehabilitation to minimize disability.

INTRODUCTION

Luigi Luciani initiated the study of cerebellar dysfunction in late 1800s, and later Gordon Holmes built and enhanced it in the early 1900s (**Tables 1** and **2**). The cerebellum is located in the posterior fossa of the brain. It controls the rate, direction, range, and force of voluntary movement through its vestibular connections (in the brainstem), and corrects and adjusts an individual's upright position in space. The cerebellum can be divided into 3 parts: midline, intermediate, and lateral. The midline cerebellum includes the cerebellar vermis and the fastigial, flocculus, and nodulus nuclei. The lateral cerebellum consists of 2 hemispheres, including the dentate nuclei. Damage to 1 hemisphere leads to symptoms that are most notable in the ipsilateral limbs.

Three cerebellar peduncles connect the cerebellum with the brainstem. The inferior cerebellar peduncle connects the cerebellum to the medulla oblongata. The important afferent fibers in the inferior cerebellar peduncle are the dorsal spinocerebellar, cuneocerebellar, olivocerebellar, vestibulocerebellar, reticulocerebellar, and the trigeminocerebellar tracts. The efferent tracts through the inferior cerebellar peduncle are the cerebellovestibular and cerebelloreticular tracts. The middle cerebellar peduncle is the largest of the 3 peduncles and connects the pons with the cerebellum, and the pontocerebellar tract is the main afferent tract. The superior cerebellar peduncle connects the cerebellum to the midbrain, and dentatothalamic and dentatorubral are the

Department of Neurology, Louisiana State University Health Sciences Center, 1501 Kings Highway, Shreveport, LA 71103, USA
* Corresponding author.
E-mail address: delli1@lsuhsc.edu

Neurol Clin 32 (2014) 871–879
http://dx.doi.org/10.1016/j.ncl.2014.07.012
0733-8619/14/$ – see front matter © 2014 Elsevier Inc. All rights reserved.

Table 1
Cerebellar connections

Peduncles	Connections	Afferent Tracts	Efferent Tracts
Superior	Midbrain	Ventral spinocerebellar Tectocerebellar Trigeminocerebellar Cerulocerebellar	Dentatothalamic Dentatorubral
Middle	Pons	Corticopontocerebellar	
Inferior	Medulla	Dorsal spinocerebellar Cuneocerebellar Olivocerebellar Vestibulocerebellar Reticulocerebellar Trigeminocerebellar	Cerebellovestibular Cerebelloreticular

main efferent fibers. The afferent tracts in the superior cerebellar peduncle include the ventral spinal cerebellar, tectocerebellar, trigeminocerebellar, and cerulocerebellar tracts. Damage or dysfunction of these pathways or the nuclei of the cerebellum results in various clinical manifestations (**Table 3**).

The most prominent sign of cerebellar dysfunction is incoordination. It is thought to be due to disruption in the timing of the normal patterning of agonist and antagonist muscle activity in the course of movement.[1] Lesion symptom mapping based on magnetic resonance imaging (MRI) is helpful in the study of the function of the cerebellar cortex and the cerebellar nuclei. Functionally, the cerebellum can be compartmentalized into 3 sagittal zones. In patients with cerebellar cortical degeneration, ataxia of stance and gait is correlated with atrophy of the medial (and intermediate) cerebellum, oculomotor disorders with atrophy of the medial cerebellum, dysarthria with the atrophy of the intermediate section, and limb ataxia with atrophy of the intermediate and lateral cerebellum.[2]

HYPOTONIA AND WEAKNESS

Although hypotonia can occur in acute cerebellar disease, it is not usually a major feature.[3] The patient may have pendular knee jerk responses. Hypotonia has been explained as a decreased response to stretch in the muscle spindle afferents. The inability of patients to check forearm movement in the rebound test is often said to result from hypotonia but may have other explanations. Although cerebellar lesions do not cause loss of motor strength in the traditional sense, many patients experience problems with sustaining a steady force with their hands. This may be mistaken for, or described by the patient as weakness.

Table 2
Functional zones of the cerebellum

Zone	Symptoms
Medial	Ataxia of gait and stance Oculomotor disturbances
Intermediate	Ataxia of gait and stance Dysarthria Limb ataxia
Lateral	Limb ataxia

Table 3
Common signs and symptoms of cerebellar dysfunction

Symptom/Sign	Functional Picture	Examination Findings
Gait ataxia	• Uncoordinated gait, wide based stance, lurching movements, impaired ability to stop, falls easily	• Impaired freestyle walking, Unsteady tandem gait • Impaired U-turn testing • Impaired axial rebound
Limb ataxia	• Uncoordination of ipsilateral arm and/or leg	• Dysmetria on FTN and HTS • Impaired finger chase test • Dysdiadochokinesia • Deliberate, slow, and effortful fine finger movements • Impaired limb rebound
Hypotonia	• Decreased ability to maintain a steady force, weakness	• Ipsilateral hypotonia of limbs • Pendular tendon reflexes
Tremor	• Coarse intention tremor (<5 Hz)	• Side-to-side tremor of outstretched arms • End-point tremor on FTN test • Tremor of leg resting on shin
Cerebellar fits caused by acute mass lesion	• Repeated episodes of alteration of consciousness and decerebrate (extensor) posturing	• Repeated extensor stiffening in an acutely unresponsive patient
Cerebellar dysarthria, Scanning speech	• Slurred speech	• Loss of rhythm and prosody • May be staccato, hesitant, slow or garbled • Speech production is labored +/− facial grimacing
Cerebellar mutism	• Lack of speech output after surgery on posterior fossa	• Transient mutism, replaced by cerebellar dysarthria pattern
Oculomotor dysfunction nystagmus	• Oscillopsia • Blurred or double vision	• Gaze evoked, upbeat, rebound, optokinetic, periodic alternating, downbeat nystagmus • Impaired slow pursuit • Impaired shift of gaze/saccades • Inability to maintain fixation on VOR testing • Square wave jerks
Vertigo	• Spinning, dizzy	• Accompanied by ataxia
Cognitive dysfunction	• Memory problems, difficulty functioning at work or in home • Impaired communication skills • Personality changes	• Impaired executive function (planning, set-shifting, verbal fluency, abstract reasoning, working memory) • Impaired visuo-spatial function • Agrammatism, dysprodia • Blunted affect or disinhibited, inappropriate behavior

GAIT ATAXIA

Cerebellar gait ataxia and truncal ataxia are caused by cerebellar lesions involving the vermis. A wide based gait and staggering or lurching from side to side characterize it. The patient is usually afraid to stand up and will try to hold on to anything nearby. He or she will reel from side to side and fall even with support. The tandem gait test is useful for even minimal degrees of gait ataxia. It is best detected by having the patient walk on a line. After 1 or 2 steps, he or she will refuse to walk and revert back to the wide base stance. Afferent (sensory) ataxia differs from cerebellar ataxia clinically by the patient's heavy dependence on visual guidance, impaired tendon reflexes and sensory deficits, and normal speech.[4] The patient should also be tested for axial rebound while he or she is standing. To perform this test, the examiner tugs at the patient's shoulders toward the examiner, and asks the patient to catch himself or herself.

The common view that cerebellar ataxia of stance does not improve with visual feedback is true only of vestibulocerebellar lesions and not in the case for ataxia resulting from atrophy of the anterior lobe of the cerebellum.[3] Ataxic patients have great difficulty in stopping abruptly during walking. They adopt a multistep stopping strategy consisting of parallel feet in order to compensate for their inability to coordinate the upper body. Thus they generate a well-coordinated lower limb joint flexor–extensor pattern and appropriate braking forces for progressively decelerating the progression of the body in the sagittal plane.[5]

The most striking abnormalities in cerebellar disease are found during tandem gait. In 1 study, the gait disorder was characterized by a widened base, increased foot rotation angles, and relatively unchanged gait velocity and stride length. Tandem gait exaggerates dysmetria and balance problems and should be carried out in every patient with a gait disorder.[6] Gait variability, which is increased in cerebellar ataxia patients, is a good predictor of falls in elderly subjects and patients with neurodegenerative diseases.[7] Increased coactivation pattern of the antagonist muscles of the ankle and knee joints during walking in patients with cerebellar ataxia is a compensatory strategy to reduce gait instability.[8] Patients with cerebellar ataxia have difficulty in U turns also. In a recent study during U turning, the patients adopted an extended joint turning strategy, and the degree of knee flexion was found to be negatively correlated with the number of falls.[9] Turning training strategies need to be included in the rehabilitation protocol of ataxic patients.[10]

LIMB ATAXIA

Limb ataxia is manifest by dysmetria, dysdiadochokinesia, and rebound. It is caused by the failure of the brain to control movements, including speed, direction, and the ability to stop or check a movement. Limb ataxia is caused by a lesion in the lateral cerebellum, interpositus, and part of the dentate nuclei.[11] Several clinical tests have been designed to test limb incoordination and the presence of tremor. Dysmetria is an inaccuracy of movement in which the desired target is either under-reached (hypometria) or over-reached (hypermetria). Dysmetria is evident in the finger chase, finger-to-nose (FTN), and toe-to-finger tests. The FTN test involves repeatedly touching the tip of the nose and then the tip of the examiner's finger. The FTN may show a tendency to fall short or overshoot the examiner's finger (past-pointing). The finger chase test involves asking the patient to follow the examiner's finger rapidly and accurately as the examiner moves his or her finger to a different location. In the lower limbs, the heel-to-shin maneuver is done by having the patient bring the heel of the leg being tested to the opposite knee and sliding it in a straight line down the anterior aspect of the tibia to the ankle. The foot should be nearly vertical while doing this.

Dysdiadochokinesia is an impaired ability to perform rapid alternating movements. It is detected by asking the patient to supinate and pronate the forearm in the unsupported position. This can also be done by having the patient alternately tap the palm and dorsum of 1 hand on the palm of the other (stationary) hand or on the thigh.

In order to examine rebound, one should ask the patient to flex the elbow against the examiner's hand and then abrupt remove the resistance and assess the ability to arrest the sudden flexion movement. The patient's face should be protected by the examiner's hand, as patients with severe cerebellar deficit will hit themselves in the face.

CEREBELLAR TREMOR

The pathophysiology of cerebellar tremor is not fully understood, but it is thought to be related to dysfunction of the cerebellar efferent pathways. These pathways include the cerebellar nuclei (mainly the emboliform and dentate nuclei), which are under the inhibitory control of the cerebellar cortex. The dentato-rubro-olivary tract (Guillain-Mollaret triangle, including the red nucleus) is a subcortical loop that may be critically involved in tremor genesis.[12]

The following conditions have to be fulfilled for the diagnosis of cerebellar (intention) tremor as per the consensus statement of the Movement Disorder Society on tremor:

1. A pure or dominant intention tremor
2. Uni- or bilateral
3. Tremor frequency mainly below 5 Hz
4. Postural tremor may be present, but not rest tremor[13]

The most common cerebellar tremors are intention (action, kinetic) tremors that only become evident on purposeful movement. The tremor often increases in amplitude as the target is reached (the end-point tremor). To-and-fro oscillations appear to result from instability at the proximal rather than distal portions of the limb and are typically perpendicular to the axis of motion. Action tremor can be examined by placing the arms in the outstretched position or observed during the FTN test. Having the patient rest the heel on the opposite knee for period of time can elicit tremor in the leg. Titubation is another tremor that is probably a result of pathology of the cerebellum or its connections, and the head or trunk can be affected.[13] The red nucleus could be a potential target for drug-refractory cerebellar tremor.[12] The intentional tremor is more likely a cerebellar tremor if it is associated with other cerebellar signs like dysmetria and a correlating lesion on MRI.[14]

CEREBELLAR FITS

John Hughlings Jackson first described cerebellar fits in 1871. These are episodes of alteration of consciousness and decerebrate rigidity (extensor posturing), and they may progress to respiratory compromise and death. This is usually seen with a large midbrain/cerebellar mass lesion (often a large hemorrhage) or other posterior fossa pathology.[14] It is important not to confuse the semiology of cerebellar fits with status epileptics, which ultimately wastes precious time as the health care team tries to get the seizures under control.

CEREBELLAR SPEECH PATTERNS

Dysarthria in cerebellar disease is characterized by disruption of articulation and prosody (rhythm and melody or pitch). Cerebellar dysarthria is described as scanning, slurred, staccato, explosive, hesitant, slow altered accent, and garbled.[15] Speech production is labored with occasional excessive facial grimacing. The cerebellum affects the autoregulation of the breath and particularly its integration with speech. A recent study demonstrated that articulatory movements of the tongue and orofacial muscles are involved in the activation of the rostral paravermal area of the anterior lobe, and this location corresponds to the area involved in cerebellar ischemia in patients with dysarthria.[16] A functional MRI (fMRI) study done by Letchenberg in 1978 with cerebellar dysarthric patients showed predominately left hemispheric lesions. Cerebellar mutism is associated with midline structures, mostly seen in children after posterior fossa surgery. The onset of mutism becomes apparent within 48 hours after surgery and usually resolves within 2 months. This transient mutism is followed by more typical cerebellar dysarthria.[17] In children who undergo surgery for medulloblastoma, the incidence of cerebellar mutism syndrome was reported to be 24%. Significant risk factors include brainstem involvement and midline location of the tumor. The dentato-thalamo-cortical tracts and lesions that affect their integrity, especially the tract that originates in the right cerebellar hemisphere,[18] may play a role in cerebellar mutism.

OCULOMOTOR ABNORMALITIES

Nystagmus is a frequent oculomotor disturbance seen in cerebellar disease. Nystagmus is generally named according to the direction of the fast phase (corrective component). Numerous types of nystagmus are seen in patients with cerebellar disease. Patients with midline cerebellar lesions can present with gaze-evoked, upbeat, rebound and abnormal optokinetic nystagmus. With lesions of the uvula, nodulus, or with their connections to the vestibular nuclei, periodic alternating nystagmus is seen. Posterior midline cerebellar lesions involving the vestibulocerebellum are associated with downbeat nystagmus.[19]

Gaze-evoked nystagmus results in the inability to maintain an eccentric position of gaze. Because of the mechanical elastic properties of the eye muscles, the eyes drift slowly toward the midline followed by a corrective saccade returning the eyeball to the eccentric position. The slow phase is to the midline, and the corrective phase (the quick jerk) is to the side. Asymmetric gaze-evoked nystagmus is usually caused by an ipsilateral lesion of the cerebellum or brainstem. Rebound nystagmus is also seen in cerebellar disease. Rebound nystagmus occurs after a few seconds following gaze-evoked nystagmus. When the patient is asked to saccade back to the primary position, the nystagmus reverses in direction (slow phase away from midline and fast phase toward the midline).

In the case of peripheral vestibular lesions, there is a slow drift toward the paretic side (slow phase) and a corrective fast component (fast phase) away from the paretic side. The nystagmus may be more pronounced in attempting to gaze away from the paretic side. The 2 main features of nystagmus, which differentiate central from peripheral-induced vestibular nystagmus, are (1) the effects of fixation and (2) the direction of the nystagmus. Peripheral vestibular nystagmus is suppressed by fixation. One may have to use Frenzel (+20 diopters) glasses during the examination to inhibit fixation. Pure vertical or torsional nystagmus suggests a central cause.

The posterior vermis and the caudal fastigial nucleus provide a signal during horizontal saccades to make them fast, accurate, and consistent. The caudal fastigial nucleus and the flocculus/paraflocculus are necessary for the normal smooth eye movements.[20]

Hence disorders of the cerebellum can result in both saccadic and pursuit extraocular movement disorders.

Smooth pursuit eye movements allow the eyes to closely follow (and fixate on) a moving object, whereas saccades eye movements occur when the patient shifts gaze quickly between 2 objects. These are examined by asking the patient to follow the examiner's slowly moving finger or target (slow pursuit) and having the patient shift gaze quickly between an eccentrically held finger and the examiner's nose.

Although small square-wave movements of the eyes are often seen even in normal individuals during fixation, macrosquare-wave jerks of large amplitude (>10°) are highly specific for cerebellar disease. Cerebellar disease slows down pursuit movements, requiring catch-up saccades to keep up with a moving target. The velocity of the saccade is normal in cerebellar disease, but the accuracy is impaired so that both hypometric and hypermetric saccades are seen. Such saccades are followed by a corrective saccade in the appropriate direction[21] producing the so-called square wave jerk. Saccadic intrusions such as ocular flutter differ from square-wave jerks in that square wave jerks are separated by the intersaccadic interval, whereas saccadic intrusions are not.

The flocculonodular lobe of the cerebellum is involved in the vestibulo-ocular reflex (VOR). The VOR is responsible for counter-rotating the eyes in response to head movements. This allows the gaze to stay fixed on a specific point. In a rotary chair, normal individuals can suppress the VOR and keep their eyes on an object moving slowly with the chair. In a patient with cerebellar disease, the eyes drift away from the object and make catch-up saccades as the chair is rotated.

A recent study has shown that oculomotor features may aid in the differential diagnosis of the spinocerebellar ataxias. Perverted head shaking nystagmus and saccadic intrusions or oscillations are the most sensitive parameters for SCA6 and SCA3, respectively,[22] and a paucity of gaze-evoked nystagmus and dysmetric saccades is more indicative of spinocerebellar ataxia type 2.[22]

DIZZINESS AND VERTIGO

Dizziness is a vague and nonspecific symptom. It refers to an abnormal sensation in relation to space and position. Vertigo is a specific type of dizziness, defined as the pathologic illusion of things rotating around patient or that patient is rotating around things. Vertigo could be either from a peripheral (labyrinth and vestibular nerve) or a central disorder (brain stem, cerebellum). Lesions in patients with central vertigo are often found dorsolateral to the fourth ventricle or in the dorsal vermis.[23] It can be challenging to differentiate cerebellar vertigo from peripheral vertigo, because the 2 syndromes share many features.

In cerebellar vertigo, patient will have severe ataxia (dysdiadochokinesia, dysmetria), while in peripherally induced vertigo, ataxia is only mild or moderate.[23] Nystagmus can be present in peripheral and cerebellar vertigo; however, the characteristics of the 2 syndromes are different. In cerebellar vertigo, the nystagmus is purely vertical, or torsional, and not inhibited by fixation. Cerebellar nystagmus may change direction with gaze toward fast phase called direction changing (bidirectional gaze-evoked nystagmus). Such patients have nystagmus that changes directions according to the patient's gaze. For example, if the patient looks to the right, it beats to the right, and when the patient looks left, it beats to the left.[24] Nystagmus in peripheral vertigo is combined horizontal and torsional; it is inhibited by fixation of eye onto an object. It does not change direction with gaze to either side. In peripheral vertigo, hearing loss and tinnitus are common, while it is absent in cerebellar vertigo. The duration of symptoms is days to weeks, with improvement over time in peripheral dysfunction, whereas symptoms are more chronic with central dysfunction.

NONMOTOR DISTURBANCES

Evidence for a cerebellar role in nonmotor functions has been demonstrated by clinical and neuroimaging research.[25] In addition to connections with the motor cortices, the cerebellum communicates with prefrontal and parietal association cortices via cerebellothalamo-cortical and cortico-ponto-cerebellar loops in nonhuman primates.[26] Schmahmann and Sherman[27] introduced the clinical entity cerebellar cognitive affective syndrome. The core features of this syndrome consist of executive dysfunctions (disturbances in planning, set-shifting, verbal fluency, abstract reasoning, working memory), visuo-spatial deficits (impaired visuo-spatial organization and memory), mild language symptoms (agrammatism and dysprodia), and personality changes (blunting of affect, disinhibition, and inappropriate behavior).[27]

Recent work implicates the cerebellum in cognition and emotion, and it has been argued that cerebellar dysfunction contributes to non-motor conditions such as autism spectrum disorders.[28] Certain cerebellar ataxias are associated with neuropsychiatric symptoms such as distractibility, hyperactivity, compulsive obsessive behavior, anxiety, depression, aggression, hallucinations, lack of empathy, and avoidant behavior.[29]

Experimental and clinical data suggest that the cerebellum is actively involved in the regulation of visceromotor functions.[30] It fine-tunes the activity of the autonomic centers in the brain. Patients with cerebellar dysfunction can have abnormal vasomotor responses to voluntary movements, such as pupil dilatation and flushing of the face, hyperventilation, or bradycardia. These subtle signs are frequently overlooked.[31]

SUMMARY

Clinical manifestations of cerebellar disease include ataxia and tremor as being the most prominent clinical signs, as well as nystagmus, dysarthria, and cognitive dysfunction. Recognition of the cerebellar pattern of disease can aid in the prompt and correct diagnosis and lead to appropriate treatment and rehabilitation to minimize disability.

REFERENCES

1. Hallett M, Shahani BT, Young RR. EMG analysis of patients with cerebellar deficits. J Neurol Neurosurg Psychiatry 1975;38:1163–9.
2. Timmann D, Konczak J, Ilg W, et al. Current advances in lesion-symptom mapping of the human cerebellum. Neuroscience 2009;162:836–51.
3. Diener HC, Dichgans J. Pathophysiology of cerebellar ataxia. Mov Disord 1992;7: 95–109.
4. Sghirlanzoni A, Pareyson D, Lauria G. Sensory neuron diseases. Lancet Neurol 2005;4:349–61.
5. Serrao M, Conte C, Casali C, et al. Sudden stopping in patients with cerebellar ataxia. Cerebellum 2013;12:607–16.
6. Stolze H, Klebe S, Petersen G, et al. Typical features of cerebellar ataxic gait. J Neurol Neurosurg Psychiatry 2002;73:310–2.
7. Schniepp R, Wuehr M, Schlick C, et al. Increased gait variability is associated with the history of falls in patients with cerebellar ataxia. J Neurol 2014;261: 213–23.
8. Mari S, Serrao M, Casali C, et al. Lower limb antagonist muscle co-activation and its relationship with gait parameters in cerebellar ataxia. Cerebellum 2014;13: 226–36.
9. Serrao M, Mari S, Conte C, et al. Strategies adopted by cerebellar ataxia patients to perform U-turns. Cerebellum 2013;12:460–8.
10. Mari S, Serrao M, Casali C, et al. Turning strategies in patients with cerebellar ataxia. Exp Brain Res 2012;222:65–75.
11. Timmann D, Brandauer B, Hermsdörfer J, et al. Lesion-symptom mapping of the human cerebellum. Cerebellum 2008;7:602–6.

12. Lefranc M, Manto M, Merle P, et al. Targeting the red nucleus for cerebellar tremor. Cerebellum 2014. http://dx.doi.org/10.1007/s12311-013-0546-z.
13. Deuschl G, Bain P, Brin M. Consensus statement of the Movement Disorder Society on Tremor. Ad Hoc Scientific Committee. Mov Disord 1998;13(Suppl 3): 2–23.
14. Pandey A, Robinson S, Cohen AR. Cerebellar fits in children with Chiari I malformation. Neurosurg Focus 2001;11:E4.
15. Urban PP. Speech motor deficits in cerebellar infarctions. Brain Lang 2013;127: 323–6.
16. Urban PP, Marx J, Hunsche S, et al. Cerebellar speech representation: lesion topography in dysarthria as derived from cerebellar ischemia and functional magnetic resonance imaging. Arch Neurol 2003;60:965–72.
17. Sherman JH, Sheehan JP, Elias WJ, et al. Cerebellar mutism in adults after posterior fossa surgery: a report of 2 cases. Surg Neurol 2005;63:476–9.
18. Pitsika M, Tsitouras V. Cerebellar mutism. J Neurosurg Pediatr 2013;12:604–14.
19. Biller J, Brazis PW. The Localization of Lesions Affecting the Cerebellum. In: Brazis PW, Masdeu JC, Biller J, editors. Localization in clinical neurology. 5th edition. Philadelphia: Lippincott Williams & Wilkins; 2006.
20. Robinson FR, Fuchs AF. The role of the cerebellum in voluntary eye movements. Annu Rev Neurosci 2001;24:981–1004.
21. Munoz DP. Commentary: saccadic eye movements: overview of neural circuitry. Prog Brain Res 2002;140:89–96.
22. Kim JS, Kim S, Youn J, et al. Ocular motor characteristics of different subtypes of spinocerebellar ataxia: distinguishing features. Mov Disord 2013;28:1271–7.
23. Büttner U, Helmchen C, Brandt T. Diagnostic criteria for central versus peripheral positioning nystagmus and vertigo: a review. Acta Otolaryngol 1999;119:1–5.
24. Lee H, Kim HA. Nystagmus in SCA territory cerebellar infarction: pattern and a possible mechanism. J Neurol Neurosurg Psychiatry 2013;84:446–51.
25. Tomlinson SP, Davis NJ, Bracewell RM. Brain stimulation studies of non-motor cerebellar function: a systematic review. Neurosci Biobehav Rev 2013;37:766–89.
26. Kelly RM, Strick PL. Cerebellar loops with motor cortex and prefrontal cortex of a nonhuman primate. J Neurosci 2003;23:8432–44.
27. Schmahmann JD, Sherman JC. The cerebellar cognitive affective syndrome. Brain 1998;121(Pt 4):561–79.
28. Reeber SL, Otis TS, Sillitoe RV. New roles for the cerebellum in health and disease. Front Syst Neurosci 2013;7:83.
29. Marmolino D, Manto M. Past, present and future therapeutics for cerebellar ataxias. Curr Neuropharmacol 2010;8:41–61.
30. Haines DE, Dietrichs E, Mihailoff GA, et al. The cerebellarhypothalamic axis: basic circuits and clinical observations. Int Rev Neurobiol 1997;41:83–107.
31. Pandolfo M, Manto M. Cerebellar and afferent ataxias. Continuum (Minneap Minn) 2013;19:1312–43.

Acute Ataxias

Differential Diagnosis and Treatment Approach

Vijayakumar Javalkar, MD, MCh[a], Roger E. Kelley, MD[b],
Eduardo Gonzalez-Toledo, MD, PhD[c], Jeanie McGee, DHEd, MSHS[a],
Alireza Minagar, MD[a],*

KEYWORDS

- Ataxia • Cerebellum • Infection • Wernicke encephalopathy • Stroke
- Decompression • Hydrocephalus • Abscess

KEY POINTS

- Acute ataxia is recognized by its mode of onset within hours to days.
- Ataxia is often a primary manifestation of cerebellar disease, and clinicians must seek its cause (one can see ataxia with spinal disease, and sensory ataxia related to peripheral neuropathy may also be present).
- The most frequent causes of ataxia include excessive alcohol consumption, an adverse effect or overdose of particular medications, or pathology of the posterior fossa such as stroke, trauma, infection, or neoplasm.
- Two presentations to keep in mind with acute ataxia are Wernicke encephalopathy characterized by ataxia, ophthalmoparesis, and confusion, as well as Miller-Fisher syndrome, characterized by ophthalmoparesis, loss of deep tendon reflexes, and ataxia.
- All patients with cerebellar ataxia of acute onset should be thoroughly evaluated in the emergency room, with the intention to exclude acute ischemic or hemorrhagic stroke in order to provide thrombolytic treatment or neurosurgical decompressive procedures.
- Patients with clinical suspicion of Wernicke encephalopathy should be treated first with thiamine and then intravenous glucose-containing fluids.
- Patients with sensory ataxia stemming from Miller-Fisher syndrome should be carefully assessed and constantly monitored for impending respiratory failure and intubated when indicated.
- Correct diagnosis and urgent treatment of patients with acute ataxia can save the patient's life.

[a] Department of Neurology, Louisiana State University Health Sciences Center, 1501 Kings Highway, Shreveport, LA 71130, USA; [b] Department of Neurology, Tulane University School of Medicine, 1430 Tulane Avenue 8065, New Orleans, LA 70112, USA; [c] Department of Radiology, Louisiana State University Health Sciences Center, 1501 Kings Highway, Shreveport, LA 71130, USA
* Corresponding author. Department of Neurology, Louisiana State University Health Sciences Center, 1501 Kings Highway, Shreveport, LA 71130.
E-mail address: aminag@lsuhsc.edu

Neurol Clin 32 (2014) 881–891
http://dx.doi.org/10.1016/j.ncl.2014.07.004   neurologic.theclinics.com

The term ataxia stems from the Greek verb taseein, which means "placing or arranging things in order." The word ataxia, which indicates absence of coordination, usually suggests the presence of poorly organized movements and points to cerebellar diseases or dysfunction of cerebellar connections to other areas of human brain, such as abnormalities affecting spinocerebellar or pontocerebellar neuroanatomic pathways. A unique form of ataxia known as sensory ataxia stems from loss of input from the peripheral nervous system and represents involvement of primary sensory neurons or the posterior columns. Acute ataxia is defined by the loss of coordinated movement, which can be axial, resulting in an ataxic gait, or appendicular, involving the extremities, within a 72-hour timeframe. Acute ataxia may also be of vestibular, epileptic, or psychogenic origin. In adults, the most common acquired causes of acute ataxia include alcohol intoxication, posterior fossa trauma, stroke, and infective processes involving the posterior fossa. In the pediatric population, the most frequent etiologies for acute ataxia consist of infections, trauma, medicinal effects, and toxicity.

Other frequent, but less severe, causes of acute ataxia include migraine, benign positional paroxysmal vertigo, and vestibular neuronitis and labyrinthitis. Certain clinical features of these conditions are presented in **Box 1**.

CLINICAL PRESENTATIONS

Ataxia is a sign, while the accompanying symptom, as reported by the patient, might include: "dizzy", "like rocking on a boat", "drunk-like sensation", or "uncoordinated." Because ataxia commonly originates from cerebellar dysfunction, one should also search for accompaniments such as dysarthria, swallowing difficulty, abnormalities of ocular movements, or intention tremor. Clinically, ataxia presents with slurred speech, limb and gait ataxia, loss of coordination, stumbling, and movement-associated tremor. A history of headaches, nausea, and vomiting should be assessed.

Neurologic examination of patients with ataxia should include measurements of blood pressure in supine, sitting, and standing positions to determine the presence of orthostatic hypotension. A focus on nonataxic neurologic manifestations is of great significance, because it points to the correct diagnosis of the cause of ataxia. In general, ipsilateral neurologic deficits stem from unilateral cerebellar lesions, while more widespread deficits indicate a pancerebellar disease. The combination of visual loss and ataxia in a young individual raises the possibility of a demyelinating disease, such as multiple sclerosis (MS). Risk factor profile, including age, vascular disease, and smoking history can help in identifying stroke or a tumor as more likely etiology. The astute clinician should also seek the presence of other neurologic manifestations associated with the ataxia, including diplopia, difficulty with visual fixation, facial weakness, inequality of pupillary size, dysarthria, dysphonia, deviation of tongue to one side, dysdiadochokinesia, dysmetria, excessive rebound phenomenon, tremor, and head or truncal titubation, along with gait instability.

The presence of ocular dysmetria, ocular flutter, opsoclonus, and ophthalmoplegia all indicate more widespread cerebellar disease with brainstem involvement. Another diagnostic clue on neurologic examination in support of a cerebellar process for acute ataxia is scanning type dysarthria. Patients with acute ataxia of cerebellar origin often have hypotonia and dysdiadochokinesia. Dysdiadochokinesia is defined as an impaired ability to perform and coordinate rapid alternating movements. In ataxic patients, examination of repetitive supination and pronation for each upper extremity is performed to determine a decompensation of normally coordinated movement. Each lower extremity can be examined separately by swift rhythmic tapping of the heel and then the toes of either foot. Dysdiadochokinesia of articulation indicates an impaired

---

Box 1
Disorders causing acute ataxia

Cerebrovascular causes

- Ischemic stroke
- Hemorrhagic stroke

Neoplasms

- Primary or metastatic tumors
- Paraneoplastic syndromes

Metabolic disorders

- Hypoglycemia
- Hyponatremia
- Hyperammonemia
- Wernicke encephalopathy
- Malnutrition causing thiamine deficiency

Medicines—adverse effects or toxicity

Acute alcohol intoxication

Posterior fossa trauma and hydrocephalus

Immune-mediated diseases

- Multiple sclerosis
- Acute disseminated encephalomyelitis

Infections

- AIDS and opportunistic infections associated with AIDS
- Other viral infections such as HSV and EBV

Polyradiculoneuropathy

- Acute inflammatory demyelinating polyradiculoneuropathy
- Miller Fisher syndrome

Miscellaneous

- Migraine
- Labyrinthitis and vestibular neuronitis
- Benign positional paroxysmal vertigo

---

ability to alternate between distinct syllables even if syllables could separately be articulated effectively. Dysmetria is a term for cerebellar dysfunction, which refers to the impaired ability to judge accurate and appropriate distance or measurement. At bedside, finger-nose-finger or finger-chin-finger maneuvers (with the eyes open and then closed) and past-pointing maneuvers (with the eyes closed) are used to determine limb overshoot or undershoot. Kinetic tremor is recognized by rhythmic contraction of reciprocally innervated agonist and antagonist muscles associated with uninterrupted movement of the affected body part. This form of tremor possesses a sinusoidal appearance and is usually intensified in amplitude as the patient is approaching the target.

Patients with sensory ataxia usually suffer from impaired proprioception, decreased or absent deep tendon reflexes, presence of a Romberg sign, typically swaying to and fro with the eyes closed, reflecting loss of visual compensation, and autonomic system abnormalities.[1]

CAUSES OF ACUTE ATAXIA

Several medical conditions cause acute ataxia and demand emergent assessment and treatment (see **Box 1**). These include ischemic and hemorrhagic stroke, cerebellar space occupying lesions, toxicity with certain medications such as antiepileptics, and trauma to the cerebellum or spinal cord. Less severe etiologies consist of exposure to toxins, solvents, and heavy metals, acute alcohol intoxication, Wernicke Korsakoff syndrome,[2] infections, transient ischemic attack, tumor without mass effect, immune-mediated diseases, and congenital and familial disorders of the cerebellum.

Patients with acute ischemic or hemorrhagic cerebellar strokes present with acute ataxia, and the cranial nerves may or may not be affected (**Figs. 1** and **2**).[3] The presentation of a patient with a relatively small cerebellar infarct can be fairly subtle, comprised of only a sense of unsteadiness, with the patient often using the term "dizziness," for which the patient may not seek medical attention. It might often be attributed to an inner ear process and may not indicate the necessity of a brain scan. It is not uncommon to see incidental cerebellar infarcts on the brain scan, especially the magnetic resonance imaging (MRI) brain scan, in patients with risk factors for stroke with no clinical correlate identified. These are most commonly of the lacunar type and are typically associated with longstanding hypertension and increasing age. Cerebellar hematomas are most commonly hypertensive in etiology, but can be seen with vascular anomalies of the posterior fossa.

Finite cerebellar-related ataxia from a localized cerebellar infarct or hematoma can be a very stable process without the need for surgical intervention. However, an important clinical point is that progression of an initial finite neurologic deficit, such as truncal or appendicular ataxia, to involvement of brainstem nuclei and/or long tract signs, reflects the potential for tonsillar herniation with death. Thus, neurosurgical consultation is advisable for all patients in case such a progression occurs. Naturally, large cerebellar infarcts or hematomas, with such brainstem compression, necessitate

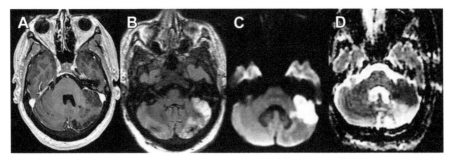

Fig. 1. Magnetic resonance, axial slices. ADC, apparent diffusion coefficient; DWI, diffusion weighted imaging. From left to right: (A) T1WI showing hypointense lesions in the left cerebellar hemisphere. (B) Fluid-attenuated inversion recovery (FLAIR) sequence with abnormal hyperintensity in both cerebellar hemispheres. The brighter lesion on the left corresponds with a new infarction. The other lesions, older, show traces of iron (old hemorrhage). (C) DWI. Restricted diffusion in the more anterior lesion on the left (D) ADC. Restricted diffusion (*black*) in the anterior lesion and hyperintensity in the posterior indicating old infarct.

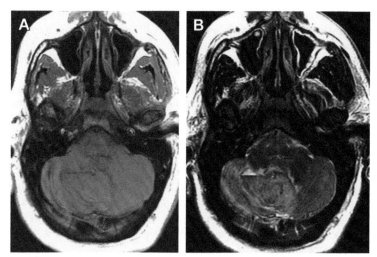

Fig. 2. Acute intracerebellar hematoma. (*A*) Left T1WI. Isointense mass formation (*B*) Right T2WI. Hypointense mass formation. It corresponds to paramagnetic blood (deoxyHb).

emergency intervention.[4,5] Patients with acute vertebrobasilar dissection, brainstem, and anterior thalamic stroke who manifest with acute ataxia will require immediate medical attention and treatment. Other clinical symptomatology associated with ataxia varies based on the affected vascular territory.

Demyelinating disorders such as acute disseminated encephalomyelitis,[6] MS (**Fig. 3**), and Miller-Fisher syndrome[7] can present with acute ataxia. Acute disseminated encephalomyelitis is most commonly seen in childhood, especially in acute exanthematous infections or following vaccinations. Acute cerebellar ataxia is most commonly associated with varicella exposure, while cerebral and spinal manifestations are more common with vaccinia and measles. MS is most commonly seen in young adults, with a predilection for women, especially in northern latitudes. The myriad manifestations reflect the multitude of demyelinating plaque locations

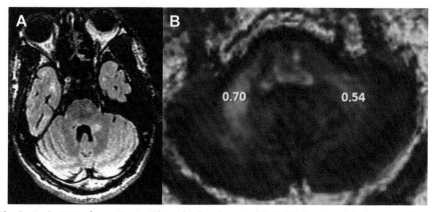

Fig. 3. Brain MRI of a patient with multiple sclerosis. (*A*) FLAIR, brain axial view, prominent plaque in left middle cerebellar peduncle. (*B*) Decreased fractional anisotropy in left middle cerebellar peduncle.

possibly seen with this disorder. Miller-Fisher syndrome, characterized by ataxia, ophthalmoparesis, and areflexia, is associated with an elevated serum anti-GQ1b antibody titer.

Primary brain tumors (eg, meningiomas and gliomas) (**Fig. 4**), as well as metastatic tumors (**Fig. 5**) such as melanoma, breast cancer, and lung cancer, may present with acute ataxia and demand neurologic and neurosurgical assessment. Other space-occupying lesions, such as cerebellar lesions abscesses and arteriovenous malformations that undergo hemorrhagic transformation, manifest with acute ataxia. Less common etiologies for mass-occupying cellebellar lesions include giant multiple sclerosis plaques and tumefactive MS lesions,[8] traumatic subdural hematoma, and progressive multifocal leukoencephalopathy (**Fig. 6**). All patients determined to have cerebellar mass-occupying lesions, with the potential for caudal and rostral herniation of cerebellum, need immediate attention, as these can be life-threatening events. Worrisome premonitory clinical manifestations of cerebellar herniation include ataxia, intractable headache, nausea and vomiting, photophobia, and decreased sensorium. As the pathologic process progresses, patients can evolve into stupor and then coma along with an ataxic respiratory pattern.

Toxicity with phenytoin, lithium, bismuth, lead, mercury, and chemotherapeutic agents such as 5-FU and cytosine arabinoside causes ataxia. Exposure to and intoxication with Toluene, and high levels of hexacarbons, bismuth, lead, and mercury also cause acute ataxia. In patients with acquired immunodeficiency syndrome (AIDS),

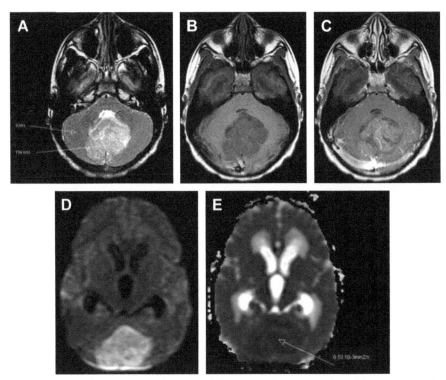

Fig. 4. Posterior fossa: Medulloblastoma. (*A*) T2WI: Prolongation of T2. (*B*) T1w/o: Hypointense mass. (*C*) T1-weight postcontrast axial view: Heterogenous enhancement. (*D*) Left DWI E. (*E*) ADC map: restricted diffusion.

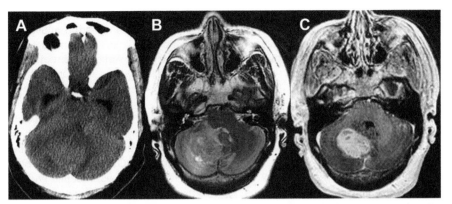

Fig. 5. Cerebellar metastatic lesion. (*A*) CT scan of brain axial view without contrast showing hyperdensity surrounded by hypodensity representing a solid mass surrounded by vasogenic edema. (*B*) MRI of brain T2-weighted axial view showing a well-defined mass in the right cerebellar hemisphere. (*C*) MRI of brain T1-weighted postcontrast axial view revealing an enhancing well-defined mass with deformation and displacement of the fourth ventricle. Vasogenic edema as hypointense rim.

acute ataxia may originate from cerebellitis due to mycoplasma pneumonia, Epstein-Barr virus (EBV), herpes simplex virus (HSV), and toxoplasmosis. Patients with Lyme disease, Whipple disease, and Creutzfeld-Jakob disease may also develop ataxia, and this can be the initial manifestation.

Autoimmune etiologies for ataxia include, but are not restricted to, paraneoplastic degeneration of the cerebellum,[9] glutamic acid decarboxylase antibody-mediated ataxia, and gluten ataxia. The anti-Yo (antipurkinje cell) antibody can be assessed with a blood test, and an elevated titer is supportive of paraneoplastic cerebellar degeneration, with ovarian cancer reported to be the most common associated malignancy.

Certain congenital and familial disorders that manifest with ataxia include Arnold-Chiari malformation and episodic ataxia (types 1 and 2). Several hereditary disorders,

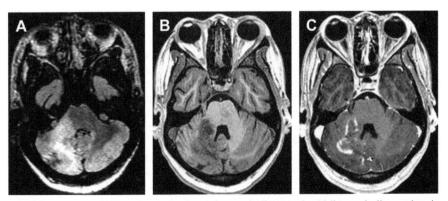

Fig. 6. AIDS patient with a lesion in the right cerebellum and middle cerebellar peduncle. (*A*) FLAIR sequence showing hyperintense area with minimal deformity and no displacement of the 4th ventricle. (*B*) T1-weighted axial view, hypointense area corresponding to the previous image (*C*) T1-weighted postcontrast axial view, peripheral enhancement of the lesion.

such as episodic ataxia, spinocerebellar ataxia, and autosomal recessive ataxia, manifest with acute ataxia as well. However, discussion of such entities is beyond the scope of this article. Other miscellaneous etiologies for ataxia included migraine attacks, termed basilar migraine, benign positional paroxysmal vertigo, and vestibular neuronitis.

DIAGNOSTIC APPROACH

In addition to obtaining a detailed history along with the performance of a comprehensive neurologic examination, neuroimaging should be performed. Ideally, MRI should be obtained, as it is clearly superior to computed tomography (CT) brain scan for posterior fossa pathology, including ischemic and hemorrhagic strokes, vascular anomalies, congenital anomalies, neoplasms, and demyelinating lesions. Assessment for alcohol toxicity, medication effect, and urinary drug screen should also be obtained. Patients should also be assessed for potential nutritional deficiencies, which may be associated with alcohol abuse, including thiamine deficiency.

The neurologic interview of a patient with ataxia should concentrate on certain features such as age, gender, pattern of onset (acute, subacute, or chronic), the distribution of ataxia (unilateral or bilateral), mode of presence (episodic, constant or progressive), and the affected area (ocular, bulbar, limbs or truncal). The speed and pattern of ataxia presentation assist the clinician to narrow the long list of differential diagnoses. An assessment of the development and progression of ataxia also assists with narrowing the vast numbers of etiologies for ataxia. For example, acute ataxia that occurs in a matter of hours to a few days more likely signifies an underlying vascular, toxic–metabolic, infectious (usually viral), or traumatic etiology.

A subacute form of ataxia that develops during weeks to months indicates the presence of an inflammatory or demyelinating, infectious, or paraneoplastic disorder. Patients who present with ataxia of slow onset with or without constant headache, along with significant unexplained weight loss, should be evaluated for primary or metastatic cancers. Ataxia of intermittent nature may stem from a vascular cause, and these patients should carefully be evaluated for transient ischemic attack and imminent stroke. In this particular group of patients, attention to other neurologic deficits secondary to brainstem ischemia is necessary. Finally, ataxia with chronic nature, which progresses over months to years, raises the possibility of an underlying genetic, or neurodegenerative, condition. An accurate family history of ataxia in search of hereditary forms of ataxia should be obtained.

Several immune-mediated diseases also cause acute ataxia. Acute disseminated encephalomyelitis is an uncommon and usually monophasic demyelinating disease that presents with altered sensorium, seizures, focal neurologic symptoms, and ataxia. Most of these patients have a recent history of vaccination or viral infections. MS, as a progressive degenerative and demyelinating disease of the human central nervous system, may manifest with acute ataxia. Miller-Fisher syndrome presents with a triad of ataxia, ophthalmoplegia, and areflexia.

All patients with acute ataxia, at presentation in an emergency setting, should undergo CT scan of the brain without contrast in search of ischemic or hemorrhagic stroke.[10] In this group of patients, the examiner should pay special attention to history of hypertension, diabetes mellitus, hyperlipidemia, and atrial fibrillation. Of course, MRI of the brain with and without contrast (stroke protocol) is a more accurate and sensitive diagnostic method to search for a vast array of cerebellar diseases. Apart from stroke or trauma, the clinician should assess the neuroimaging for the presence of mass lesions and tumors, hydrocephalus, demyelinating disorders, development anomalies, Wernicke encephalopathy, medicinal affects (eg, cerebellar atrophy associated with use of phenytoin), and cerebellitis caused by infections. In certain cases and based on clinical suspicion, other MRI procedures such as magnetic resonance spectroscopy and functional MRI may be obtained.

In all patients with acute ataxia, the clinician should obtain a complete blood count, comprehensive metabolic panel, serum lipid profile, erythrocyte sedimentation rate, C-reactive protein, antinuclear antibodies, thyroid peroxidase antibody, serum levels of folic acid, vitamin B12[11] and vitamin E, serum copper, ceruloplasmin level, serum lactate, pyruvate, serum levels of certain medications or substances that can cause ataxia such as phenytoin and alcohol, urine drug and heavy metal screens, venous ammonia level, serum human immunodeficiency virus (HIV) test, and serum electrophoresis. If the clinician suspects an immune-mediated etiology for ataxia, then relevant tests such as antithyroglobulin antibodies, antithyroid peroxidase antibodies, antinuclear antibodies, anti GAD antibodies and antigliadin antibodies should be requested. In epileptic patients, serum levels of the antiepileptic medication such as phenytoin, valproic acid, phenobarbital, or carbamazepine should be checked.

If the previously mentioned studies fail to reveal the underlying cause of acute ataxia, provided there is no contraindication, spinal tap should be performed and cerebrospinal fluid examined for protein, glucose, number and percentage of leukocytes, viral and bacterial antigens, and culture. If one suspects a demyelinating disorder, then an MS panel including the presence of oligoclonal bands, immunoglobulin G (IgG) index, and myelin basic protein should be requested. Other tests on cerebrospinal fluid based on the clinical grounds should include levels of angiotensin-converting enzyme, lactate, and protein 14-3-3. In patients with sensory ataxia, nerve conduction and electromyographic studies are indicated.

All patients with acute ataxia should undergo a detailed ophthalmologic examination, and the examiner should focus on detecting nystagmus as well as characteristic features of the nystagmus, assessing for visual fixation as well as examination of saccades and smooth visual pursuit. Assessment for benign positional vertigo may also need to be considered.

In all patients with unexplained acute or subacute ataxia, a paraneoplastic panel should be requested, and this panel consists of anti-Yo antibody (breast and ovarian cancers), anti-PQ antibody (voltage-gated calcium channel, lung cancer), anti-Tr antibody (Hodgkin disease), anti-Ri (breast cancer), and anti-Hu (lung cancer).

DIFFERENTIAL DIAGNOSIS

Differential diagnosis of acute ataxias is extensive, and a detailed list is presented in **Box 2**.

MANAGEMENT

Management of patients with acute ataxias is a vast topic, and here the focus is on the most common and urgent approaches. Patients with acute ataxia should be carefully assessed in the emergency room for ischemic or hemorrhagic stroke. Patients with acute ischemic cerebellar stroke who present with acute ataxia and are still within the 4.5 hour treatment window must be treated with alteplase (tissue plasminogen activator [TPA]) unless there is a particular contraindication for use of TPA. If TPA cannot be used, aspirin may be considered in an effort to improve outcome and for recurrent stroke prevention once the mechanism of the stroke has been addressed. These patients should be admitted to the hospital, and in certain cases intra-arterial thrombolysis or intra-arterial mechanical thrombectomy may be beneficial. Treatment

---

Box 2
Clinical features associated with less severe causes of acute ataxia

- Migraine

    Obtaining detailed history with focus on headaches features in all patients with ataxia is necessary

    Dizziness affects almost 30% of migraine sufferers, while ataxia is less common; a therapeutic response to a medication that prevents migraine headaches may assist to ratify the diagnosis

- Benign positional paroxysmal vertigo

    Clinically presents with short (5–20 s) episodes of vertigo/ataxia induced by certain movements such as flexing, extending, or rotating the head

    Manifestations frequently persist for days or weeks and then may spontaneously improve

    Dix-Hallpike test is used to diagnose BPPV

- Vestibular neuronitis/labyrinthitis

    Sudden onset of severe vertigo/ataxia

    Frequently associated with nausea and vomiting

    Not associated with hearing loss or other neurologic abnormalities

    Patients often present with ataxia and nystagmus when vertiginous

    Once the persistent vertigo resolves, the patient often shows motion-induced dizziness, which may last for days or weeks

    A group of patients may develop recurrent episodes of vestibular neuronitis over weeks or months; however, these recurrent episodes are usually not as severe as the first episode

---

of uncontrolled hypertension as well as management of diabetes mellitus is necessary. However, permissive hypertension is often the recommended approach for acute ischemic strokes. Further discussion of these treatment options is beyond the scope of this article. In addition, in patients with ischemic cerebellar, stroke clinicians should be vigilant of impending hydrocephalus. In addition, in cerebellar strokes, the clinician should be on alert for clinical manifestations of increased intracranial pressure with risk of herniation. This group of unstable patients should be moved to intensive care units for close observation and treatment.

Patients who present with transient ischemic attacks (TIAs) should be admitted and treated with antiplatelet agents such as aspirin, clopidogrel, or aspirin plus extended-release dipyridamole unless there are specific contraindications. Treating patients with recurrent or crescendo TIAs with heparin remains controversial. In certain patients with ischemic stroke caused by cervical artery dissection, cardioembolic disease, or antiphospholipid antibody syndrome, anticoagulant therapy may be indicated. Treatment of other risk factors for stroke such as hyperlipidemia and smoking cessation should also be addressed.

In cases of malnutrition, Wernicke-Korsakoff syndrome, and acute ethanol intoxication, patients should be treated with thiamine, with a loading dose of 100 mg intravenously, followed by 50 to 100 mg daily intravenously or intramuscularly until the patient is placed on a balanced diet that provides adequate amounts of thiamine.

In all patients with ataxia caused by Miller-Fisher syndrome, respiratory function should assessed carefully, and in cases when respiratory function is deteriorating, the patient should be intubated. Acute demyelinating disorders are treated with intravenous corticosteroids, and certain forms of immune-mediated ataxias, such as Miller Fisher syndrome, are managed with intravenous immunoglobulin or plasmapheresis.

In patients with cerebellar space occupying lesions, which raise the possibility of abscess or tumor, infectious disease and neurosurgical consultations should be obtained, respectively. These patients should be closely monitored for manifestations and complications of increased intracranial pressure, and, if indicated, treatment with antibiotics or corticosteroids should be considered.

SUMMARY

In many cases, acute ataxia presents a neurologic emergency that must be assessed and treated effectively in order to save a patient's life and protect the patient from potential permanent complications and disabilities. A thorough knowledge of cerebellar anatomy and physiology and familiarity with common causes of acute ataxia, enable the clinician to develop a rapid and effective diagnostic approach and effective management approach.

REFERENCES

1. Ohyama K, Koike H, Masuda M, et al. Autonomic manifestations in acute sensory ataxic neuropathy: a case report. Auton Neurosci 2013;179(1–2):155–8.
2. Sechi G, Serra A. Wernicke's encephalopathy: new clinical settings and recent advances in diagnosis and management. Lancet Neurol 2007;6(5):442–55.
3. Kelly PJ, Stein J, Shafqat S, et al. Functional recovery after rehabilitation for cerebellar stroke. Stroke 2001;32(2):530–4.
4. Neugebauer H, Witsch J, Zweckberger K, et al. Space-occupying cerebellar infarction: complications, treatment, and outcome. Neurosurg Focus 2013;34: 1–13.
5. Witsch Neugebauer H, Zweckberger K, Juttler E. Primary cerebellar hemorrhage: complications, treatment and outcome. Clin Neurol Neurosurg 2013;115:863–9.
6. İncecik F, Hergüner MÖ, Altunbaşak Ş. Acute disseminated encephalomyelitis: an evaluation of 15 cases in childhood. Turk J Pediatr 2013;55(3):253–9.
7. Teener JW. Miller Fisher's syndrome. Semin Neurol 2012;32(5):512–6.
8. Nagappa M, Taly AB, Sinha S, et al. Tumefactive demyelination: clinical, imaging and follow-up observations in thirty-nine patients. Acta Neurol Scand 2013; 128(1):39–47.
9. Didelot A, Honnorat J. Paraneoplastic disorders of the central and peripheral nervous systems. Handb Clin Neurol 2014;121:1159–79.
10. Edlow JA, Newman-Toker D, Savitz SI. Diagnosis and initial management of cerebellar infarction. Lancet Neurol 2008;7(10):951–64.
11. Crawford JR, Say D. Vitamin B12 deficiency presenting as acute ataxia. BMJ Case Rep 2013;2013.

The Cerebellum and Sleep

Lourdes M. DelRosso, MD, FAASM[a],*, Romy Hoque, MD, FAASM[b]

KEYWORDS

- Cerebellum • Sleep disorders • Ataxia • Insomnia • Apnea

KEY POINTS

- The cerebellum participates in the REM/NREM sleep cycles.
- Blood flow changes have been seen in the cerebellum of patients affected by various sleep disorders.
- Sleep disturbances are reported in patients with cerebellar diseases.

INTRODUCTION

The role of the cerebellum in motor control has been established during wakefulness. During sleep, cerebellar participation in motor control also involves regulation of position, movements, and muscle tone. Early studies on cerebelloctomized cats showed a small decease in wakefulness and NREM sleep, and increase in REM sleep, possibly revealing a participation of the cerebellum in fine-tuning and regulating the sleep–wake cycle.[1] Changes in the sleep–wake cycle have also been reported after lesions in the fastigial nucleus and middle cerebellar peduncle. The thalamus, a crucial participant in NREM sleep generation, receives afferents from the cerebellum as demonstrated by the electroencephalogram (EEG) changes produced after electrical stimulation or suppression of various cerebellar nuclei.[2]

Functional magnetic resonance imaging (fMRI) has shown significantly increased activity in the cerebellum during slow wave sleep (**Fig. 1**). Further research is needed to determine whether the cerebellum actively participates in the generation or modulation of slow wave sleep, or whether it is recruited by the oscillations originated in the thalamus.[3]

During REM sleep, the cerebellum participates in the production of REM atonia and phasic activity of the lateral rectus muscles of the eyes.[4] It has been hypothesized that during REM sleep, the cerebellum regulates autonomic inputs from the amygdala, periaqueductal gray, and thalamus (ie, multisensory integration), and expresses

Disclosure: The authors do not have any conflict of interest to disclose.
[a] University of Pennsylvania School of Medicine, The Children's Hospital of Philadelphia, 34 Street and Civic Center Boulevard, Philadelphia, PA 19104, USA; [b] Louisiana State University School of Medicine, 1501 Kings Highway, Shreveport, LA 71103, USA
* Corresponding author.
E-mail address: lourdesdelrosso@me.com

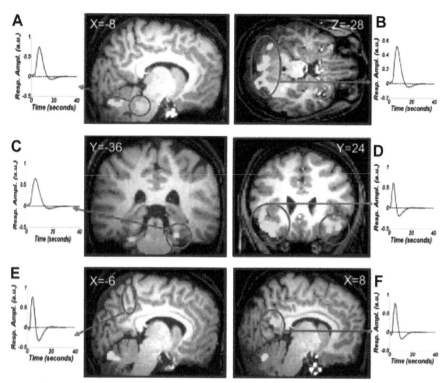

Fig. 1. fMRI results. Brain regions activated in relation to slow oscillation: common effects of both high-amplitude slow waves and delta waves. (*Middle*) Significant responses associated with both slow waves and delta waves. Functional results are displayed on an individual structural image (display at $P < 0.001$, uncorrected), at different levels of the x, y, and z axes, as indicated for each section. (*Left* and *Right*) Time course (in seconds) of fitted response amplitudes (in arbitrary units) during slow waves or delta waves in the corresponding circled brain area. All responses consist of regional increases in brain activity. (*A*) Pontine tegmentum. (*B*) Cerebellum. (*C*) Right parahippocampal gyrus. (*D*) Inferior frontal gyrus. (*E*) Precuneus. (*F*) Posterior cingulate cortex. (*From* Dang-Vu TT, Schabus M, Desseilles M, et al. Spontaneous neural activity during human slow wave sleep. Proc Natl Acad Sci U S A 2008;105(39):15162; with permission.)

parasympathetic and sympathetic outputs to the brainstem ventilatory and oculomotor neurons.[5] The fastigial nucleus may be particularly important in the inhibition of delta waves leading to the desynchronization of REM sleep and waking.[6]

THE CEREBELLUM IN SLEEP DISORDERS

Cerebellar findings in sleep disorders include

- Decreased blood blow in obstructive sleep apnea (OSA)
- Decreased gray matter in insomnia
- Atrophy in fatal familial insomnia (FFI)
- Water diffusion differences in congenital central hypoventilation syndrome (CCHS)

Obstructive Sleep Apnea

OSA has been associated with sympathetic activation, excessive daytime sleepiness, and cognitive changes, which may or may not resolve after treatment. These changes may be attributed to changes in cerebral blood flow. Positron emission tomography (PET) studies on patients with OSA demonstrate decreased blood flow in the cortico-spinal tracts, superior cerebellar peduncles, pontocerebellar fibers, and midbrain red nucleus.[7] These areas project to the cerebellum, and are involved in motor coordination and autonomic regulation.

The decrease in cerebral blood flow does not necessarily manifest as cerebral damage in magnetic resonance imaging (MRI). Newer MRI modalities like fractional inosotropy (FI) allow for a more sensitive evaluation of fiber integrity. FI studies have shown extensive white matter alteration in OSA patients. The affected areas include the internal capsule, ventral lateral thalamus, corticospinal tract, middle cerebellar peduncle, and the cerebellar deep nuclei. The postulated mechanism of damage of these areas is cytotoxicity secondary to intermittent hypoxia. The affected areas in the cerebellum, including the middle cerebellar peduncle and deep cerebellar nuclei, are important in cardiovascular control, coordination of the upper airway musculature with the diaphragm, and cognitive performance.[8]

Chronic Insomnia

Neuroimaging studies have demonstrated an increase in brain metabolism both during sleep and wakefulness in patients with chronic insomnia. A study of gray matter volume in patients with chronic insomnia demonstrated statistically significant decreases in cerebellum gray matter volume (**Fig. 2**). The clinical implications of these findings are not clear. It is unknown whether the gray matter deficit contributes to the onset of insomnia or is a consequence of the sleep disorder.

Fatal Familial Insomnia

FFI is an extremely rare autosomal-dominant prion disease characterized by insomnia, dysautonomia, somatomotor abnormalities (eg, cerebellar ataxia and dysarthria) and cognitive behavioral changes (oneiric stupor). PET studies have demonstrated severe thalamic hypometabolism, while neuropathologic data have revealed apoptotic neurons in the thalamus and medullary olives.[9] These findings suggest an initial involvement of the thalamus with progressive spread to other areas of the brain. With time, patients with FFI develop moderate atrophy of the cerebellum, with spongiform changes of the cerebellar cortex.[10] Mehta and colleagues[11] reported a case of FFI with progressive gait deterioration that required the use of a wheelchair 6 months after the onset of symptoms. The patient also had slurred speech, difficulty with manual coordination, and insomnia. An autopsy revealed marked atrophy of the cerebellum and degeneration of the thalamus. Western blot analysis confirmed the presence of abnormal protease-resistant prion protein consistent with FFI.

Congenital Central Hypoventilation Syndrome

CCHS is a syndrome characterized by hypoventilation at birth, with more severe hypoventilation during sleep compared with wakefulness. CCHS is associated with a mutation of the PHOX2B gene, which plays a role in autonomic system development. Kumar and colleagues[12] studied 12 patients with CCHS using MRI with diffusion tensor imaging (DTI) sequences. Visual inspection of T1 and T2 weighted imaging showed no obvious brainstem or cerebellar abnormalities. Compared with controls, DTI in CCHS showed significant water diffusion differences in the lateral medulla,

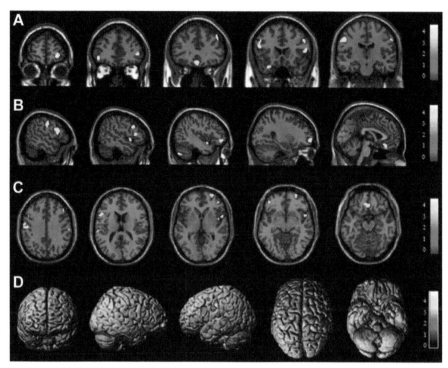

Fig. 2. A statistical brain map showing a decrease in gray matter concentration (GMC) in patients with chronic primary insomnia (PI) compared with normal controls (NCs). GMCs were significantly decreased in PI compared with NCs (uncorrected at P<.001, 2-sample t-test) in the following brain structures: right superior frontal gyrus, left orbitofrontal gyrus, right inferior frontal gyrus, right medial frontal gyrus, right middle frontal gyrus, right precentral gyrus, left postcentral gyrus (A) coronal; left postcentral gyrus, left inferior frontal gyrus, right middle frontal gyrus, right inferior frontal gyrus, right superior temporal gyrus, left middle frontal gyrus, left cerebellum, right superior frontal gyrus, left medial frontal gyrus (B) sagittal; left postcentral gyrus, right middle frontal gyrus, right precentral gyrus, left inferior frontal gyrus, right superior frontal gyrus, right inferior frontal gyrus, right superior temporal gyrus, left middle frontal gyrus, left medial frontal gyrus (C) axial. The overall areas with reduced GMCs were shown in a 3-dimensional brain surface rendering view (D). The results were displayed with the cluster threshold more than 50 voxels. Scales in the color bar are t scores. The left side of the images represents the left hemisphere of the brain. (*From* Joo EY, Noh HJ, Kim JS, et al. Brain gray matter deficits in patients with chronic primary insomnia. Sleep 2013;36(7):1004; with permission.)

dorsal midbrain, basal pons, cerebellar cortex, deep cerebellar nuclei, and the superior and inferior cerebellar peduncles. Involvement of such widespread brainstem and cerebellar regions may each contribute to the ventilatory disturbances seen in CCHS.

SLEEP DISTURBANCES IN CEREBELLAR DISEASES

Sleep complaints have been identified as part of the nonmotor symptoms found in cerebellar ataxia patients. The most frequent sleep disorders reported are restless leg syndrome (RLS), REM behavior disorder (RBD), excessive daytime sleepiness (EDS), and sleep apnea.[13] The mechanism, although still unclear, may be secondary to intrinsic cerebellar dysfunction.

Autosomal Dominant Spinocerebellar Ataxias

Dang and Cunnington[14] reported EDS in 2 patients with spinocerebellar ataxia 1 (SCA1). In the first patient, a 50-year-old woman, polysomnography revealed a total sleep time apnea–hypopnea index of 20.3. Despite compliance with continuous positive airway pressure (CPAP) therapy, EDS persisted. The second patient was a 48-year-old woman whose polysomnography did not reveal sleep-disordered breathing, but did show a periodic limb movement index of 95.8. She was treated with the dopamine receptor agonist pergolide. Leg movements and sleep restlessness improved, but EDS persisted.

RLS has been reported in up to 30% of patients with SCA, compared with 2% to 9% in the general population. The mechanism of RLS has been attributed to dysregulation of the dopaminergic system. Dopamine receptor availability was not reduced in patients with early stages of SCA1, SCA2, and SCA3 who had RLS symptoms.[15]

REM sleep without atonia and generalized myoclonic jerks have been seen in polysomnographic recordings of patients with SCA2.[16] Full-blown dream enacting behavior has been reported in patients with SCA3 (Joseph Machado disease), and in some patients, this may precede the onset of cerebellar symptoms by more than 10 years.[17,18] The mechanism may be related to midbrain cholinergic or pontine noradrenergic involvement.[19]

SCA6 is predominantly a cerebellar syndrome with only mild pyramidal signs. The lack of brainstem findings in SCA6 makes it an ideal type of SCA in which to study the effects of the cerebellum on sleep. Increased EDS has been noted on questionnaire-based studies into SCA6, but polysomnogram (PSG)-based studies are lacking.[6]

Autosomal-Recessive Ataxias

Friedreich ataxia (FA) is the most common recessive ataxia worldwide; however, data on sleep disorders are scarce. Corben and colleagues[20] studied 80 patients with FA; 21 patients underwent PSG scored in accordance with Rechtschaffen and Kales criteria, and 17 patients had sleep-disordered breathing based on respiratory disturbance index (RDI). Four patients had no OSA on PSG (RDI <5/h); 9 patients had mild OSA (RDI 5–20/h), and 3 patients had moderate OSA (RDI 20–30/h). Five patients had severe OSA (RDI >30/h). Mean RDI plus or minus standard deviation for all patients who underwent PSG was 18.6 plus or minus 18.2, with a range from 0 to 59.4. In those with PSG-verified OSA, RDI severity had a positive correlation with both disease severity and duration. Neither fragmentary myoclonus nor periodic leg movements were mentioned in the study.

Joubert syndrome is an autosomal-recessive disorder clinically associated with ataxia, hypotonia, developmental delay, and static encephalopathy. MRI of the brain shows hypoplasia of the cerebellar vermis, elongation of the superior cerebellar peduncles, and widening of the interpeduncular fossa, all-resulting in the molar tooth-like appearance of the midbrain. Patients with Joubert syndrome have demonstrated abnormal breathing patterns consisting of tachypnea followed by apnea. The mechanism is thought to be secondary to brainstem involvement. Wolfe and colleagues[21] described a 25-year-old man with Joubert syndrome whose diagnostic polysomnography revealed severe central apneas with periodic breathing and a central apnea hypopnea index of 48 events per hour of sleep. Central apneas were unresponsive to adaptive servoventilation, but resolved with bilevel positive airway pressure in spontaneous/timed mode.

Ataxia–telangiectasia (A-T) is an autosomal-recessive disease characterized by ataxia, cutaneous telangiectasias, and immunodeficiency. In a polysomnographic study of 12 adolescents with A-T, decreased sleep efficiency was noted without an increase in sleep-disordered breathing.[22]

Sleep complaints in patients with cerebellar disorders may include

- Excessive sleepiness
- Restless leg syndrome
- Obstructive apnea
- Central apnea
- Rapid eye movement behavior disorder

CASE STUDY

The case is a 6 year-old boy with Dandy-Walker syndrome and hydrocephalus status after ventriculo-peritoneal shunt and seizures. A prior report of Dandy-Walker syndrome in the literature did not reveal sleep architecture changes in sleep stages.[23]

This case differs in that sleep and wake could not be identified based on EEG criteria. The authors postulate that the degree of hydrocephalus and the degree of aplasia/hypoplasia of the cerebellum may correlate with the preservation of sleep EEG architecture.

The boy's sleep complaints included snoring.

The polysomnogram report included

- Apnea hypopnea index: 9.3 events per hour of sleep
- Oxyhemoglobin saturation nadir: 74%
- Periodic leg movement index: 0
- Electroencephalography: no sleep stage differentiation (see representative epoch **Fig. 3**)

No tonsilar/adenoid hypertrophy was found during otolaryngology consultation, and continuous positive airway pressure therapy was initiated.

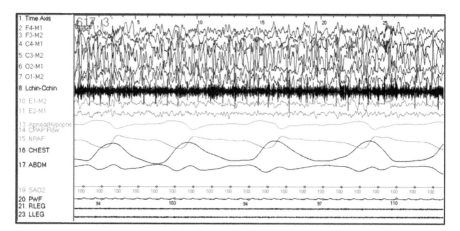

Fig. 3. 30-s polysomnogram epoch from a patient with Dandy-Walker syndrome. Electroencephalography channels show generalized slow wave, making sleep–wake differentiation impossible. Video monitoring was used to aid in estimating sleep and wake. NREM and REM sleep stages were not distinguished.

SUMMARY

The cerebellum has an important role in sleep. Certain sleep disorders have demonstrated decreased activity in the cerebellum, and sleep complaints are common in patients with cerebellar diseases.

REFERENCES

1. Cunchillos JD, De Andres I. Participation of the cerebellum in the regulation of the sleep–wakefulness cycle. Results in cerebellectomized cats. Electroencephalogr Clin Neurophysiol 1982;53(5):549–58.
2. de Andres I, Garzon M, Reinoso-Suarez F. Functional anatomy of non-REM sleep. Front Neurol 2011;2:70.
3. Dang-Vu TT, Schabus M, Desseilles M, et al. Spontaneous neural activity during human slow wave sleep. Proc Natl Acad Sci U S A 2008;105(39):15160–5.
4. Gadea-Ciria M, Fuentes J. Analysis of phasic activities in the lateral rectus muscle of the eyes (PALRE) during paradoxical sleep in chronic cerebellectomized cats. Brain Res 1976;111(2):416–21.
5. Dharani NE. The role of vestibular system and the cerebellum in adapting to gravitoinertial, spatial orientation and postural challenges of REM sleep. Med Hypotheses 2005;65(1):83–9.
6. Howell MJ, Mahowald MW, Gomez CM. Evaluation of sleep and daytime somnolence in spinocerebellar ataxia type 6 (SCA6). Neurology 2006;66(9):1430–1.
7. Yadav SK, Kumar R, Macey PM, et al. Regional cerebral blood flow alterations in obstructive sleep apnea. Neurosci Lett 2013;555:159–64.
8. Macey PM, Kumar R, Woo MA, et al. Brain structural changes in obstructive sleep apnea. Sleep 2008;31(7):967–77.
9. Pedroso JL, Pinto WB, Souza PV, et al. Complex movement disorders in fatal familial insomnia: a clinical and genetic discussion. Neurology 2013;81(12):1098–9.
10. Cortelli P, Fabbri M, Calandra-Buonaura G, et al. Gait disorders in fatal familial insomnia. Mov Disord 2014;29(3):420–4.
11. Mehta LR, Huddleston BJ, Skalabrin EJ, et al. Sporadic fatal insomnia masquerading as a paraneoplastic cerebellar syndrome. Arch Neurol 2008; 65(7):971–3.
12. Kumar R, Macey PM, Woo MA, et al. Diffusion tensor imaging demonstrates brainstem and cerebellar abnormalities in congenital central hypoventilation syndrome. Pediatr Res 2008;64(3):275–80.
13. Pedroso JL, Braga-Neto P, Felicio AC, et al. Sleep disorders in cerebellar ataxias. Arq Neuropsiquiatr 2011;69(2A):253–7.
14. Dang D, Cunnington D. Excessive daytime somnolence in spinocerebellar ataxia type 1. J Neurol Sci 2010;290(1–2):146–7.
15. Reimold M, Globas C, Gleichmann M, et al. Spinocerebellar ataxia type 1, 2, and 3 and restless legs syndrome: striatal dopamine D2 receptor status investigated by [11C]raclopride positron emission tomography. Mov Disord 2006;21(10): 1667–73.
16. Boesch SM, Frauscher B, Brandauer E, et al. Disturbance of rapid eye movement sleep in spinocerebellar ataxia type 2. Mov Disord 2006;21(10):1751–4.
17. Syed BH, Rye DB, Singh G. REM sleep behavior disorder and SCA-3 (Machado-Joseph disease). Neurology 2003;60(1):148.
18. D'Abreu A, Friedman J, Coskun J. Non-movement disorder heralds symptoms of Machado-Joseph disease years before ataxia. Mov Disord 2005;20(6):739–41.

19. Pedroso JL, Braga-Neto P, Felicio AC, et al. Sleep disorders in Machado-Joseph disease: frequency, discriminative thresholds, predictive values, and correlation with ataxia-related motor and non-motor features. Cerebellum 2011;10(2):291–5.

20. Corben LA, Ho M, Copland J, et al. Increased prevalence of sleep-disordered breathing in Friedreich ataxia. Neurology 2013;81(1):46–51.

21. Wolfe L, Lakadamyali H, Mutlu GM. Joubert syndrome associated with severe central sleep apnea. J Clin Sleep Med 2010;6(4):384–8.

22. McGrath-Morrow SA, Sterni L, McGinley B, et al. Polysomnographic values in adolescents with ataxia telangiectasia. Pediatr Pulmonol 2008;43(7):674–9.

23. Kohyama J, Watanabe S, Iwakawa Y, et al. A case of Dandy-Walker malformation: consideration on the teratogenic period and sleep structures. Brain Dev 1988; 10(6):392–6.

Toxic-Metabolic, Nutritional, and Medicinal-Induced Disorders of Cerebellum

Nadejda Alekseeva, MD[a], Jeanie McGee, DHEd, MSHS[b],
Roger E. Kelley, MD[c], Amir Hadi Maghzi, MD[d],
Eduardo Gonzalez-Toledo, MD, PhD[e], Alireza Minagar, MD[a],*

KEYWORDS

- Cerebellum • Ataxia • Atrophy • Thiamine deficiency • Phenytoin • Ethanol

KEY POINTS

- A number of toxic, metabolic, nutritional, and medicinal insults may affect the cerebellum.
- Acute alcohol intoxication, chronic alcoholism, anticonvulsant therapy, and thiamine deficiency are among the more common causes of cerebellar dysfunction.
- Metabolic explanations for cerebellar dysfunction can include hypoglycemia and hypothyroidism, as well as pronounced electrolyte disturbance.
- Illicit drugs such as cocaine, heroin, and phencyclidine can result in cerebellar damage.
- Poisoning with a number of agents, including carbon monoxide and insecticides, can affect the cerebellum.
- Rapid assessment and management of patients with toxin- and metabolic-induced disorders of the cerebellum can have an important impact on outcome.

INTRODUCTION

The human cerebellum is situated behind the pons and medulla within the posterior cranial fossa and is composed of 2 vastly convoluted hemispheres and a narrow medial section known as the vermis. The cerebellar vermis (derived from Latin word for worm) is situated in the corticonuclear zone of the cerebellum (**Fig. 1**). Three pairs of dense fiber bundles known as peduncles connect the cerebellum to the brain. Despite extensive research into the role of the cerebellum in human

[a] Department of Psychiatry, Overton Brooks VA Medical Center, 510 East Stoner Avenue, Shreveport, LA 71101, USA; [b] Department of Neurology, LSU Health Sciences Center, 1501 Kings Highway, Shreveport, LA 71103, USA; [c] Department of Neurology, Tulane University, 1430 Tulane Avenue, #8065, New Orleans, LA 70112, USA; [d] Department of Neurology, University of California, 350 Parnassus Avenue, San Francisco, CA 94117, USA; [e] Department of Radiology, LSU Health Sciences Center, Shreveport - 1501 Kings Highway, Shreveport, LA 71103, USA
* Corresponding author. LSUHSC-Shreveport, 1501 Kings Highway, Shreveport, LA 71130.
E-mail address: aminag@lsuhsc.edu

Neurol Clin 32 (2014) 901–911
http://dx.doi.org/10.1016/j.ncl.2014.07.001
0733-8619/14/$ – see front matter © 2014 Elsevier Inc. All rights reserved.

neurologic.theclinics.com

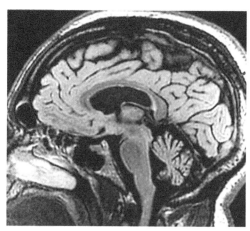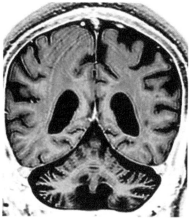

Fig. 1. (*Left*) Magnetic resonance imaging, fluid-attenuated inversion recovery sequence, coronal view showing a remarkable decrease in volume of the cerebellar vermis. (*Right*) Coronal inverted T2 weighted image shows decreased volume of the cerebellum, and hypoplastic vermis.

motor control and cognition, the exact mechanisms of its activities are only marginally understood. The cerebellum receives significant input from cerebral cortical and subcortical regions as well as the spinal cord. Such circuitry allows the cerebellum to have extensive information from the somesthetic, vestibular, visual, and auditory sensory systems, as well as from motor and nonmotor regions of the cerebral cortex.

Although the afferent connections are more substantial the efferent projections, the cerebellum possesses widespread outgoing connections to many regions of the brainstem, midbrain, and cerebral cortex. The cerebellum does not initiate motor activity; however, it does interact with many regions of the brain where movements are initiated to ensure that such motor activity is performed in a coordinated fashion. Like other components of the human brain, the cerebellum is sensitive and vulnerable to a wide gamut of pathologic processes that can lead to cerebellar dysfunction. In addition, a number of pathologies specifically affect the cerebellum. Insult to the cerebellum can result in a constellation of neurologic deficits, including:

- Ataxia (truncal, limb, and gait);
- Hypotonia;
- Dysarthria; and
- Ocular motility problems (including nystagmus and tremor).

The cerebellum is particularly susceptible to the toxic effects of metabolic and medicinal insults; the cerebellar cortex and Purkinje neurons are particularly vulnerable.[1] In susceptible individuals, the most frequent etiology for a toxic abnormality of the cerebellar function stems from acute alcohol poisoning as well as alcoholism. The cerebellum is potentially sensitive to drug exposure, such as anticonvulsants, antineoplastics, lithium salts, and calcineurin inhibitors; to illicit drugs, such as cocaine, heroin, phencyclidine; and to environmental poisons, such as mercury, lead, manganese, and toluene/benzene derivatives. Thus, the astute clinician must be aware of the multiple potential factors that can adversely affect cerebellar function. This will obviously guide timely and effective management with efforts to prevent long-standing disability or even death.

TOXIC AND METABOLIC DISORDERS
Alcohol and Ethanol

Alcohol (ethanol) can promote toxic effects on both the central and peripheral nervous systems. The damaging effects of alcohol on the nervous system stem from acute intoxication and withdrawal syndrome owing to abrupt cessation of alcohol intake. Acute and subacute disorders that can affect the cerebellum include nutritional deficiencies. A direct toxic effect on the components of the brain affects the vermis of the cerebellum and the mamillary bodies. Indirect effects can be from a brain injury-related propensity to falling.

After ingestion, alcohol rapidly crosses the blood–brain barrier. It directly interacts with a number of neurochemical receptors. Clinically, depending on the amount ingested, as well as the buildup of tolerance, the patient can present with behavioral effects of ethanol such as euphoria, social disinhibition, and drowsiness, as well as aggression in combination with slurred speech and gait ataxia. At particularly high serum concentrations of ethanol, subjects can develop progressive lethargy that can evolve into stupor and coma with the potential for death related to respiratory depression or cardiovascular collapse.

Ethanol, by itself or in combination with thiamine deficiency, can exert deleterious effects on the cerebellum. Ethanol-induced changes in cerebellar activity causes impairment of motor coordination and ataxia. In addition, alcohol-related cerebellar dysfunction may play a role in cognitive deficits associated with alcoholism.

Pathophysiology

The exact pathophysiology of the deleterious impact of ethanol on the human cerebellum remains marginally understood. As a psychoactive drug, ethanol diffusely affects the γ-aminobutyric acid (GABA)ergic transmission in brain via the facilitation of presynaptic interneuron firing.[2,3] Recent scientific observations show that alcohol consumption impairs motor coordination by increasing the tonic inhibition of granule cells, which are mediated by a specific extrasynaptic GABA A receptor subtype.[4] The excitability of the cerebellar granule cells is in part modulated by the GABAergic output from the Golgi cells. GABAergic input is received from the granule cells in tonic currents mediated by extrasynaptic receptors, as well as from phasic currents. These phasic currents are mediated by synaptic receptors.[5] The input received from both type of currents results in a filtering effect of the mossy fibers, which represent the most significant input to the cerebellum. This suppressive input profoundly alters cerebellar information and storage capacity.[5] This specific combination of α-6 and δ extrasynaptic subunit in this specific combination of α-6 and δ extrasynaptic subunits in the GABA A receptor is only found in these types of cerebellar granule cells, and the unique combination seems to direct the firing power of these cells by producing tonic inhibition.[4] Studies have demonstrated that alcohol indirectly enhances GABAergic transmission to the cerebellar granule cells via an increase in GABA release from the Golgi cells.[5] Concentrations of alcohol in the blood high enough to produce behavioral changes have been shown to enhance the tonic inhibition of cerebellar granule cells mediated by the extrasynaptic GABA receptors.[4] The greatest effect of this increased GABA inhibition is impaired motor coordination.[4]

Neuropathologically, direct adverse effects of ethanol on the human central nervous system include both cerebral atrophy and cerebellar degeneration. Alcoholic cerebellar degeneration is recognized by atrophy and loss of granule cells, mainly in the anterior superior section of the vermis.

Metabolic Disorders

A number of metabolic disorders, such as metachromatic leukodystrophy, Refsum disease, and mitochondrial disorders such as Leigh syndrome and Kearns–Sayre syndrome, affect the cerebellum and result in ataxia and other neurologic manifestations of cerebellar dysfunction. A detailed discussion of these disorders is beyond the scope of this article.

In patients with epilepsy, anticonvulsants, particularly diphenylhydantoin, carbamazepine, and primidone, can cause ataxia. In children, a constellation of ataxia, papilledema, and drowsiness can be seen with lead poisoning. Rare metabolic causes of cerebellar ataxia include Maple syrup urine disease, Hartnup disease, and ataxia-telangiectasia.

CARBON MONOXIDE AND HYPERTHERMIA

The cerebellar cortex is susceptible to oxygen deprivation and, at its resting state, consumes one of the highest amounts of the oxygen within the human central nervous system. In the human central nervous system, the cerebellar Purkinje cells and the hippocampal neurons are the most vulnerable groups to the adverse effects of hypoxia. In postanoxic animals, there is loss of Purkinje cells with resultant ataxia.[6] In humans, such vulnerability is even more pronounced and in many cases the postanoxic neurologic syndrome manifests with clinical features of cortical, pyramidal, extrapyramidal abnormalities as well as cerebellar ataxia.[7,8]

Carbon Monoxide Poisoning

Carbon monoxide (CO) poisoning as well as severe hyperthermia can have a profound effect on cerebellar function. CO has a high affinity for the oxygen-binding site of hemoglobin and can promote cardiopulmonary arrest. Because CO results in hypoxia, most of the clinical manifestations of CO poisoning stem from this hypoxic insult, which primarily affects the nervous system and heart. CO poisoning can be acute or chronic. The most common neurologic presentations of acute CO poisoning include headache, dizziness, and visual impairment. Severe CO poisoning may result in seizures and coma as well as respiratory impairment. Long-term residual neurologic deficits stemming from CO poisoning include behavioral disturbance with cognitive impairment, parkinsonism, and cerebellar abnormalities.[9,10]

Hyperthermia

Hyperthermia is associated with insufficient or inappropriate reactions of heat-regulating circuits. Hyperthermia can be seen during heat waves, resulting in heat stroke. Older individuals who have a limited ability to adjust to the temperature, athletes having inappropriate exposure to temperature extremes, and children left in cars during the summer months seem to be the most susceptible. Illicit drug use (especially amphetamines and cocaine) and the use of agents that can be associated with neuroleptic malignant syndrome identify other populations at greater risk. Neurologic manifestations can include cerebellar dysarthria, gait ataxia or a pan-cerebellar syndrome.[11] Symptoms may resolve within 3 to 10 days in those individuals with a reversible injury. Cerebellar deficits may also be part of a diffuse encephalopathy, which includes seizure, disorientation, dizziness, and severe fatigue.[12] Up to 20% of patients affected with heat stroke experience residual neurologic deficits and neuroimaging of brain has shown cerebellar atrophy may follow months after the initial event of hyperpyrexia.[13]

Purkinje cells are for the most part susceptible to heat-induced pathology. Neuropathologic studies have demonstrated significant and widespread loss of Purkinje cells along with expression of heat shock protein 70 by Bergmann glia.[14] Based on the findings of the study by Bazille and colleagues,[14] loss of Purkinje cell axons leads to appearance of myelin pallor of the white matter of the folia and the hilum of the dentate nuclei. DNA internucleosomal breakages were observed by utilizing in situ end-labeling in the dentate nuclei and centromedian nuclei of the thalamus. This observation was associated with degeneration of the cerebellar efferent pathways, including the superior cerebellar peduncles, and decussation of the superior cerebellar peduncles and dentatothalamic tract. According to these investigators, Ammon's horn and other areas that are vulnerable to the deleterious effects of hypoxia were not affected.[14]

NUTRITIONAL DEFICIENCIES

It is well recognized that a balanced and adequate diet is necessary for the development and normal functioning of the human nervous system. Nutritional inadequacies, particularly vitamin deficiency states, can exert adverse effects on central and peripheral components of the nervous system, resulting in a spectrum of neurologic presentations that can include mental retardation, altered sensorium, psychosis, seizures, cerebellar ataxias, and peripheral neuropathies. A number of nutritional inadequacies that cause cerebellar disorders are discussed herein.

THIAMINE DEFICIENCY

Neurologic disorders associated with thiamine deficiency include beriberi, Wernicke encephalopathy, and Korsakoff syndrome. Potential causes of thiamine dietary insufficiency can include recurrent vomiting, gastric surgery, alcoholism, severe dieting, and elevated demand with insignificant nutritional intake.[15] Thiamine deficiency associated with alcoholism is more common in males, whereas thiamine deficiency stemming from gastric–bariatric surgery is more frequent in females.[16] Wernicke encephalopathy manifests with subacute onset of ocular abnormalities, gait ataxia, and alteration of mental status. Ocular abnormalities consist of horizontal and vertical nystagmus, ophthalmoparesis, and conjugate gaze palsy. Gait and trunk ataxia originate from cerebellar and vestibular dysfunction. Cerebellar involvement also presents with dysarthria. Patients with Wernicke encephalopathy can progress to develop Korsakoff syndrome, which is characterized by severe anterograde and retrograde amnesia as well as confabulation.

MEDICINES

A number of medications at toxic levels can result in neurologic abnormalities. Cerebellar dysfunction may stem from the direct impact of toxic levels of these medications or may be part of a more global phenomenon, such as toxic encephalopathy. Once a clinician encounters medicinal-induced cerebellar syndromes, certain features in the patient's clinical picture should be carefully sought. The development of medicinal-induced cerebellar disorders usually initially affects the patient's gait, and this may or may not be followed by involvement of the extremities. The cerebellar involvement, particularly ataxia with nystagmus, may occur with either acute or chronic use of the offending medicine and can occur when the serum levels of the medicine are "subtherapeutic, therapeutic, or toxic." In general, the cerebellar disorder usually improves with cessation of the offending medicine; however, certain cerebellar findings may persist.

An interesting practical concept is that patients who chronically take a particular medication may develop acute cerebellar deficits with no alteration of their dosage.

Antiepileptics

Antiepileptics, as a family, are well recognized for their potential for toxicity and causing cerebellar ataxia. Certain antiepileptics, such as phenytoin, carbamazepin, and barbiturates, are well known for causing ataxia, whereas benzodiazepines are most often associated with excessive sedation before patients develops ataxia. Valproic acid is commonly associated with the onset of a tremor that closely imitates intention tremor of the cerebellar origin.

Phenytoin

Patients with epilepsy who take relatively higher doses of phenytoin may develop permanent ataxia and cerebellar atrophy. This has impacted on the decision-making process in the choice of older versus newer anticonvulsant agents. Of interest, there is a correlation between the dose of phenytoin and development of ataxic symptoms with a tendency for patients at a lower dose to develop nystagmus and truncal ataxia, whereas appedicular ataxia becomes more prominent at higher dosing. These clinical manifestations can slowly progress, but may improve by lowering the dose or cessation of phenytoin. In clinical practice, certain patients tolerate high doses without developing any ataxia. Such patients do not necessarily have to be switched from phenytoin to an alternative agent, at least in the shorter run, if expense and tolerability, along with the ready ability to check blood levels to ensure compliance, make this a reasonable choice.

Patients with epilepsy who have a CYP2C mutation (*2 or *3) show a reduction in phenytoin metabolism that in turn is associated with cerebellar atrophy with mainly loss of cerebellar white matter.[17] Of note, cerebellar abnormalities may develop a number of years after initiation of treatment despite therapeutic blood levels. As an indicator of compliance with medication, most patients on phenytoin at a therapeutic level have nystagmus and this tends to become increasingly prominent as the serum level exceeds 20 μg/mL. It is important to recognize that, with cessation of treatment with phenytoin, some patients recover completely with resolution of the cerebellar dysfunction, whereas some may suffer from permanent cerebellar impairment.[18] It is also important to recognize that the serum phenytoin level, because of its binding characteristics, needs to be corrected if the serum albumin level is low.

Certain patients with previous, clinically asymptomatic cerebellar injury or with myoclonic-type epilepsy may be more prone to phenytoin toxicity. An important clinical point is that certain medicines may increase the half-life of phenytoin and increase the chance of toxicity. These drug–drug interactions are not necessarily uncommon with phenytoin and have impacted on its attractiveness as a choice for anticonvulsant therapy. Neuroimaging studies may demonstrate various degrees of cerebellar atrophy in patients with permanent cerebellar dysfunction after chronic exposure to phenytoin (see **Fig. 1**).

Neuropathologic examinations of these patients have demonstrated widespread loss of Purkinje cells, a decline in the population of granule cells, and Bergmann gliosis with relative sparing of basket cell axons.[19] Urgent admission and treatment of patients with acute intoxication with phenytoin and ataxia is necessary to avoid possible long-term neurologic deficits.

Carbamazepine

Carbamazepine, another still commonly used antiepileptic, can be associated with dose-dependent ataxic manifestations. Affected patients manifest gaze-evoked nystagmus, action tremor, and gait ataxia.[1,11,20] Elderly patients and those with pre-existing cerebellar atrophy are at greater risk for developing cerebellar damage at lesser serum concentrations. Of clinical pertinence is that carbamazepine is also used in the treatment of painful entities such as trigeminal neuralgia and may also be used to stabilize the mood in patients with bipolar (manic–depressive) disorder. In the latter scenario, the combination of carbamazepine and lithium salt—2 toxic agents for the cerebellum—requires familiarity with this issue and close observation.[21] Treatment of psychiatric patients suffering from mood disorders with a combination of lithium compounds and carbamazepine may cause cerebellar toxicity even when serum concentrations of both medicines are within therapeutic range. Clinicians should also be aware that certain medicines that are CYP 3A4 inhibitors suppress carbamazepine metabolism and increase its serum concentration. Some of the more common agents include clarithromycin, fluoxetine, verapamil, oxybutynin, valproic acid, and loratadine. Toxicity with carbamazepine is a potential medical emergency, because it can lead to a decrease in the level of consciousness and coma. It is significant to recognize that in certain patients the total serum concentration of carbamazepine is therapeutic; however, the free drug level is actually elevated. Patients with clinical manifestations of severe carbamazepine toxicity need to be admitted and treated in monitored units because toxicity with carbamazepine may cause coma and death.

Phenobarbital
Phenobarbital is another commonly used antiepileptic that can cause ataxic signs, including gaze-evoked nystagmus, tremor, and gait ataxia. Based on our own observations of epileptic patients, a significant number of them suffer from cerebellar abnormalities.

Gabapentin
Gabapentin (Neurontin, Pfizer, New York, NY) augments GABAergic suppression and can cause ataxia. This ataxic side effect is generally readily treated with either reduction in the dose or, if necessary, discontinuation. Of interest, gabapentin may ameliorate ataxia in patients with isolated cerebellar atrophy.[22] Vigabatrin suppresses GABA transaminase and may cause ataxia when it is used for treatment of drug-resistant epilepsy. This potential side effect tends to be observed during initiation of the therapy.[23]

NICOTINE

Nicotine is a well-recognized cerebellar toxin[24,25] and, in the adult rat, chronic exposure to nicotine causes a decrease in the number of Purkinje cells in the cerebellar vermis.[26] Clinical reports indicate that nicotine may at least temporarily worsen ataxia in patients with multiple system atrophy[27] and in patients with spinocerebellar ataxia, cigarette smoking can transiently aggravate dysarthria, limb ataxia, and truncal titubation.[28]

Although a number of scientific observations have assessed the deleterious effects of chronic nicotine exposure on the various cells and layers of cerebellum, 1 particular study concentrated on the effects of long-term nicotine exposure on cerebellar white matter.[29] The investigators administered oral nicotine via cannula for 60 days, using dose rates of 5 and 10 mg/d to male Drukrey rats. At the conclusion of the study, the cerebellum was removed and neuropathologic study demonstrated that long-term nicotine exposure had caused significant loss of the white core of cerebellum.

ANTINEOPLASTIC MEDICINES

Treatment of cancer patients with a number of antineoplastic medicines such as 5-fluorouracil, methotrexate, cytarabine, cisplatin, oxaliplatin, paclitaxel, capecitabine, and epothilone D can be associated with neurologic side effects, particularly ataxia. At high doses, 5-fluorouracil may induce a pancerebellar syndrome.[30,31] Intrathecal administration of methotrexate may cause damage to cerebellar structures and induce ataxia.[32] Administration of cytarabine at doses greater than 3 g/m^2 may cause intoxication, which presents with nystagmus and other cerebellar deficits.[33] Cisplatin, oxaliplatin, and paclitaxel, which are used in the treatment of cancer, may induce polyneuropathy with a significant component of sensory ataxia.[34] Capecitabine, an antimetabolic agent, is utilized for the treatment of metastatic colorectal and breast cancers and may cause widespread toxic encephalopathy as well as diffuse white matter lesions that affect both supratentorial and infratentorial structures.[35,36] Epothilone D, which is used for treatment of prostate cancer, may demonstrate neurologic toxic effects including ataxia.[37]

AMIODARONE

Amiodarone is an antiarrhythmic medicine with a thyroxinelike structure, and is used for treatment of both atrial and cardiac arrhythmias. As a class III antiarrhythmic medicine, amiodarone prolongs phase 3 of the cardiac action potential. Amiodarone can have a number of unfavorable side effects, such as interstitial lung disease, skin rash, hypothyroidism or hyperthyroidism, corneal microdeposits, ataxia (particularly gait ataxia), tremor, dizziness, cognitive impairment, and peripheral neuropathy.[38] Up to 5% to 7% of patients treated with amiodarone manifest a cerebellar disorder.[39] The neurologic side effects of amiodarone, particularly cerebellar ataxia, may improve once the patient stops taking the medication, but may continue for a number of years, perhaps reflective of the long half-life of elimination of amiodarone.

Procainamide hydrochloride is another antiarrhythmic medicine used for treatment of ventricular tachycardia that may induce cerebellar ataxia at high doses with a significant increase in serum level. The ataxia resolves after cessation of the medicine.[40]

Bismuth preparations are used for treatment of gastrointestinal and skin disorders. Bismuth can induce a progressive toxic neurologic syndrome that is recognized by encephalopathic features, such as confusion, seizures, delirium, myoclonus, and cerebellar deficits, including tremor and gait ataxia.[41,42]

Lithium salts, which are still used extensively for the treatment of acute mania and prophylaxis of recurrent bipolar and unipolar affective disorders, may cause toxicity during maintenance treatment or acutely. Such neurologic toxicity manifests with tremor and ataxia. The hypothyroidism induced by lithium salts may intensify the ataxia. Acute lithium intoxication can be associated with a constellation of neurologic symptoms, including altered sensorium, seizures, hypokinesia, tremor, and enhanced deep tendon reflexes; it can also include coma in severe cases. Although these neurologic deficits associated with acute lithium toxicity resolve, some patients may demonstrate a cerebellar disorder with dysarthria, tremor, and gait ataxia.[11]

ILLICIT DRUGS

Use of illicit drugs such as phencyclidine, cocaine, and heroin can cause neurologic damage with a predilection for cerebellar ataxia.

Phencyclidine

Phencyclidine (also known as PCP or angel dust), is a member of the dissociative anesthetics and primarily functions as a noncompetitive N-methyl-D-aspartate receptor antagonists.[43] Utilization of this illicit drug at toxic doses may cause cerebellar ataxia, tremor, and nystagmus. It has been shown that phencyclidine in rats is toxic to the cerebellar Purkinje cells. Näkki and colleagues[43] assessed the expression of Fos protein in the cerebellum and functionally related nuclei of the brainstem. These investigators observed that PCP induced Fos immunostaining in neurons of the inferior olive, cerebellar granule cell layer, and deep cerebellar and vestibular nuclei. They concluded that high doses of PCP cause toxicity to the Purkinje cells at least partially via excessive activity of climbing fibers, which represent the excitatory neural input that arises from the inferior olive and synapses on Purkinje cell dendrites.

Cocaine

Cocaine use can cause seizures, delirium, altered mental status, and cerebellar ataxia. As a psychomotor stimulant, cocaine is particularly notorious for causing both ischemic and hemorrhagic strokes[44] and the ischemic stroke may leave the patient with cerebellar ataxia. The proposed underlying pathophysiologic mechanisms for cocaine-induced strokes include hypertension, embolism, vasospasm, and vasculitis.

Heroin

Another illicit, often dangerous, agent is heroin, which can result in serious neurologic complications. Inhalation[45] or ingestion of heroin can uncommonly be associated with a toxic spongiform leukoencephalopathy.[46,47] Clinically, patients may present with lethargy, inattention, forgetfulness, and personality changes as well as dysarthria, ataxia, dementia, coma, and even death.[48] Neuropathologic study of the brains of chronic heroin addicts has demonstrated loss of Purkinje cell layer along with a reactive proliferation of Bergman glia.[49]

SUMMARY

A large number of toxic and metabolic insults, nutritional deficiencies, and commonly used medications can have toxic and injurious effects on cerebellum. Clinicians' familiarity with this subject and search for the insulting agent can have a significant on patients' lives.

REFERENCES

1. Manto M. Toxic agents causing cerebellar ataxias. Handb Clin Neurol 2012;103: 201–13.
2. Siggins GR, Roberto M, Nie Z. The tipsy terminal: presynaptic effects of ethanol. Pharmacol Ther 2005;107(1):80–98.
3. Weiner JL, Valenzuela CF. Ethanol modulation of GABAergic transmission: the view from the slice. Pharmacol Ther 2006;111(3):533–54.
4. Hanchar HJ, Dodson PD, Olsen RW, et al. Alcohol-induced motor impairment caused by increased extrasynaptic GABA(A) receptor activity. Nat Neurosci 2005;8(3):339–45.
5. Carta M, Mameli M, Valenzuela CF. Alcohol enhances GABAergic transmission to cerebellar granule cells via an increase in Golgi cell excitability. J Neurosci 2004; 24(15):3746–51.

6. Auer RN, Siesjö BK. Biological differences between ischemia, hypoglycemia, and epilepsy. Ann Neurol 1988;24(6):699–707.

7. Ginsberg MD. Delayed neurological deterioration following hypoxia. Adv Neurol 1979;26:21–44.

8. Plum F, Posner JB, Hain RF. Delayed neurological deterioration after anoxia. Arch Intern Med 1962;110:18–25.

9. Savoldi F, Mazzella GL, Bo P, et al. Cerebellar ataxia due to acute carbon monoxide poisoning. Riv Neurobiol 1973;19(3–4):197–206 [in Italian].

10. Kułakowska A, Drozdowski W, Halicka D, et al. Neurologic and psychiatric sequelae of carbon monoxide poisoning. Neurol Neurochir Pol 2000;34(3): 587–95.

11. Manto MU, Topka H. Reversible cerebellar gait ataxia with postural tremor during episodes of high pyrexia. Clin Neurol Neurosurg 1996;98:227–30.

12. Lawden MC, Blunt S, Matthews T, et al. Recurrent confusion and ataxia triggered by pyrexia in a case of occult multiple sclerosis. J Neurol Neurosurg Psychiatr 1994;57(11):1436.

13. Mohapatro AK, Thomas M, Jain S, et al. Pancerebellar syndrome in hyperpyrexia. Australas Radiol 1990;34(4):320–2.

14. Bazille C, Megarbane B, Bensimhon D, et al. Brain damage after heat stroke. J Neuropathol Exp Neurol 2005;64(11):970–5.

15. Kumar N. Neurologic presentations of nutritional deficiencies. Neurol Clin 2010; 28(1):107–70.

16. Kumar N. Acute and subacute encephalopathies: deficiency states (nutritional). Semin Neurol 2011;31(2):169–83.

17. Twardowschy CA, Werneck LC, Scola RH, et al. The role of CYP2C9 polymorphisms in phenytoin-related cerebellar atrophy. Seizure 2013;22(3):194–7.

18. Chatak NR, Santoso RA, McKinney WN. Cerebellar degeneration following long term phenytoin therapy. Neurology 1976;26:818–20.

19. Crooks R, Mitchell T, Thom M. Patterns of cerebellar atrophy in patients with chronic epilepsy: a quantitative neuropathological study. Epilepsy Res 2000; 41(1):63–73.

20. Seymour JF. Carbamazepine overdose. Features of 33 cases. Drug Saf 1993; 8(1):81–8.

21. Rittmannsberger H, Leblhuber F. Asterixis induced by carbamazepine therapy. Biol Psychiatry 1992;32(4):364–8.

22. Gazulla J, Tintoré MA. The P/Q-type voltage-dependent calcium channel as pharmacological target in spinocerebellar ataxia type 6: gabapentin and pregabalin may be of therapeutic benefit. Med Hypotheses 2007;68:131–6.

23. Browne TR, Mattson RH, Penry JK, et al. A multicentre study of vigabatrin for drug-resistant epilepsy. Br J Clin Pharmacol 1989;27(Suppl 1):95S–100S.

24. Manto MU, Jacquy J. Other cerebellotoxic agents. In: Manto MU, Pandolfo M, editors. The cerebellum and its disorders. Cambridge (England): Cambridge University Press; 2002. p. 342–66.

25. Slotkin TA, Greer N, Faust J, et al. Effects of maternal nicotine injections on brain development in the rat: ornithine decarboxylase activity, nucleic acids and proteins in discrete brain regions. Brain Res Bull 1986;17(1):41–50.

26. Chen WJ, Edwards RB, Romero RD, et al. Long term nicotine exposure reduces Purkinje cell number in the adult rat cerebellar vermis. Neurotoxicol Teratol 2003; 25(3):329–34.

27. Johnsen JA, Miller VT. Tobacco intolerance in multiple system atrophy. Neurology 1986;36(7):986–8.

28. Houi K, Oka H, Mochio S. The effects of nicotine on a patient with spinocerebellar degeneration whose symptoms were temporarily exacerbated by cigarette smoking. Rinsho Shinkeigaku 1993;33:774–6.
29. Tewari A, Hasan M, Sahai A, et al. White core of cerebellum in nicotine treated rats - a histological study. J Anat Soc India 2010;59:150–3.
30. Murray P. Cerebellar toxicity with capecitabine in a patient with metastatic breast cancer. Clin Oncol (R Coll Radiol) 2008;20(5):382–3.
31. Pirzada NA, Ali II, Dafer RM. Fluorouracil-induced neurotoxicity. Ann Pharmacother 2000;34(1):35–8.
32. Oliff A, Bleyer WA, Poplack DG. Acute encephalopathy after initiation of cranial irradiation for meningeal leukaemia. Lancet 1978;2(8079):13–5.
33. Marsot Dupuch K. Acute cerebellar syndrome following intermediate-dose cytarabine. Br J Haematol 2001;113(4):846.
34. Pasetto LM, D'Andrea MR, Rossi E, et al. Oxaliplatin-related neurotoxicity: how and why? Crit Rev Oncol Hematol 2006;59(2):159–68.
35. Renouf D, Gill S. Capecitabine-induced cerebellar toxicity. Clin Colorectal Cancer 2006;6:70–1.
36. Fantini M, Gianni L, Tassinari D, et al. Toxic encephalopathy in elderly patients during treatment with capecitabine: literature review and a case report. J Oncol Pharm Pract 2011;17(3):288–91.
37. Beer TM, Higano CS, Saleh M, et al. Phase II study of KOS-862 in patients with metastatic androgen independent prostate cancer previously treated with docetaxel. Invest New Drugs 2007;25(6):565–70.
38. Willis MS, Lugo AM. Amiodarone-induced neurotoxicity. Am J Health Syst Pharm 2009;66(6):567–9.
39. Garretto NS, Rey RD, Kohler G, et al. Cerebellar syndrome caused by amiodarone. Arq Neuropsiquiatr 1994;52(4):575–7.
40. Schwartz AB, Klausner SC, Yee S, et al. Cerebellar ataxia due to procainamide toxicity. Arch Intern Med 1984;144(11):2260–1.
41. Gordon MF, Abrams RI, Rubin DB, et al. Bismuth toxicity. Neurology 1994;44(12):2418.
42. Gordon MF, Abrams RI, Rubin DB, et al. Bismuth subsalicylate toxicity as a cause of prolonged encephalopathy with myoclonus. Mov Disord 1995;10(2):220–2.
43. Näkki R, Sharp FR, Sagar SM. FOS expression in the brainstem and cerebellum following phencyclidine and MK801. J Neurosci Res 1996;43(2):203–12.
44. Fonseca AC, Ferro JM. Drug abuse and stroke. Curr Neurol Neurosci Rep 2013;13:325.
45. Au-Yeung K, Lai C. Toxic leucoencephalopathy after heroin inhalation. Australas Radiol 2002;46(3):306–8.
46. Weber W, Henkes H, Möller P, et al. Toxic spongiform leucoencephalopathy after inhaling heroin vapour. Eur Radiol 1998;8(5):749–55.
47. Bega DS, McDaniel LM, Jhaveri MD, et al. Diffusion weighted imaging in heroin-associated spongiform leukoencephalopathy. Neurocrit Care 2009;10(3):352–4.
48. Filley CM, Kleinschmidt-DeMasters BK. Toxic leukoencephalopathy. N Engl J Med 2001;345:425.
49. Oehmichen M, Meissner C, Reiter A, et al. Neuropathology in non-human immunodeficiency virus-infected drug-addicts: hypoxic brain damage after chronic intravenous drug abuse. Acta Neuropathol 1996;91:642–6.

Neuro-oncological Disorders of the Cerebellum

Thomas J. Pfiffner, MD[a], Ronak Jani, MD[a], Laszlo Mechtler, MD[b],*

KEYWORDS

- Brain tumors • Magnetic resonance imaging (MRI) • Neuro-oncology • Cerebellum
- Neuroimaging • Paraneoplastic syndrome

KEY POINTS

- Nonspecific symptoms of cerebellar disease, such as dystaxia, vertigo, nausea, headaches, and loss of developmental milestones, should prompt the neurologist to screen for posterior fossa tumors, especially in children.
- The most common pediatric cerebellar neoplasms are pilocytic astrocytomas, medulloblastomas, or ependymomas, whereas in adults, metastatic disease is the most common.
- The role of conventional neuroimaging in the diagnosis of brain tumors is essential regarding localization, characterization, and establishing a treatment plan.
- Newer magnetic resonance imaging techniques, such as susceptibility-weighted imaging, diffusion-weighted imaging/apparent diffusion coefficient, diffusion tensor imaging, and perfusion-weighted imaging provide additional presurgically important information.

INTRODUCTION

After leukemia, central nervous system tumors are the second most common neoplasm in children, making up the most common solid neoplasms in children. They account for the greatest mortality from cancer in children.[1] These tumors occur with an annual incidence of approximately 3 per 100,000. Supratentorial tumors are more common in infants and children up to the age of 3 years and after the age of 10 years; from 4 to 10 years of age, infratentorial tumors predominate.[2] In contrast to children, intra-axial posterior fossa tumors in adults are rare, and most commonly consist of metastasis from an extracranial site. Most posterior fossa tumors in adult patients are extra-axial and include schwannomas, meningiomas, epidermoid, and metastatic leptomeningeal disease. This article provides an overview of the intra-axial tumors that affect the cerebellum, which can be categorized by location and age (**Table 1**). For each tumor, we review conventional neuroimaging findings and discuss the value of

[a] DENT Neurologic Institute, 3980 Sheridan Drive, Amherst, NY 14226, USA; [b] DENT Neurologic Institute, Roswell Park Cancer Institute, 3980 Sheridan Drive, Buffalo, NY 14226, USA
* Corresponding author.
E-mail address: lmechtler@dentinstitute.com

Neurol Clin 32 (2014) 913–941
http://dx.doi.org/10.1016/j.ncl.2014.07.011
0733-8619/14/$ – see front matter © 2014 Elsevier Inc. All rights reserved.

neurologic.theclinics.com

Table 1
Cerebellar tumors based on age

Tumor	Age
Ependymoma	2–4 y
Classic medulloblastoma	Usually <10 y of age
Choroid plexus papilloma	18–25 y for 4th ventricle choroid plexus papilloma
Central nervous system lymphoma	Immunocompromised <40 Immunocompetent >60
Pilocytic astrocytoma	1st 2 decades of life
Hemangioblastoma	Sporadic: 5th and 6th decades of life Associated with von Hippel-Lindau disease: 3rd or 4th decade of life
Glioblastoma	Primarily in elderly patients
Lhermitte-Duclos disease	3rd and 4th decades of life
Metastases	Usually >50 y

more advanced neuroimaging techniques. Current management strategies are also briefly discussed. Finally, cerebellar paraneoplastic disorders, are discussed.

The clinical presentation is often dictated by the age of the patient and the location of the tumor. Brain tumors in infants often have relatively nonspecific symptoms initially, which may include irritability, listlessness, vomiting, failure to thrive, loss of developmental milestones, and progressive macrocephaly.[3,4] Although older children are more likely to manifest localizing neurologic findings, these are by no means uniformly present. Instead, many patients have recurrent bouts of headache, nausea, and vomiting, often occurring early in the morning, along with insidiously progressive ataxia. This symptom complex suggests the presence of increased intracranial pressure and is particularly common for posterior fossa tumors.[5–7] In some benign tumors, such as cerebellar pilocytic astrocytomas (PA), ataxia may be the primary symptom, and parents will sometimes comment that the child has been "clumsy" for years before the initial detection of a brain tumor.[6]

The current standard of neuroimaging for brain tumor evaluation is anatomic magnetic resonance imaging (MRI) with gadolinium-based intravenous contrast agent, providing highly sensitive tumor detection and characterization far superior to any other imaging modality. MRI has been found to be more sensitive than computed tomography (CT) in the detection of asymptomatic progression of disease. However, conventional MRI suffers from nonspecificity with respect to vastly different pathologic processes that appear to be similar on imaging. In the past decade, the development and application of various functional imaging techniques have increased, such as proton MR spectroscopy, diffusion-weighted (**Fig. 1**) and perfusion-weighted MRI (DWI/PWI). These advances, along with refinements in surgical techniques and adjuvant management approaches, have contributed to marked improvements in the outcomes of brain tumors. **Table 2** summarizes the characteristic findings of the most common cerebellar tumors.[8]

MEDULLOBLASTOMA

Medulloblastoma (MB) is the most common malignant central nervous system (CNS) tumor in children. All MBs, regardless of the subtype, are designated as World Health Organization (WHO) grade IV neoplasms. MB usually occurs more frequently in male individuals and usually before 10 years of age. Although uncommon, it can occur in

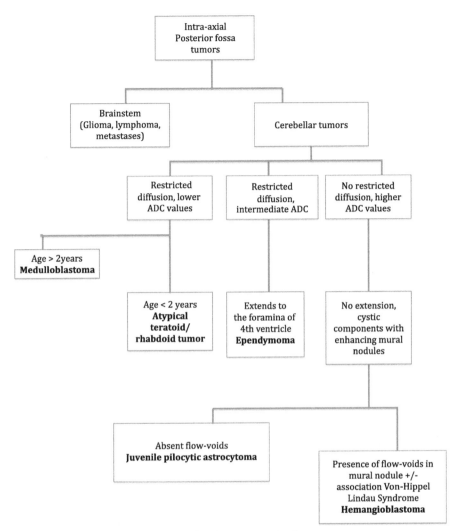

Fig. 1. DWI and ADC characteristics of pediatric posterior fossa tumors.

adults in the third or fourth decade of life. It is thought to arise from primitive cells of the external granular layer of the cerebellum, which persist until the second year of life.[9]

Pathology

The most common location is midline. MBs are located most often within the fourth ventricle and focally infiltrate the dorsal brainstem. Posterior inferior extension into the cisterna magna is common. Unlike ependymoma, lateral extension into the cerebellopontine angle is rare.[10] Paramedian location is more common in adults and in the desmoplastic variant (cerebellar hemisphere), as well as the MB with extensive nodularity variant (cerebellar hemisphere).[11] Microscopically, classic MBs are highly cellular tumors. The typical appearance is that of dense sheets comprised of uniform cells with round or oval hyperchromatic pleomorphic nuclei surrounded by scanty cytoplasm ("small round blue-cell tumor"). Neuroblastic (Homer-Wright) rosettes (radial arrangements of tumor cells around fibrillary processes) are found in 40% of cases.[10,12]

Table 2
Differential imaging findings amongst medulloblastoma, ependymoma, astrocytoma, and hemangioblastoma within the posterior fossa

Feature	Medulloblastoma	Ependymoma	Astrocytoma	Hemangioblastoma
Unenhanced CT	Hyperdense	Isodense	Hypodense	Hypodense cyst, isodense nodule
Enhancement	Moderate	Minimal	Nodule enhances, cyst does not	Nodule enhances, cyst dose not
Calcification	Uncommon (10%–21%)	Common (40%–50%)	Uncommon (<10%)	Absent
Origin	Vermis	Fourth-ventricle ependyma	Hemispheric	Hemispheric
T2WI	Intermediate	Intermediate	Bright	Bright
Site	Midline	Midline	Eccentric	Eccentric
Subarachnoid seeding	15%–50%	Uncommon	Rare	Absent
Age, y	5–12	2–10	10–20	Sporadic: 5th and 6th decade. VHL associated: 3rd and 4th decades
Cyst formation	10%–20%	15%	60%–80%	60%
Foraminal spread	No	Yes (Luschka, Magendie)	No	No
Hemorrhage	Rare	10%	Rare	Absent
MRS metabolite				
NAA	Low	Intermediate	Intermediate	
Lactate	Absent	Often present	Often present	
Choline	High	Less elevated	High	
ADC values	Low	Intermediate	High	High

Abbreviations: CT, computed tomography; MR, magnetic resonance; MRS, magnetic resonance spectroscopy; NAA, N-acetyl aspartate; T2WI, T2-weighted image; VHL, von Hippel-Lindau disease.
Adapted from Yousem DM, Zimmerman RD, Grossman RI. Neuroradiology: the requisites. Philadelphia: Mosby Elsevier; 2010.

Four MB variants have been described in the 2000 WHO classification:

- Type I: Desmoplastic MB
- Type II: MB with extensive nodularity
- Type III: Anaplastic MB
- Type IV: Large-cell MB

Clinical

Clinical manifestations depend on the age and extension of the disease. MB located in the fourth ventricle can cause obstructive hydrocephalus and increased intracranial pressure, and leads to vomiting, headache, and papilledema. Vermian location of the tumor can cause ataxia. Hemispheric location of the tumor, which is more common in older children and adults, manifests as limb ataxia and dysdiadochokinesis. Pressure from the hydrocephalus on the dorsal brain stem can lead to Parinaud syndrome, vertical gaze palsy, and pupils reactive to light but not to without accommodation. Abducens nerve palsy is common. Metastases to the spinal canal can lead to spinal cord compression and cerebral hemispheric spread can lead to seizures.[9]

Imaging

On noncontrast CT, MB appears moderately hyperdense due to its high cellularity. 22% of cases show calcification and 90% show contrast enhancement.

On T1-weighted MRI it appears hypointense, and on T2-weighted images (T2WI) signal ranges from hypointense to hyperintense. The tumor may enhance homogeneously after contrast administration, although calcified and necrotic areas can contribute to a more heterogeneous or poor enhancement pattern.[13,14] A "grapelike" pattern is associated with anaplastic MB.[9,15] The densely cellular nature of MB and the high nuclear-to-cytoplasm ratio lead to restriction of the water diffusion, resulting in high signal on DWI and low apparent diffusion coefficient (ADC) values (**Fig. 2**).[16] Magnetic resonance spectroscopy (MRS) shows elevated choline levels, higher than those of other posterior fossa masses, indicative of high turnover of tumor cells. There is also marked decrease in the N-acetyl aspartate (NAA), resulting in high choline/NAA ratio, and marked increase of choline/creatine ratio and significant decrease of NAA/creatine ratio.[13,17,18] Perfusion imaging has its main application in preoperative tumor grading. Relative cerebral blood volume (rCBV) is significantly higher in high-grade than in low-grade tumors due to tumor neovascularization. Perfusion also has the potential to identify disease progression, characterized by increased rCBV values compared with stable lesions in which rCBV does not change significantly.[19]

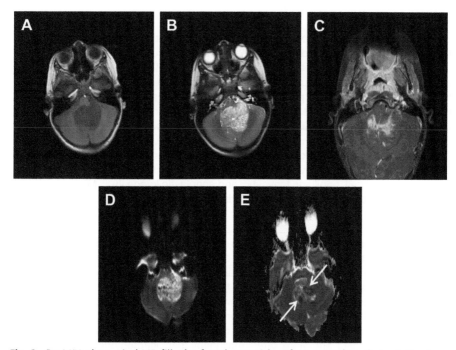

Fig. 2. On MRI, the typical MB fills the fourth ventricle, often extending through the foramen of Magendie into the cisterna magna. (*A*) Most MBs are heterogeneously hypointense to gray matter on T1WI. (*B*) Signal on T2WI varies from hypointense to hyperintense. Contrast enhancement is variable. (*C*) Moderately intense enhancement is typical but heterogeneous enhancement is the rule. DWI (*D*) shows restricted diffusion, whereas the ADC (*E*) map reveals that the mass is hypointense to normal cerebellar parenchyma, consistent with decreased diffusion (*arrows*).

Treatment and Prognosis

Several prognostic factors are considered. Complete surgical resection is considered the best prognostic variable. Residual tumor smaller than 1.5 cm^2 is considered average risk, whereas residual tumor larger than 1.5 cm^2 is high risk.[9,20] Children younger than 3 have a poorer prognosis, due to the extension of the tumor, which makes excision more difficult, and also because of the difficulty of giving radiotherapy at this age.[9,17] Presence of metastasis at the diagnosis is associated with poorer prognosis.[9,21]

Treatment includes surgical resection, radiotherapy, and chemotherapy for children older than 3 years. For children younger than 3 years (in whom MB is rare), radiotherapy is not advisable because of side effects.[9,22] Studies in which chemotherapy was administered during and after radiotherapy with drug regimens such as cisplatin, N-(2-chloroethyl)-N-cyclo-hexyl-N-nitrosourea (CCNU), and vincristine, or cyclophosphamide, cisplatin, vincristine, and etoposide have demonstrated survival rates as high as 85% in children with average-risk disease and 60% or better for those with poor-risk disease. Reported 5-year progression-free survival and overall survival in patients treated with radiotherapy alone have been remarkably consistent in studies performed over the past 25 years, at approximately 60%. Survival rates in adults have been in the range of 50% to 60%, similar to that in children treated with radiotherapy alone and inferior to that in patients younger than 21 years receiving adjuvant radiotherapy and chemotherapy.[23]

EPENDYMOMA

Ependymomas are glial neoplasms derived from differentiated ependymal cells lining the ventricles of the brain and central canal of the spinal cord. They represent the third most common intracranial tumors in children (after MB and astrocytoma). Sixty percent to 70% of them occur infratentorially and 30% to 40% occur supratentorially. Ependymomas involving the posterior fossa generally present in young children with a mean age of diagnosis of 4 years, yet 25% to 40% of patients are younger than 2 years. Of the infratentorial tumors, 95% are located within the floor of the fourth ventricle and the remaining 5% are seen in the cerebello-pontine angle.[24] Cerebrospinal fluid (CSF) dissemination occurs in up to 17% of patients.[25,26] According to WHO classification, histologic variants include myxopapillary ependymoma (grade I); classic (grade II) and its variants: clear cell, papillary, tanycytic; and anaplastic (grade III).[10] Microscopically, perivascular pseudorosettes are characteristic.

Clinical

Symptoms are location-dependent. Fourth-ventricle ependymomas commonly cause intraventricular obstructive hydrocephalus and present with headache, vomiting, and papilledema. Ataxia is common. The classic (or grade II) and its variants (clear cell, tanycytic, and papillary) when compared to anaplastic (grade III) tumors, have not been linked to a significant different outcome.[27] Because of its intraventricular location, infratentorial ependymomas will become clinically symptomatic earlier, secondary to increased intracranial pressure and obstructive hydrocephalus. Supratentorial ependymomas (85%) are more often malignant than infratentorial ependymomas (50%).[28]

Neuroimaging

On T1WI, these tumors are usually isointense/hypointense and will commonly squeeze through the fourth ventricular foramina into cisterns (**Fig. 3**). Generally, posterior fossa ependymomas have an indistinct interface with floor of the fourth ventricle. On CT

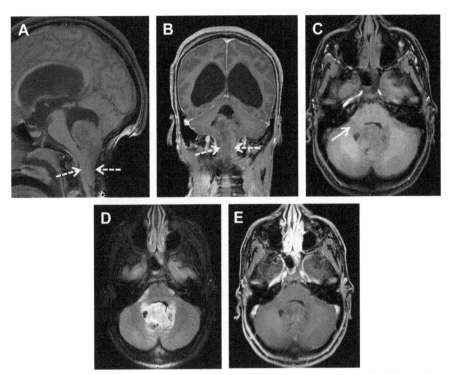

Fig. 3. T1WI show a heterogeneously hypointense fourth ventricle mass extruding poster-oinferiorly through the foramen of Magendie (*C, solid arrow*) into the cisterna magna and upper cervical canal (*A, B, dashed arrows*). These tumors are generally hyperintense on T2/FLAIR (*D*). (*E*) A heterogeneously enhancing fourth ventricle mass. A mass in the fourth ventricle that extrudes through the outflow foramina is characteristic of ependymoma. Ependymoma characteristically lacks restricted diffusion on DWI.

imaging, calcium is a common (50%) finding and typically is punctate. On T2* gradient echo (GRE) or susceptibility-weighted imaging (SWI) sequences, "blooming" or hypo-intensity of calcium or hemosiderin, is often seen. Posterior fossa cysts occur uncommonly (15%) and are small, whereas supratentorially, they are most often associated with large cysts (80%). Mild to moderate enhancement is seen.[8,29]

Most ependymomas do not restrict on DWI, although some cases may show foci of restricted diffusion. On MRS, elevated choline and lactate levels, as well as reduced NAA, are the most common findings. Perfusion MR shows markedly elevated cerebral blood volume with poor return to the baseline. The primary utility of MRS in the setting of ependymoma is to evaluate for tumor recurrence and posttreatment changes. Leptomeningeal seeding is seen in fewer than 10% and MR staging of the spine should be considered.[13,29,30]

Treatment and Prognosis

The most important prognostic factor is the extent of surgical resection. The goal of the treatment is total gross resection.[31] However, complete resection of posterior fossa ependymomas is usually difficult because of close proximity to the vital structures. Thus, radiation is considered as standard adjuvant treatment of ependymomas in older children. Although chemotherapy with cisplatin and carboplatin has activity in inducing tumor regression,[32] a role of chemotherapy in adjuvant management is controversial.[33] Five-year survival rates exceed 60% after gross total resection, but are below 30% after subtotal removal.[34,35] Five-year survival rates are above 80% when both extensive resection and irradiation are used.[36,37] The histology also influences prognosis, with anaplastic (grade III) ependymoma having markedly worse outcomes than grade II tumors.[34,38,39]

CHOROID PLEXUS PAPILLOMA AND CARCINOMA

WHO grading indicates that 80% are CPPs (WHO grade I), 15% are atypical papillomas (WHO grade II), and fewer than 5% are papillary carcinomas (WHO grade III).[40] Choroid plexus tumors are rare neoplasms that arise from the choroid plexus epithelium, comprising 0.3% to 0.6% of all intracranial tumors and account for 4.0% of pediatric intracranial tumors.[41] Median age at presentation is 1.5 years for lateral and third-ventricular choroid plexus papillomas (CPPs), 22.5 years for fourth-ventricle CPPs, and 35.5 years for cerebello-pontine angle CPPs. There is a very slight male predominance.

Choroid plexus carcinomas (CPCa) occur in patients with Li-Fraumeni syndrome, a cancer predisposition syndrome caused by TP53 germline mutation. However, most CPCa do not have a germline TP53 mutation. It is also associated with Aicardi syndrome, an X-linked dominant syndrome that occurs almost exclusively in female individuals. Aicardi syndrome is defined by the triad of infantile spasms, corpus callosum agenesis, and pathognomonic chorioretinal abnormalities. The prevalence of CPPs in Aicardi syndrome is estimated at 3% to 5%.[42,43]

Pathology

Fifty percent of choroid plexus tumors are found in the lateral ventricles, 40% are in the fourth ventricle, and 5% in the third ventricle. The trigone is the most common overall site. CPPs are occasionally found as primary cerebellopontine angle tumors (CPA), in which tufts of choroid plexus extrude through the foramina of Luschka into the adjacent CPA cisterns. Extraventricular CPPs are extremely rare. They have been reported in the brainstem, cerebellum, pituitary fossa, and septi pellucidi.[41,43]

Clinically, CPPs usually present with headaches due to hydrocephalus caused by overproduction of CSF by the tumor, but also can be due to obstructive hydrocephalus.[40]

Microscopically, CPPs are composed of fibrovascular cores lined by a single layer of uniform cuboidal to columnar epithelial cells with round or oval, basally situated monomorphic nuclei. CPCa are typically characterized by increased mitotic activity, nuclear and cellular atypia, necrosis, loss of papillary differentiation, and invasion of adjacent brain tissue.[44]

Imaging

Most CPPs on noncontrast CT are isodense to hyperdense compared with brain. Calcifications are seen in 25% of cases. Hydrocephalus, either obstructive or caused by CSF overproduction, is common. On MRI, a sharply marginated lobular mass that is isointense to slightly hypointense relative to brain is seen on T1WI. CPPs are isointense to hyperintense on T2WI and fluid-attenuated inversion recovery (FLAIR). Linear and branching internal "flow voids" reflect the increased vascularity common in CPPs. GRE or SWI may show hypointense foci secondary to calcification or intratumoral hemorrhage. Intense homogeneous enhancement is seen after contrast administration (**Fig. 4**). CPPs generally do not restrict on DWI. MRS may show elevated myoinositol.[10,43,45]

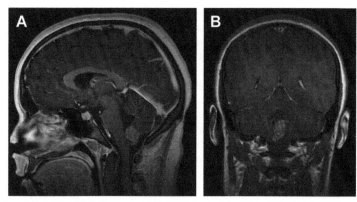

Fig. 4. T1-weighted sagittal (*A*) and coronal (*B*) images with gadolinium enhancement of a fourth ventricular choroid plexus papilloma in an 11-year-old girl. (*From* Weeks A, Fallah A, Rutka JT. Posterior fossa and brainstem tumors in children. In: Ellenbogen RG, Abdulrauf SI, Sekhar LN, editors. Principles of neurological surgery. Philadelphia: Elsevier, 2012; with permission.)

Treatment and Prognosis

CPPs are best managed by total gross resection via a ventricular approach, which is usually curative. Adjuvant chemotherapy or radiotherapy is not indicated for uncomplicated CPP. In patients with CPCa, total gross resection should be followed by radiation therapy. However, it should be avoided in young children because of long-term side effects. Chemotherapy can be an option in these patients; however, there is limited experience with this modality with a lack of evidence for an impact on long-term outcome.[46] Histology is the most important prognostic factor as 1-year, 5-year, and 10-year projected survival rates are 90%, 81%, and 77% in CPP compared with only 71%, 41%, and 35% in CPCa, respectively.[47]

PILOCYTIC ASTROCYTOMA

PA, or juvenile PA, is a slowly growing glioma, classified as grade I by WHO, occurring typically in children and young adults.[48] PAs commonly occur in the first 2 decades of life, with few cases being reported in the older than 30-year age group, whereas occurrence beyond 50 years is exceptional.[49] PA is the most common pediatric cerebellar neoplasm and the most common pediatric glioma, constituting 85% of all cerebellar astrocytomas and 10% of all cerebral astrocytomas in the age group.[50] The cerebellum is the most common location, accounting for nearly 60% of all PAs. No gender predilection has been shown.[50,51] The occurrence of PAs in neurofibromatosis type 1 (NF1) is well known, occurring in approximately 15% of individuals with this autosomal-dominant genetic disorder.[10] The most common of which are found in the optic tract and hypothalamus, followed in frequency by brainstem and cerebellar PAs.[52,53] PAs tend to have a more benign clinical course, especially when they occur in individuals with NF1.[8]

Pathology

In a study of 101 children with cerebellar PA, the most frequent primary location was in the cerebellar hemisphere at 34% of the time, 29% occurred in the vermis, fourth ventricle 27% of the time, and cerebellar peduncle 11%.[54] The macroscopic appearance of PA varies with its location within the CNS. Tumors of the cerebellum are typically well-circumscribed, cystlike masses with a discrete mural nodule. Microscopically, the classic finding of PA is a biphasic pattern of 2 distinct astrocyte populations. The dominant type is composed of compact, hairlike ("pilocytic") bipolar cells with Rosenthal fibers, which are electron-dense glial fibrillary acidic protein (GFAP)-positive cytoplasmic inclusions. Intermixed are loosely textured, hypocellular, GFAP-negative areas that contain multipolar cells with microcysts. Immunohistochemistry with MIB-1 is typically less than 1%, indicating low proliferative potential.[50,55] Clinical presentation of patients with a cerebellar PA often present with headache, morning nausea, gait disturbance, blurred vision, diplopia, and neck pain. Clinical signs usually include hydrocephalus, papilledema, truncal ataxia, appendicular dysmetria, head tilt, cranial nerve palsies, and nystagmus.[50]

Imaging

The most common appearance of a cerebellar PA is a well-delineated cerebellar cyst with a mural nodule (**Fig. 5**). CT scan usually reveals a mixed cystic/solid mass in the cerebellar hemisphere or vermis and little, if any, edema, and variable mass effect. Calcification is seen in 10% to 20%, and hemorrhage is uncommon. Almost all (94%) mural nodules enhance, typically intensely, with contrast.[50,56] On MRI, PAs are usually well delineated and appear slightly hyperintense to CSF on T1WI and T2WI. The mural nodule is typically isointense to hypointense relative to normal brain on T1WI, and hyperintense compared with normal brain with T2WI. It usually shows a well-delineated cyst with a typical peripheral mural nodule that enhances strongly with contrast.[50,56] However, the MRI appearance of PAs may be variable in terms of contrast uptake of both the solid part and the cyst wall. Most cyst walls do not, but

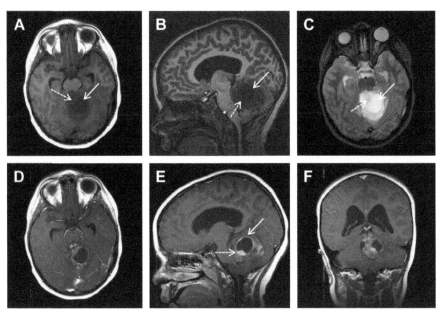

Fig. 5. A 6-year-old with headache demonstrates a large mass of the vermis with a cyst and characteristic enhancing mural nodule. Cystic PAs are usually well-delineated and appear slightly hyperintense to CSF on both T1WI (*A, B*) and T2WI (*C*) (*solid arrows*). The mural nodule is isointense to hypointense on T1WI (*A, B*) and isointense/hyperintense on T2WI (*C*) (*dashed arrows*). T1 C+ scan (*D–F*) shows enhancement of the cyst wall (*arrow*) and mural nodule (*dashed arrow*). Early hydrocephalus is seen due to mass affect on the aqueduct.

some may enhance strongly. However, cyst wall enhancement is not necessarily indicative of tumor involvement.[56] MRS in PAs often shows elevated choline, low NAA, and a lactate peak, paradoxic findings that are more characteristic of malignant neoplasms than this clinically benign-behaving tumor.[50] This lactate elevation most likely reflects alterations in mitochondrial metabolism or represents variability in glucose utilization rates among low-grade astrocytomas, as opposed to necrosis, which is a rare histologic feature in PA.[57] Perfusion MR shows low rCBV. Paradoxic fluorodeoxyglucose positron emission tomography (FDG PET) findings of increased uptake of glucose might reflect the unusual vascularity of pilocytic tumors.[58]

Treatment and Prognosis

The overall prognosis of cerebellar astrocytoma is excellent, with a 10-year survival rate of 100%, and recurrence-free or progression-free rate of 71%, in one series.[54] Almost half of residual tumors show spontaneous regression or arrested growth over time.[54] Many studies noted that the recurrence rate in PA in any location is highly dependent on the success of surgical resection.

HEMANGIOBLASTOMA

Hemangioblastoma (HB) is also known as capillary hemangioma, and are designated WHO grade I tumors. Cerebellar hemangioblastomas are highly vascular benign tumors that comprise 2% of all intracranial tumors.[59,60] They account for 7% to 12% of all infratentorial tumors in adults, and the cerebellar hemisphere is by far the most common site.[61] It is the second most common infratentorial parenchymal mass in adults, following metastasis.[61] They may occur sporadically, but have been found in association with von Hippel-Lindau (VHL) disease in approximately 30% of cases.[60] Multiple HBs are almost always associated with VHL disease.[62] Sporadic tumors occur in the fifth and sixth decades of life, whereas VHL-associated tumors manifest in the third or fourth decades.[62] Symptoms are nonspecific, consisting of headache most of the time. Other symptoms consist of dizziness and vomiting.[60]

Pathology

Grossly, the common appearance is that of a beefy-red, vascular-appearing nodule that abuts a pial surface. Macroscopically, hemangioblastomas are well circumscribed and very often cystic; they sometimes consist solely of a small, mural nodule attached to the wall of a considerably larger cyst. Paradoxic FDG PET findings of increased uptake of glucose might reflect the unusual vascularity of pilocytic tumors. The histologic picture of hemangioblastoma is highly characteristic, consisting of numerous capillary blood vessels of different sizes, separated by trabeculae or sheets of clear cells with round or elongated nuclei. The cyst wall of most HBs is non-neoplastic, composed of compressed brain with fibrillary neuroglia devoid of tumor cells. The intratumoral cyst fluid shares a proteomic fingerprint with normal serum and has no proteins in common with HB tumor tissue. Cyst formation in HBs is therefore a result of vascular leakage from tumor vessels, not tumor liquefaction or active secretion. Mitoses are rare.[63]

Imaging

Histologically and radiologically, cerebellar HBs are traditionally described as 4 types:

- Type 1 (5%) is a simple cyst without a macroscopic nodule
- Type 2 is a cyst with a mural nodule (60%)
- Type 3 HBs are solid tumors (26%)

- Type 4 HBs are solid tumors with internal cysts (9%)[62]

The most common appearance on CT is a well-delineated isodense to slightly hyperdense nodule associated with a hypodense cyst. Calcification and gross hemorrhage are absent. The nodule enhances strongly and uniformly after contrast administration.[10] MR findings (**Fig. 6**) consist of an isointense nodule with prominent "flow voids" seen on T1WI. If an associated peritumoral cyst is present, it is typically hypointense to parenchyma on T1WI but hyperintense compared with CSF. The tumor nodule is moderately hyperintense on T2WI and FLAIR compared with brain parenchyma. Intratumoral cysts and prominent "flow voids" are common. The cyst fluid is very hyperintense on both T2WI and FLAIR. If present, blood products "bloom" on T2*.[10] Intense enhancement of the nodule, but not the cyst itself, is typical. Cyst wall enhancement should raise the possibility of tumor involvement as compressed, non-neoplastic brain does not enhance. Noncystic HBs enhance strongly but often heterogeneously.[10] On angiography, the most common appearance is that of an intensely vascular tumor nodule that shows a prolonged vascular "blush." "Early draining" veins are common. If a tumor-associated cyst is present, vessels appear displaced and "draped" around an avascular mass.[10]

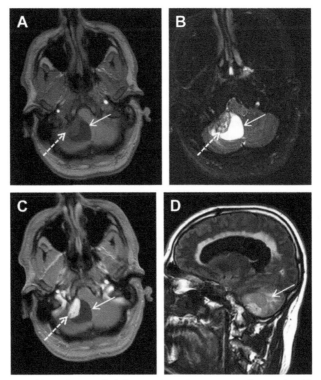

Fig. 6. A 40-year-old with a well-delineated cystic structure (*arrows*) with a peripheral nodule (*dashed arrows*) within the right cerebellar hemisphere. The tumor cyst is hypointense to parenchyma on T1WI but hyperintense compared with CSF (*A*), and very hyperintense on T2WI (*B*). T1 C+ MR axial image (*C*) shows that the tumor nodule (*dashed arrow*) enhances intensely, whereas the cyst wall (*solid arrow*) does not. Peritumoral edema is seen (*arrow, D*). The sagittal FLAIR image shows resulting hydrocephalus with CSF parenchymal extension (*D*). Hemangioblastoma was confirmed after surgical resection.

Treatment and Prognosis

Asymptomatic hemangioblastomas may be managed conservatively with serial MRI scans. Surgery is generally reserved for patients with symptomatic tumors, where complete surgical excision is the only curative therapy for these tumors. Total resection eliminates tumor recurrence although new hemangioblastomas may develop in the setting of VHL.[59,60,62] In these cases, the cumulative effects of multiple tumors and procedures may lead to significant morbidity.[59]

ATYPICAL TERATOID/RHABDOID TUMOR

Atypical teratoid/rhabdoid tumors (AT/RT) of the CNS are aggressive childhood neoplasms that are located most commonly in the posterior fossa, preferentially in the cerebellar hemispheres.[10,64–67] However, AT/RTs occur in both supratentorial and infratentorial compartments.[10] These tumors are rare, accounting for only 1% to 2% of central nervous system tumors in children of all ages, but 10% to 20% of tumors in patients younger than 3 years old, a period during which AT/RT approaches primitive neuroectodermal tumor (PNET) in frequency.[10,64,68] Primary CNS AT/RT was recognized as a separate entity and added to the WHO classification of tumors in 1993 as a grade IV embryonal tumor.[64,65] The clinical presentation of AT/RT typically depends on the age of onset and the location of the tumor. Children younger than 3 years usually present with nonspecific signs and symptoms, such as vomiting, lethargy, irritability, weight loss, enlarging head circumference, and failure to thrive. Older patients commonly present with increased intracranial pressure or localizing signs. Cranial nerve palsies, headache, and hemiplegia are common.[66,69]

Pathology

The gross pathologic appearance of AT/RT is that of a large, soft, fleshy, hemorrhagic, necrotic mass, similar to that of CNS PNETs.[10] Microscopically, AT/RTs have morphologic features of MB/PNET, with epithelial, primitive neuroepithelial, and mesenchymal differentiation, together with prominent rhabdoid cells.[67] AT/RTs are characterized by a loss of the long arm of chromosome 22, which results in the deletions in the *INI1/hSNF5/BAF47* gene. This is considered pathognomonic of AT/RT, differentiating this tumor from MB/PNET by the absence of INI-1 immunohistochemical staining.[10,65,67]

Imaging

The imaging features of AT/RT are nonspecific, sharing many imaging features of other embryonal tumors, given that they are densely cellular neoplasms that frequently contain hemorrhage, necrosis, cysts, and calcification (**Fig. 7**).[10,66] On nonenhanced CT (NECT), these tumors are solid or mixed lesions. The solid portion is commonly hyperdense on NECT, a feature attributed to the tumor's high cellularity and high nuclear/cytoplasmic ratio.[66] Calcification and obstructive hydrocephalus are common. Enhancement is typically strong but heterogeneous.[10] AT/RTs are heterogeneously hypointense to isointense to brain on T1WI and isointense to hyperintense on T2WI. "Blooming" foci on T2* are common, and usually show mild to moderate restricted diffusion. MRS shows elevated choline and decreased or absent NAA.[10] Moderate to marked enhancement with gadolinium is seen. Extensive vasogenic edema can be expected.[66] Leptomeningeal spread is present in approximately 20% of patients at diagnosis according to the AT/RT registry.[64,65,68] Therefore, a contrast-enhanced MRI of the entire neuro-axis is essential at the time of presentation and on follow-up because of the high rate of recurrence and leptomeningeal spread.[65,66]

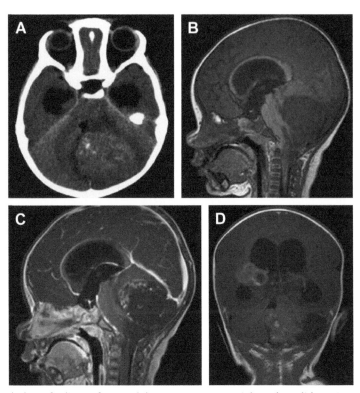

Fig. 7. Radiologic findings of AT/RT. (*A*) On noncontrast axial CT, the solid portion of the tumor is hyperdense. (*B, C*) T1-weighted sagittal MRI without and with gadolinium enhancement, shows a hypointense lesion in the cerebellar vermis that enhances heterogeneously and is associated with perilesional edema. (*D*) Postcontrast coronal MRI showing a metastatic AT/RT with a lesion in the posterior fossa and one in the right lateral ventricle. (*From* Jung TY, Rutka JT. Posterior fossa tumors in the pediatric population: multidisciplinary management. In: Quiñones-Hinojosa, editor. Schmidek and Sweet's operative neurosurgical techniques. Philadelphia: Elsevier, 2012; with permission.)

Treatment and Prognosis

There is no satisfactory treatment for AT/RT. Overall, patients usually succumb to their disease between 6 months and 1 year from diagnosis of local tumor relapse or of leptomeningeal dissemination.[68] Tekautz and colleagues[70] reported that children younger than 3 years have a more dismal prognosis than those older than 3 years. The purpose of surgery initially is to make the diagnosis and to reduce the tumor bulk.[66] Hilden and colleagues[68] recommended an aggressive approach to these tumors with the use of a combination of chemotherapy, radiotherapy, stem-cell rescue, and intrathecal chemotherapy, and have shown a median survival of 16.75 months and median disease-free survival of 10 months.

LHERMITTE-DUCLOS DISEASE

Lhermitte-Duclos disease (LDD), or dysplastic cerebellar gangliocytoma is a rare benign cerebellar mass composed of dysplastic ganglion cells.[71] Other names for this disease are granular cell hypertrophy, granulomolecular hypertrophy of the cerebellum, cerebellar hamartoma, ganglioneuroma, and gangliomatosis of the cerebellum.[71] LDD is classified as WHO grade I, but has the propensity to progress or to recur after surgery.[72] There is considerable controversy over the cause of LDD, whether it has a hamartomatous, neoplastic, or congenital malformative origin. LDD may occur as part of the multiple hamartoma syndrome called Cowden syndrome, an autosomal-dominant condition characterized by multiple hamartomas and neoplastic lesions in skin and internal organs, favoring a hamartomatous origin of LDD.[10,71,73] The prevalence of LDD is unknown. LDD is most commonly diagnosed in the third and fourth decades. The average age is 34 years. There is no gender predilection.[71] Patients may be asymptomatic or present with symptoms of increased intracranial pressure, such as headache, nausea, and vomiting. Cranial nerve palsies, cerebellar symptoms, and visual abnormalities also are common.[10,71]

Pathology

The gross appearance of LDD is a tumorlike mass that expands and replaces the normal cerebellar architecture. On cut section, the cerebellar folia are markedly widened and have a grossly "gyriform" appearance.[10] Histologic examination reveals marked disruption of the normal cerebellar cortical cell layers with dysplastic hypertrophied ganglion cells leading to expansion of the granule layer and increased myelination in the molecular layer, causing it to widen. There is loss of Purkinje cells and white matter. Mitotic activity, necrosis, and endothelial proliferation are absent.[71]

Imaging

Most cases of LDD are hypodense on unenhanced CT images. Mass effect with compression of the fourth ventricle, effacement of the cerebellopontine angle cistern, and hydrocephalus are common. Calcification is uncommon. No appreciable enhancement is seen on contrast-enhanced CT.[71] MRI is the modality of choice (Fig. 8). MRI reveals an expansile mass with the typical striated, corduroy, or "tiger-stripe" folial pattern that consists of alternating bands on both T1WI and T2WI. The bands are hyperintense and isointense relative to gray matter on T2WI and isointense and hypointense on T1WI. Calcification is uncommon. T2* demonstrates prominent venous channels surrounding the grossly thickened folia. Most dysplastic gangliocytomas do not enhance; however, enhancement has been reported and is probably due to the presence of these anomalous veins.[71] DWI may show restricted diffusion, likely reflecting the hypercellularity and increased axonal density characteristic of LDD.[10] PWI shows increased rCBV, regional cerebral blood-flow (rCBF), and mean transit time within the lesion, correlating to the prominent dilated interfolial veins, not malignancy.[72,74] With MRS, Thomas and colleagues[74] found slight reductions in choline, creatine, NAA, and myo-inositol (MI) on the affected side with a prominent lactate peak within the lesion. The choline/creatine ratio was not elevated.

Treatment and Prognosis

Shunting or surgical debulking are options for symptomatic patients with hydrocephalus, and the surgical procedure should be as radical as possible. Because LDD is not encapsulated and blends gradually into normal cerebellar tissue, incomplete removal of the lesion is not rare.[10,71,75] Intraoperative MRI may lead to safe and complete removal of these lesions.[75] The prognosis is favorable and the mortality low.[75,76]

GLIOBLASTOMA

Although glioblastoma, WHO grade IV tumor, is the most common primary brain tumor, occurrence of glioblastoma in the cerebellum is extremely rare, with a frequency

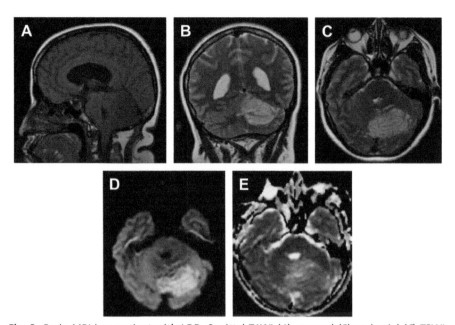

Fig. 8. Brain MRI in a patient with LDD. Sagittal T1WI (*A*), coronal (*B*) and axial (*C*) T2WI, axial DWI (*D*), and correspondent ADC map (*E*). The mass-lesion in the left cerebellar hemisphere is hyperintense on T2WI, with alternating hyperintense and isointense bands, referred to as a "tiger-striped" appearance (*B, C*). The lesion demonstrates high signal intensity on DWI (*D*), with patchy mixed diffusion pattern on corresponding ADC map (*E*). (*From* Cianfoni A, Wintermark M, Piludu F, et al. Morphological and functional MR imaging of Lhermitte–Duclos disease with pathology correlate. J Neuroradiol 2008;35(5):297–300; with permission.)

of 0% to 3.4%.[77–79] Glioblastomas may develop de novo (primary) or from a previous low-grade astrocytoma (secondary).[77,80,81] Martin and colleagues[82] reported a case of secondary glioblastoma 5 years after treatment of MB. Secondary glioblastomas develop more frequently in younger patients and often contain TP53 mutation (65%), whereas primary glioblastomas occur in elderly patients and are generally characterized by loss of heterozygosity 10q (loss of heterozygosity [LOH] 10q) (70%), epidermal growth factor receptor (eGFR) amplification (63%) and TP53 mutation at a frequency lower than 30%.[81]

Treatment and Prognosis

The treatment of cerebellar glioblastomas does not differ much from treatment of glioblastomas at other locations. It is usually palliative and encompasses surgery, radiotherapy, and chemotherapy.[77] The median survival for cerebellar glioblastoma is known to be approximately 19 months.[83,84]

PRIMARY CENTRAL NERVOUS SYSTEM LYMPHOMA

Primary central nervous system lymphoma (PCNSL) accounts for 1% to 5% of all brain tumors. The incidence rates of PCNSL are increasing among immunocompetent patients, but immunocompromised patients have an increased risk of developing PCNSL. However, with the introduction of highly active antiretroviral therapy, the incidence of PCNSL in the HIV population has declined. The brain stem or cerebellum or both are affected in 9% to 13%.[85] Although PCNSLs can occur in all age groups, they are generally tumors of middle-aged and older adults. The peak age in immuno-competent patients is 60 years, and the mean age at onset in patients with HIV/AIDS is 40 years. Lymphomas in transplant recipients generally occur between the ages of 35 and 40. Mean age of onset in children with inherited immunodeficiencies is 10 years. There is an overall 3:2 male predominance.[10]

Imaging

PCNSL typically has a characteristic appearance on both CT and MRI (**Fig. 9**) due to its hypercellularity, high nuclear/cytoplasmic ratio, disruption of the blood-brain barrier, and its predilection for the periventricular and superficial regions, often in contact with ventricular or meningeal surfaces. Unenhanced CT typically reveals hyperdens or isodens lesions, and virtually all lesions show contrast enhancement. On unenhanced T1-weighted MRI, lesions are typically hypointense or isointense, and on T2-weighted MRI, isointense to hyperintense but often hypointense to gray matter. Most lesions show moderate-to-marked contrast enhancement on CT and MRI.[85–89] Non-AIDS PCNSL typically presents as a solitary homogeneously enhancing parenchymal

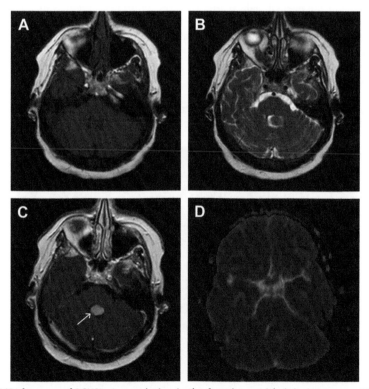

Fig. 9. MRI features of PCNSL. A mass lesion in the fourth ventricle is isointense on T1WI (*A*), and hypointense to cortex on T2WI (*B*). The lesion (*arrow*) enhances strongly with gadolinium (*C*). Diffusion restricted is seen as hypointensity on the ADC map (*D*) due to the hyper-cellularity of this lesion (*arrow*). (*From* Zacharia TT, Law M, Naidich TP, et al. Central nervous system lymphoma characterization by diffusion-weighted imaging and MR spectroscopy. J Neuroimaging 2008;18(4):411–7; with permission.)

mass, but multiple lesions are reported in 20% to 40% of non-AIDS PCNSLs.[85,86,90,91] Linear enhancement along perivascular spaces is highly suggestive of PCNSL.[85,88] Perifocal edema is usually present but less prominent than that in malignant gliomas or metastases.[85,90,92] Because CNS lymphomas are highly cellular tumors, more than 95% of PCNSLs show mild to moderate diffusion restriction and low ADC values.[10] On perfusion MR, rCBV is relatively low compared with glioblastoma.[10,85] Diffusion tensor imaging (DTI) is a sensitive tool for the detection of alterations in white matter structure.[85,93] A quantitative fractional anisotropy (FA) map shows hypointensity corresponding to decreased FA values in most brain tumors. Different degrees of cellularity and cellular organization also may affect the FA value, and FA values of PCNSLs are significantly lower than those of glioblastoma.[85,93] In PCNSL, proton MRS (**Fig. 10**) has demonstrated elevated lipid peaks combined with high choline/creatine ratios (**Table 3**).[85,91]

Treatment and Prognosis

Treatment options for PCNSL include corticosteroids, radiation, and chemotherapy with agents such as methotrexate and rituximab.[10,94] Approximately 70% of PCNSLs initially respond to treatment, but relapse is very common. Only 20% to 40% of patients experience prolonged progression-free survival. PCNSL is an aggressive tumor with a median survival of only a few months, untreated. Even with conventional chemotherapy and radiation therapy, the 5-year survival rate is less than 10%.[10] Immunocompromised patients have significantly poorer prognosis compared with immunocompetent patients.

METASTASIS

Brain metastasis is a leading cause of mortality and morbidity in patients with cancer. Metastases represent the most common cancer of the brain, outnumbering primary

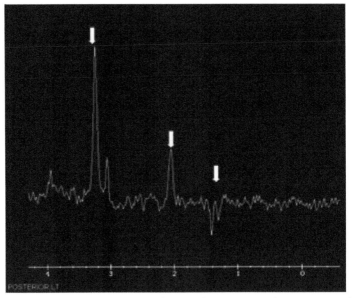

Fig. 10. Proton MRS in PCNSL. From left to right, *arrows* indicate increased choline, decreased NAA, and high lipid peak, consistent with a hypercellular neoplasm.

Table 3
Main magnetic resonance spectroscopy markers of brain tumors

Compound	Location, ppm	Metabolic Marker of...	Change in Tumors
NAA	2.0	Neuronal activity mostly	↓(All)
Cr/Pcr	3.0	Energy cascade	=/↓
Cho	3.2	Cellular membranes, density, turnover	↑(All)
Lac	1.33	Necrosis, malignancy	(PA, malignant)
Lip (short TE)	0.9/1.3	Necrosis, malignancy	↑(Malignant)
ml (short TE)	3.6	Cellularity, astrocytes	↑↑(CPP)
Tau (short TE)	3.36	Cerebellar development	↑(MB)

Abbreviations: ↑, increase; ↓, decrease; =, no change; Cho, choline; CPP, choroid plexus papilloma; Cr/Pcr, creatinine/phosphocreatinine; Lac, lactate; Lip, lipid; MB, medulloblastoma/PNET; ml, myo-inositol; NAA, n-acetylcysteine; PA, pilocytic astrocytoma; Tau, taurine; TE, echo time.
Adapted from Barkovich A, Raybaud C. Pediatric Neuroimaging. 5th edition. Philadelphia: Wolters Kluwer/Lippincott Williams and Wilkins; 2012.

brain tumors 10-fold, and 20% to 40% of all patients with cancer will develop metastatic spread to the brain.[95,96] The brain parenchyma is the most common site, the vast majority located in the cerebral hemispheres. Only 15% of metastases are found in the cerebellum.[10] In one retrospective study, the median age at diagnosis of cerebellar metastases was 57 years, with an almost 2-to-1 ratio favoring men over women.[97] Lung carcinoma was the primary site in almost 50% and breast in 25%. Other reported primary sites include gastrointestinal tract carcinoma, endometrial/ovarian, melanoma, and esophageal carcinoma.[97–99] Although most investigators report no predisposition for systemic neoplasms to metastasize to the cerebellum, a study from Memorial Sloan-Kettering Cancer Center suggested that abdominal and pelvic neoplasms have a disproportionate tendency to involve the cerebellum compared with the cerebral hemispheres.[98] However, evidence for this phenomenon is scarce, and a more recent review found no evidence that pelvic and gastrointestinal tumors metastasize preferentially to the posterior fossa.[100]

Presentation

Initial clinical symptoms generally include signs of increased intracranial pressure, such as severe headache, gait disturbance, nausea, and vomiting.[97,98] Because cerebellar metastasis may cause obstructive hydrocephalus and brain stem compression, survival of patients with cerebellar metastasis has been reported as more disappointing than that reported for cerebral hemispheric metastasis.[97,98,101,102]

Imaging

Brain metastases on CT appear as solitary or multiple mass lesions with variable surrounding vasogenic edema.[103] Acutely hemorrhagic metastases appear hyperdense to brain tissue. Melanoma metastases tend to be hyperdense to brain even in the absence of hemorrhage.[104,105] With the exception of treated metastases, calcification is rare.[106] The vast majority of parenchymal metastasis enhances strongly after contrast administration. Solid, punctate, nodular, or ring patterns can be seen.[10] On MRI, metastases are usually isointense or hypointense on T1, hyperintense on T2, and exhibit avid enhancement. Some metastases, such as melanoma, are T1 hyperintense due to the paramagnetic effects of melanin. Hemorrhagic metastases also may demonstrate T1 signal hyperintensity, depending on the age of hemorrhage.[107] Signal intensity on T2WI can vary widely depending on tumor type, lesion cellularity, presence of hemorrhage, and amount of peritumoral edema. Many metastases are very cellular neoplasms with high nuclear-to-cytoplasmic ratios and thus appear hypointense on T2WI and FLAIR. Exceptions are mucinous tumors, cystic metastases, and tumors with large amounts of central necrosis, all of which can appear moderately hyperintense.[10] Vasogenic edema can be substantial, and is unrelated to lesion size, although some metastases show little or no surrounding edema.[103,107] Both subacute hemorrhage and melanin cause prominent signal intensity loss ("blooming") on GRE, or SWI sequences. Contrast-enhanced FLAIR that may improve sensitivity compared with contrast-enhanced inversion recovery (IR) and IR-prepared fast spoiled gradient echo sequences.[10,108]

With the exception of highly cellular neoplasms, such as MB, lymphoma, and high-grade gliomas, most primary brain tumors do not show restriction on DWI. Metastases tend to demonstrate facilitated diffusion in the form of elevated ADC values.[109] However, the behavior of metastases on DWI may be unpredictable. Lymphoma tends to exhibit lower ADC values compared with high-grade glial neoplasms and metastases.[110] DTI with a combination of FA and ADC calculations may be helpful in distinguishing metastasis from glioblastoma, showing higher anisotropy from the enhancing region in glioblastoma compared with both brain metastases and primary CNS lymphoma.[10,111] Brain metastases are often highly vascular lesions that tend to exhibit elevated rCBV compared with contralateral normal white matter, as do many high-grade glial neoplasms, and most glioblastomas in particular. Comparison of rCBV of the enhancing component of the tumor is not able to accurately differentiate between these 2 groups.[110,112–114] The rCBV within peritumoral T2-hyperintense component is higher in glioblastoma, compared with metastases.[113–116] Perfusion MRI may help distinguish CNS lymphoma from metastases and high-grade glioma, as lymphoma demonstrates lower rCBV compared with these 2 entities.[112,117] Prominent lipid signal is the dominating peak on MRS in most brain metastases. However, lipid signal also is common in many cellular processes, including inflammation and necrosis. Choline is generally elevated, and creatine is decreased or absent in most metastases.[10] The enhancing components of both brain metastases and high-grade gliomas demonstrate increased choline/creatine peak ratios compared with normal brain.[109,113,118,119] In the spectroscopic examination, choline levels are high in peritumoral areas of gliomas and low in metastasis.[83,116,120] Choline peak is reduced in infections compared to tumors.[120]

Treatment and Prognosis

Survival of patients with cerebellar metastases has been limited by development of obstructive hydrocephalus and brain stem compression.[97,121–124] Most reports have indicated that cerebellar metastases have shown poor prognosis in general. Surgical resection followed by radiation therapy has been shown to increase the mean duration of survival in patients with cerebellar metastases when compared with radiation alone,[97,99] and shortens the need for corticosteroid therapy, provides immediate symptomatic relief, and many times avoids the requirement of a ventricular peritoneal shunt. Radiosurgery is being used more often in the treatment of brain metastases with encouraging results.[99]

PARANEOPLASTIC SYNDROME

Paraneoplastic syndromes are a group of rare disorders that are triggered by an abnormal immune system response to an underlying (usually undetected) malignant tumor. Patients with paraneoplastic neurologic syndrome (PNS) most often present with neurologic symptoms before an underlying tumor is detected. PNSs include many neurologic disorders, such as paraneoplastic cerebellar degeneration (PCD) caused by an immune-mediated mechanism. Any part of the nervous system can be involved depending on the type of primary malignancy. These syndromes affect 1% to 3% of all patients with cancer.[125] In one study, PCD was observed in 25% of PNSs, occurring in 2 of every 1000 patients with cancer.[126]

PCD occurs predominantly in patients with cancer of the ovary, uterus, or adnexa; cancer of the breast; small-cell carcinoma of the lung; or Hodgkin lymphoma. Both sexes are affected, but PCD is far more common in women than in men. PCD associated with anti-Yo antibody occurs in middle-aged women with occult ovarian or breast cancer that is usually indolent. PCD associated with anti-Hu antibody occurs in middle-aged men and women or patients with risk factors for lung cancer. When it is associated with Hodgkin lymphoma, patients are usually young men, and the cerebellar disease often follows the diagnosis of lymphoma. The development of PCD is quite rapid and patients are severely disabled in days to weeks. Because most of the patients have occult malignancy, patients are less likely to develop symptoms of PCD if they have a known history of malignancy. A common clinical presentation is mild dizziness and nausea followed by vertigo and nystagmus that may suggest a peripheral vestibular problem. These symptoms are followed by ataxia of the limbs and midline, oscillopsia, dysarthria, tremor, and sometimes dysphagia and blurry vision. The ocular motor and bulbar abnormalities suggest some degree of brain stem involvement. Mild memory and cognitive deficits, as well as affective symptoms, can occur in approximately 20% of patients with PCD. This is known as cerebellar cognitive affective syndrome.[127]

Findings that are inconsistent with a diagnosis of PCD include the following:

- Severely altered mental status with myoclonus and ataxia
- Predominantly corticospinal tract dysfunction
- Unilateral cerebellar dysfunction
- Familial cerebellar degeneration

Two major patterns of antibody response have been described: anti-Hu (type IIa, antineuronal nuclear antibodies type 1) and anti-Yo (type 1, anti-Purkinje cell antibodies). Both anti-Yo and anti-Hu antibodies are believed to be elicited by tumor antigens that are cross-reactive with neuronal antigens.

Table 4 describes all the antibodies associated with PCD.

Diagnosis and Treatment

CSF may show lymphocytic pleocytosis, elevated protein, increased CSF immunoglobulin G relative to serum, and oligoclonal banding. In some cases, CSF studies are normal. Initially, MRI of brain is typically normal. Some cases demonstrate transient cerebellar enlargement with focal or diffuse hyperintensity on FLAIR. Mild cortical-meningeal enhancement may be present. Later in the course of illness, cerebellar atrophy may be seen, along with hypometabolism on PET. Definitive diagnosis can be

Table 4
Antibodies associated with PCD

	Predominant Syndrome	Associated Cancer
Antibodies predominantly associated with PCD[a]		
Anti-Yo (PCA-1) antibodies	PCD	Ovarian Breast cancers
Anti-Tr antibodies	PCD	Hodgkin lymphoma
Anti-mGluR1 antibodies[b]	PCD	Hodgkin lymphoma
Anti-Zic4 antibodies[c]	PCD	Small-cell lung cancer
Sometimes associated with PCD		
Anti-VGCC antibodies	Eaton-Lambert syndrome, PCD	Small-cell lung cancer Lymphoma
Anti-Hu (ANNA-1) antibodies	Encephalomyelitis, PCD, sensory neuronopathy	Small-cell lung cancer Other cancers
Anti-Ri (ANNA-2) antibodies	PCD, brain-stem encephalitis, paraneoplastic opsoclonus- myoclonus	Breast cancer Gynecologic cancer Small-cell lung cancer
Anti-CV2/CRMPS antibodies	Encephalomyelitis, PCD, chorea, peripheral neuropathy, uveitis	Small-cell lung cancer Thymoma Other cancers
Anti-Ma protein antibodies[d]	Limbic, hypothalamic, brain-stem encephalitis (infrequently PCD)	Testicular cancer Lung cancer
Anti-amphiphysin antibodies	Stiff-person syndrome, encephalomyelitis, PCD	Breast cancer Small-cell lung cancer

Abbreviation: PCD, paraneoplastic cerebellar degeneration.

[a] There is no uniform nomenclature for some of these antibodies; variant names appear in parentheses. mGluR1: metabotropic glutamate receptor 1, Zic4: zing finger of the cerebellum 4, and VCGG: voltage-gated calcium channel.

[b] Anti-mGluR1 antibodies have been identified in only 2 patients.

[c] Anti-Zic4 antibodies are predominantly associated with PCD only when no other paraneoplastic antibodies are detectable.

[d] Ma proteins include Ma1 and Ma2. Patients with brain-stem and cerebellar dysfunction usually have antibodies against both MA1 and Ma2.

Adapted from Dalmau J, Gonzalez RG, Lerwill MF. Case 4-2007- A 56-year-old woman with rapidly progressive vertigo and ataxia. N Engl J Med 2007;356(6):612–20.

made with detection of antineuronal antibodies in serum or CSF.[10,128] No effective treatments have been found for PCD. Early detection and removal of the malignancy does not reliably improve the course of the neurologic syndrome. There are isolated reports of improvement with intravenous immunoglobulin, plasma exchange, and rituximab, but evidence-based treatment recommendations do not exist. The largest case series demonstrate overall ineffectiveness of immunosuppressive therapies.[129,130]

SUMMARY

Brain tumors are the most common form of solid tumors in children, normally occurring in the infratentorial region, usually the cerebellum or fourth ventricle. Intra-axial posterior fossa tumors in adults are rare, and generally caused by metastasis from an extracranial site. The potential for herniation and hydrocephalus increases the seriousness of tumors in this region. Symptoms related to these findings should prompt the neurologist to screen for posterior fossa tumors, especially in children. Modern neuroimaging has led to earlier diagnosis and better understanding of the anatomy of such lesions, and has allowed the neurosurgeon to more safely excise posterior fossa tumors, particularly fourth-ventricular tumors, in a manner not possible in the past. Recent advances in imaging, neurosurgical techniques, chemotherapy approaches, and radiation oncology have resulted in some improvement in overall survival and morbidity. However, the prognosis for many children with high-grade and malignant brain tumors remains guarded in terms of mortality and long-term morbidity. Further developments, such as molecular and functional imaging, may give important specific information about tumor histology and biological behavior, which will improve clinical outcomes.

REFERENCES

1. Levy AS. Brain tumors in children: evaluation and management. Curr Probl Pediatr Adolesc Health Care 2005;35(6):230–45.
2. Paldino MJ, Faerber EN, Poussaint TY. Imaging tumors of the pediatric central nervous system. Radiol Clin North Am 2011;49(4):589–616, v.
3. Sakamoto K, Kobayashi N, Ohtsubo H, et al. Intracranial tumors in the first year of life. Childs Nerv Syst 1986;2(3):126–9.
4. Pollack IF. Brain tumors in children. N Engl J Med 1994;331(22):1500–7.
5. Halperin EC, Watson DM, George SL. Duration of symptoms prior to diagnosis is related inversely to presenting disease stage in children with medulloblastoma. Cancer 2001;91(8):1444–50.
6. Viano JC, Herrera EJ, Suarez JC. Cerebellar astrocytomas: a 24-year experience. Childs Nerv Syst 2001;17(10):607–10 [discussion: 611].
7. Alston RD, Newton R, Kelsey A, et al. Childhood medulloblastoma in northwest England 1954 to 1997: incidence and survival. Dev Med Child Neurol 2003; 45(5):308–14.
8. Mechtler L. Neuroimaging in neuro-oncology. Neurol Clin 2009;27(1):171–201, ix.
9. Martinez Leon MI. Review and update about medulloblastoma in children. Radiologia 2011;53(2):134–45 [in Spanish].
10. Osborn AG. Osborn's brain: imaging, pathology, and anatomy. 1st edition. Salt Lake City (UT): Amirsys Pub; 2013. p. 1272, xi.
11. Fruehwald-Pallamar J, Puchner SB, Rossi A, et al. Magnetic resonance imaging spectrum of medulloblastoma. Neuroradiology 2011;53(6):387–96.
12. Castillo M. Stem cells, radial glial cells, and a unified origin of brain tumors. AJNR Am J Neuroradiol 2010;31(3):389–90.
13. Panigrahy A, Bluml S. Neuroimaging of pediatric brain tumors: from basic to advanced magnetic resonance imaging (MRI). J Child Neurol 2009;24(11):1343–65.
14. Koeller KK, Rushing EJ. From the archives of the AFIP: medulloblastoma: a comprehensive review with radiologic-pathologic correlation. Radiographics 2003;23(6):1613–37.
15. Giangaspero F, Perilongo G, Fondelli MP, et al. Medulloblastoma with extensive nodularity: a variant with favorable prognosis. J Neurosurg 1999;91(6): 971–7.
16. Kotsenas AL, Roth TC, Manness WK, et al. Abnormal diffusion-weighted MRI in medulloblastoma: does it reflect small cell histology? Pediatr Radiol 1999;29(7): 524–6.
17. Dhall G. Medulloblastoma. J Child Neurol 2009;24(11):1418–30.
18. Panigrahy A, Krieger MD, Gonzalez-Gomez I, et al. Quantitative short echo time 1H-MR spectroscopy of untreated pediatric brain tumors: preoperative diagnosis and characterization. AJNR Am J Neuroradiol 2006;27(3):560–72.

19. Rossi A, Gandolfo C, Morana G, et al. New MR sequences (diffusion, perfusion, spectroscopy) in brain tumours. Pediatr Radiol 2010;40(6):999–1009.
20. Saunders DE, Hayward RD, Phipps KP, et al. Surveillance neuroimaging of intracranial medulloblastoma in children: how effective, how often, and for how long? J Neurosurg 2003;99(2):280–6.
21. Harisiadis L, Chang CH. Medulloblastoma in children: a correlation between staging and results of treatment. Int J Radiat Oncol Biol Phys 1977;2(9–10): 833–41.
22. Gururangan S, Krauser J, Friedman H, et al. Efficacy of high-dose chemotherapy or standard salvage therapy in patients with recurrent medulloblastoma. Neuro Oncol 2008;10(5):745–51.
23. Packer RJ, Vezina G. Management of and prognosis with medulloblastoma: therapy at a crossroads. Arch Neurol 2008;65(11):1419–24.
24. McGuire CS, Sainani KL, Fisher PG. Incidence patterns for ependymoma: a surveillance, epidemiology, and end results study. J Neurosurg 2009;110(4): 725–9.
25. Foreman NK, Bouffet E. Ependymomas in children. J Neurosurg 1999;90(3):605.
26. Figarella-Branger D, Civatte M, Bouvier-Labit C, et al. Prognostic factors in intracranial ependymomas in children. J Neurosurg 2000;93(4):605–13.
27. Godfraind C. Classification and controversies in pathology of ependymomas. Childs Nerv Syst 2009;25(10):1185–93.
28. Mermuys K, Jeuris W, Vanhoenacker PK, et al. Best cases from the AFIP: supratentorial ependymoma. Radiographics 2005;25(2):486–90.
29. Yuh EL, Barkovich AJ, Gupta N. Imaging of ependymomas: MRI and CT. Childs Nerv Syst 2009;25(10):1203–13.
30. Plaza MJ, Borja MJ, Altman N, et al. Conventional and advanced MRI features of pediatric intracranial tumors: posterior fossa and suprasellar tumors. AJR Am J Roentgenol 2013;200(5):1115–24.
31. Tihan T, Zhou T, Holmes E, et al. The prognostic value of histological grading of posterior fossa ependymomas in children: a Children's Oncology Group study and a review of prognostic factors. Mod Pathol 2008;21(2):165–77.
32. Gaynon PS, Ettinger L, Baum E, et al. Carboplatin in childhood brain tumors. A Children's Cancer Study Group Phase II trial. Cancer 1990;66(12):2465–9.
33. Needle MN, Goldwein JW, Grass J, et al. Adjuvant chemotherapy for the treatment of intracranial ependymoma of childhood. Cancer 1997;80(2):341–7.
34. Horn B, Heideman R, Geyer R, et al. A multi-institutional retrospective study of intracranial ependymoma in children: identification of risk factors. J Pediatr Hematol Oncol 1999;21(3):203–11.
35. Robertson PL, Zeltzer PM, Boyett JM, et al. Survival and prognostic factors following radiation therapy and chemotherapy for ependymomas in children: a report of the Children's Cancer Group. J Neurosurg 1998;88(4):695–703.
36. Merchant TE, Mulhern RK, Krasin MJ, et al. Preliminary results from a phase II trial of conformal radiation therapy and evaluation of radiation-related CNS effects for pediatric patients with localized ependymoma. J Clin Oncol 2004; 22(15):3156–62.
37. Merchant TE, Zhu Y, Thompson SJ, et al. Preliminary results from a Phase II trail of conformal radiation therapy for pediatric patients with localised low-grade astrocytoma and ependymoma. Int J Radiat Oncol Biol Phys 2002;52(2):325–32.
38. Merchant TE, Jenkins JJ, Burger PC, et al. Influence of tumor grade on time to progression after irradiation for localized ependymoma in children. Int J Radiat Oncol Biol Phys 2002;53(1):52–7.

39. Merchant TE, Li C, Xiong X, et al. Conformal radiotherapy after surgery for paediatric ependymoma: a prospective study. Lancet Oncol 2009;10(3):258–66.
40. Koeller KK, Sandberg GD, Armed Forces Institute of Pathology. From the archives of the AFIP. Cerebral intraventricular neoplasms: radiologic-pathologic correlation. Radiographics 2002;22(6):1473–505.
41. Jinhu Y, Jianping D, Jun M, et al. Metastasis of a histologically benign choroid plexus papilloma: case report and review of the literature. J Neurooncol 2007; 83(1):47–52.
42. Gozali AE, Britt B, Shane L, et al. Choroid plexus tumors; management, outcome, and association with the Li-Fraumeni syndrome: the Children's Hospital Los Angeles (CHLA) experience, 1991-2010. Pediatr Blood Cancer 2012; 58(6):905–9.
43. Ogiwara H, Dipatri A Jr, Alden T, et al. Choroid plexus tumors in pediatric patients. Br J Neurosurg 2012;26(1):32–7.
44. Zhang TJ, Yue Q, Lui S, et al. MRI findings of choroid plexus tumors in the cerebellum. Clin Imaging 2011;35(1):64–7.
45. Severino M, Schwartz ES, Thurnher MM, et al. Congenital tumors of the central nervous system. Neuroradiology 2010;52(6):531–48.
46. McEvoy AW, Galloway M, Revesz T, et al. Metastatic choroid plexus papilloma: a case report. J Neurooncol 2002;56(3):241–6.
47. Wolff JE, Sajedi M, Brant R, et al. Choroid plexus tumours. Br J Cancer 2002; 87(10):1086–91.
48. Cyrine S, Sonia Z, Mounir T, et al. Pilocytic astrocytoma: a retrospective study of 32 cases. Clin Neurol Neurosurg 2013;115(8):1220–5.
49. Malik A, Deb P, Sharma MC, et al. Neuropathological spectrum of pilocytic astrocytoma: an Indian series of 120 cases. Pathol Oncol Res 2006;12(3):164–71.
50. Koeller KK, Rushing EJ. From the archives of the AFIP: pilocytic astrocytoma: radiologic-pathologic correlation. Radiographics 2004;24(6):1693–708.
51. Murray RD, Penar PL, Filippi CG, et al. Radiographically distinct variant of pilocytic astrocytoma: a case series. J Comput Assist Tomogr 2011;35(4):495–7.
52. Hsieh MS, Ho JT, Lin LW, et al. Cerebellar anaplastic pilocytic astrocytoma in a patient of neurofibromatosis type-1: case report and review of the literature. Clin Neurol Neurosurg 2012;114(7):1027–9.
53. Dunn IF, Agarwalla PK, Papanastassiou AM, et al. Multiple pilocytic astrocytomas of the cerebellum in a 17-year-old patient with neurofibromatosis type I. Childs Nerv Syst 2007;23(10):1191–4.
54. Ogiwara H, Bowman RM, Tomita T. Long-term follow-up of pediatric benign cerebellar astrocytomas. Neurosurgery 2012;70(1):40–7 [discussion: 47–8].
55. Tabrizi RD, Mittelbronn M, Marquardt G, et al. Radiologically typical pilocytic astrocytoma with histopathological signs of atypia. Childs Nerv Syst 2012;28(10): 1791–4.
56. Beni-Adani L, Gomori M, Spektor S, et al. Cyst wall enhancement in pilocytic astrocytoma: neoplastic or reactive phenomena. Pediatr Neurosurg 2000;32(5): 234–9.
57. Hwang JH, Egnaczyk GF, Ballard E, et al. Proton MR spectroscopic characteristics of pediatric pilocytic astrocytomas. AJNR Am J Neuroradiol 1998;19(3): 535–40.
58. Kumar VA, Knopp EA, Zagzag D. Magnetic resonance dynamic susceptibility-weighted contrast-enhanced perfusion imaging in the diagnosis of posterior fossa hemangioblastomas and pilocytic astrocytomas: initial results. J Comput Assist Tomogr 2010;34(6):825–9.

59. Newman S, Wasserberg J. A case report of the management of multiple meta-chronous haemangioblastomas in a patient with von Hippel-Lindau disease. Br J Neurosurg 2008;22(1):104–6.
60. Lee SH, Park BJ, Kim TS, et al. Long-term follow-up clinical courses of cere-bellar hemangioblastoma in von Hippel-Lindau disease: two case reports and a literature review. J Korean Neurosurg Soc 2010;48(3):263–7.
61. Yamashita K, Yoshiura T, Hiwatashi A, et al. Arterial spin labeling of hemangio-blastoma: differentiation from metastatic brain tumors based on quantitative blood flow measurement. Neuroradiology 2012;54(8):809–13.
62. Slater A, Moore NR, Huson SM. The natural history of cerebellar hemangioblasto-mas in von Hippel-Lindau disease. AJNR Am J Neuroradiol 2003;24(8):1570–4.
63. Gray F, De Girolami U, Poirier J, et al. Escourolle & Poirier manual of basic neuro-pathology. 4th edition. Philadelphia: Butterworth Heinemann; 2004. p. 400, xiv.
64. Ginn KF, Gajjar A. Atypical teratoid rhabdoid tumor: current therapy and future directions. Front Oncol 2012;2:114.
65. Udaka YT, Shayan K, Crawford JR, et al. Atypical presentation of atypical teratoid rhabdoid tumor in a child. Case Rep Oncol Med 2013;2013:815923.
66. Parmar H, Hawkins C, Bouffet E, et al. Imaging findings in primary intracranial atypical teratoid/rhabdoid tumors. Pediatr Radiol 2006;36(2):126–32.
67. Parwani AV, Stelow EB, Pambuccian SE, et al. Atypical teratoid/rhabdoid tumor of the brain: cytopathologic characteristics and differential diagnosis. Cancer 2005;105(2):65–70.
68. Hilden JM, Meerbaum S, Burger P, et al. Central nervous system atypical tera-toid/rhabdoid tumor: results of therapy in children enrolled in a registry. J Clin Oncol 2004;22(14):2877–84.
69. Rorke LB, Packer R, Biegel J. Central nervous system atypical teratoid/rhabdoid tumors of infancy and childhood. J Neurooncol 1995;24(1):21–8.
70. Tekautz TM, Fuller CE, Blaney S, et al. Atypical teratoid/rhabdoid tumors (ATRT): improved survival in children 3 years of age and older with radiation therapy and high-dose alkylator-based chemotherapy. J Clin Oncol 2005; 23(7):1491–9.
71. Shinagare AB, Patil NK, Sorte SZ. Case 144: dysplastic cerebellar gangliocy-toma (Lhermitte-Duclos disease). Radiology 2009;251(1):298–303.
72. Klisch J, Juengling F, Spreer J, et al. Lhermitte-Duclos disease: assessment with MR imaging, positron emission tomography, single-photon emission CT, and MR spectroscopy. AJNR Am J Neuroradiol 2001;22(5):824–30.
73. Nowak DA, Trost HA. Lhermitte-Duclos disease (dysplastic cerebellar ganglio-cytoma): a malformation, hamartoma or neoplasm? Acta Neurol Scand 2002; 105(3):137–45.
74. Thomas B, Krishnamoorthy T, Radhakrishnan VV, et al. Advanced MR imaging in Lhermitte-Duclos disease: moving closer to pathology and pathophysiology. Neuroradiology 2007;49(9):733–8.
75. Buhl R, Barth H, Hugo HH, et al. Dysplastic gangliocytoma of the cerebellum: rare differential diagnosis in space occupying lesions of the posterior fossa. Acta Neurochir (Wien) 2003;145(6):509–12 [discussion: 512].
76. Milbouw G, Born JD, Martin D, et al. Clinical and radiological aspects of dysplastic gangliocytoma (Lhermitte-Duclos disease): a report of two cases with review of the literature. Neurosurgery 1988;22(1 Pt 1):124–8.
77. Grahovac G, Tomac D, Lambasa S, et al. Cerebellar glioblastomas: pathophys-iology, clinical presentation and management. Acta Neurochir (Wien) 2009; 151(6):653–7.

78. Kuroiwa T, Numaguchi Y, Rothman MI, et al. Posterior fossa glioblastoma multiforme: MR findings. AJNR Am J Neuroradiol 1995;16(3):583–9.
79. Stark AM, Nabavi A, Mehdorn HM, et al. Glioblastoma multiforme—report of 267 cases treated at a single institution. Surg Neurol 2005;63(2):162–9 [discussion: 169].
80. Kleihues P, Ohgaki H. Primary and secondary glioblastomas: from concept to clinical diagnosis. Neuro Oncol 1999;1(1):44–51.
81. Ohgaki H, Kleihues P. Genetic pathways to primary and secondary glioblastoma. Am J Pathol 2007;170(5):1445–53.
82. Martin SE, Brat DJ, Vance GH, et al. Glioblastoma occurring at the site of a previous medulloblastoma following a 5-year remission period. Neuropathology 2012;32(5):543–50.
83. Hur H, Jung S, Kim IY, et al. Cerebellar glioblastoma multiforme in an adult. J Korean Neurosurg Soc 2008;43(4):194–7.
84. Kulkarni AV, Becker LE, Jay V, et al. Primary cerebellar glioblastomas multiforme in children. Report of four cases. J Neurosurg 1999;90(3):546–50.
85. Haldorsen IS, Espeland A, Larsson EM. Central nervous system lymphoma: characteristic findings on traditional and advanced imaging. AJNR Am J Neuroradiol 2011;32(6):984–92.
86. Coulon A, Lafitte F, Hoang-Xuan K, et al. Radiographic findings in 37 cases of primary CNS lymphoma in immunocompetent patients. Eur Radiol 2002;12(2):329–40.
87. Gliemroth J, Kehler U, Gaebel C, et al. Neuroradiological findings in primary cerebral lymphomas of non-AIDS patients. Clin Neurol Neurosurg 2003;105(2):78–86.
88. Go JL, Lee SC, Kim PE. Imaging of primary central nervous system lymphoma. Neurosurg Focus 2006;21(5):E4.
89. Koeller KK, Smirniotopoulos JG, Jones RV. Primary central nervous system lymphoma: radiologic-pathologic correlation. Radiographics 1997;17(6):1497–526.
90. Haldorsen IS, Krakenes J, Krossnes BK, et al. CT and MR imaging features of primary central nervous system lymphoma in Norway, 1989-2003. AJNR Am J Neuroradiol 2009;30(4):744–51.
91. Kuker W, Nagele T, Korfel A, et al. Primary central nervous system lymphomas (PCNSL): MRI features at presentation in 100 patients. J Neurooncol 2005;72(2):169–77.
92. Schlegel U, Schmidt-Wolf IG, Deckert M. Primary CNS lymphoma: clinical presentation, pathological classification, molecular pathogenesis and treatment. J Neurol Sci 2000;181(1–2):1–12.
93. Toh CH, Castillo M, Wong AM, et al. Primary cerebral lymphoma and glioblastoma multiforme: differences in diffusion characteristics evaluated with diffusion tensor imaging. AJNR Am J Neuroradiol 2008;29(3):471–5.
94. Chou AP, Lalezari S, Fong BM, et al. Post-transplantation primary central nervous system lymphoma: a case report and review of the literature. Surg Neurol Int 2011;2:130.
95. Nussbaum ES, Djalilian HR, Cho KH, et al. Brain metastases. Histology, multiplicity, surgery, and survival. Cancer 1996;78(8):1781–8.
96. Serres S, Soto MS, Hamilton A, et al. Molecular MRI enables early and sensitive detection of brain metastases. Proc Natl Acad Sci U S A 2012;109(17):6674–9.
97. Yoshida S, Takahashi H. Cerebellar metastases in patients with cancer. Surg Neurol 2009;71(2):184–7 [discussion: 187].
98. Fadul C, Misulis KE, Wiley RG. Cerebellar metastases: diagnostic and management considerations. J Clin Oncol 1987;5(7):1107–15.

99. Ghods AJ, Munoz L, Byrne R. Surgical treatment of cerebellar metastases. Surg Neurol Int 2011;2:159.

100. van der Sande JJ, van Tinteren H, Brandsma D, et al. Brain metastases in patients with pelvic or abdominal malignancy do not prevail in the posterior fossa: a retrospective study. J Neurol 2009;256(9):1485–7.

101. Schoenwaelder M, Waugh J, Russell P. Cerebellar metastases from prostatic carcinoma. Australas Radiol 2004;48(3):430–3.

102. Soffietti R, Ruda R, Mutani R. Management of brain metastases. J Neurol 2002; 249(10):1357–69.

103. Potts DG, Abbott GF, von Sneidern JV. National Cancer Institute study: evaluation of computed tomography in the diagnosis of intracranial neoplasms. III. Metastatic tumors. Radiology 1980;136(3):657–64.

104. Ginaldi S, Wallace S, Shalen P, et al. Cranial computed tomography of malignant melanoma. AJR Am J Roentgenol 1981;136(1):145–9.

105. McGann GM, Platts A. Computed tomography of cranial metastatic malignant melanoma: features, early detection and unusual cases. Br J Radiol 1991; 64(760):310–3.

106. Nakase H, Sakaki T, Fujita T, et al. Multiple calcified metastatic brain tumor—case report. Neurol Med Chir (Tokyo) 1991;31(12):787–91.

107. Fink KR, Fink JR. Imaging of brain metastases. Surg Neurol Int 2013;4(Suppl 4): S209–19.

108. Chen W, Wang L, Zhu W, et al. Multicontrast single-slab 3D MRI to detect cerebral metastasis. AJR Am J Roentgenol 2012;198(1):27–32.

109. Al-Okaili RN, Krejza J, Wang S, et al. Advanced MR imaging techniques in the diagnosis of intraaxial brain tumors in adults. Radiographics 2006;26(Suppl 1):S173–89.

110. Calli C, Kitis O, Yunten N, et al. Perfusion and diffusion MR imaging in enhancing malignant cerebral tumors. Eur J Radiol 2006;58(3):394–403.

111. Wang S, Kim S, Chawla S, et al. Differentiation between glioblastomas, solitary brain metastases, and primary cerebral lymphomas using diffusion tensor and dynamic susceptibility contrast-enhanced MR imaging. AJNR Am J Neuroradiol 2011;32(3):507–14.

112. Bendini M, Marton E, Feletti A, et al. Primary and metastatic intraaxial brain tumors: prospective comparison of multivoxel 2D chemical-shift imaging (CSI) proton MR spectroscopy, perfusion MRI, and histopathological findings in a group of 159 patients. Acta Neurochir (Wien) 2011;153(2):403–12.

113. Chiang IC, Kuo YT, Lu CY, et al. Distinction between high-grade gliomas and solitary metastases using peritumoral 3-T magnetic resonance spectroscopy, diffusion, and perfusion imaging. Neuroradiology 2004;46(8):619–27.

114. Hakyemez B, Erdogan C, Gokalp G, et al. Solitary metastases and high-grade gliomas: radiological differentiation by morphometric analysis and perfusion-weighted MRI. Clin Radiol 2010;65(1):15–20.

115. Cha S, Lupo JM, Chen MH, et al. Differentiation of glioblastoma multiforme and single brain metastasis by peak height and percentage of signal intensity recovery derived from dynamic susceptibility-weighted contrast-enhanced perfusion MR imaging. AJNR Am J Neuroradiol 2007;28(6):1078–84.

116. Law M, Cha S, Knopp EA, et al. High-grade gliomas and solitary metastases: differentiation by using perfusion and proton spectroscopic MR imaging. Radiology 2002;222(3):715–21.

117. Hakyemez B, Erdogan C, Bolca N, et al. Evaluation of different cerebral mass lesions by perfusion-weighted MR imaging. J Magn Reson Imaging 2006; 24(4):817–24.

118. Bulakbasi N, Kocaoglu M, Ors F, et al. Combination of single-voxel proton MR spectroscopy and apparent diffusion coefficient calculation in the evaluation of common brain tumors. AJNR Am J Neuroradiol 2003;24(2):225–33.

119. Fan G, Sun B, Wu Z, et al. In vivo single-voxel proton MR spectroscopy in the differentiation of high-grade gliomas and solitary metastases. Clin Radiol 2004;59(1):77–85.

120. Demir MK, Hakan T, Akinci O, et al. Primary cerebellar glioblastoma multiforme. Diagn Interv Radiol 2005;11(2):83–6.

121. Datta R, Hakan T, Akinci O, et al. Survival in relation to radiotherapeutic modality for brain metastasis: whole brain irradiation vs. gamma knife radiosurgery. Am J Clin Oncol 2004;27(4):420–4.

122. Lutterbach J, Bartelt S, Stancu E, et al. Patients with brain metastases: hope for recursive partitioning analysis (RPA) class 3. Radiother Oncol 2002;63(3):339–45.

123. Weinberg JS, Rhines LD, Cohen ZR, et al. Posterior fossa decompression for life-threatening tonsillar herniation in patients with gliomatosis cerebri: report of three cases. Neurosurgery 2003;52(1):216–23 [discussion: 223].

124. Winfree CJ, Mack WJ, Sisti MB. Solitary cerebellar metastasis of malignant pleural mesothelioma: case report. Surg Neurol 2004;61(2):174–8 [discussion: 178–9].

125. Lorusso L, Hart IK, Giometto B, et al. Immunological features of neurological paraneoplastic syndromes. Int J Immunopathol Pharmacol 2004;17(2):135–44.

126. Rojas I, Graus F, Keime-Guibert F, et al. Long-term clinical outcome of paraneoplastic cerebellar degeneration and anti-Yo antibodies. Neurology 2000;55(5):713–5.

127. Schmahmann JD, Sherman JC. The cerebellar cognitive affective syndrome. Brain 1998;121(Pt 4):561–79.

128. Gilmore CP, Elliott I, Auer D, et al. Diffuse cerebellar MR imaging changes in anti-Yo positive paraneoplastic cerebellar degeneration. J Neurol 2010;257(3):490–1.

129. Peterson K, Elliott I, Auer D, et al. Paraneoplastic cerebellar degeneration. I. A clinical analysis of 55 anti-Yo antibody-positive patients. Neurology 1992;42(10):1931–7.

130. Shams'ili S, Rosenblum MK, Kotanides H, et al. Paraneoplastic cerebellar degeneration associated with antineuronal antibodies: analysis of 50 patients. Brain 2003;126(Pt 6):1409–18.

Traumatic Injury to the Posterior Fossa

Menarvia Nixon, MD, Sudheer Ambekar, MD, Shihao Zhang, MD,
Cory Markham, BS, Hesam Akbarian-Tefaghi, BS, Kevin Morrow, BS,
Anil Nanda, MD, FACS, Bharat Guthikonda, MD*

KEYWORDS

- Traumatic brain injury • Posterior fossa • Intra-axial lesions • Extra-axial lesions
- Vascular injuries

KEY POINTS

- Traumatic injury to the posterior fossa is a complex pathologic condition because of the great heterogeneity of lesions present.
- As with all traumatic brain injuries, treatment of primary brain injuries and prevention of secondary brain injuries is the mainstay of management.
- It is imperative to recognize traumatic lesions of the posterior fossa early because of the occurrence of rapid neurologic decline.
- The decision regarding whether or not to proceed with surgical intervention depends on the patient's clinical condition, neurologic status, and imaging findings.
- In general, nonoperative management should be considered only if the patient is fully conscious and the associated posterior fossa lesions are small with little or no mass effect. Posterior fossa traumatic vascular injuries should also be managed either by an open surgical or endovascular approach.

INTRODUCTION

It is estimated that more than 1.7 million cases of traumatic brain injury (TBI) occur in the United States each year and nearly 3% of these cases result in fatality. Although the leading cause of TBI in the United States is injury from falls, motor vehicle accidents are the leading cause of TBI that results in mortality.[1] Trauma to the posterior cranial fossa is a subset of TBI that affects the parts of the brain located inferior to the tentorium cerebelli including the cerebellum, brainstem, major cranial blood vessels, and parts of cranial nerves III-XII (**Fig. 1**).[2] However, most studies do not distinguish between trauma to the posterior fossa and other types of TBI. Major injuries within the posterior fossa are reported in 3.3% of all head trauma.[3] Despite having

Department of Neurosurgery, LSU HSC Shreveport, 1501 Kings Highway, Shreveport, LA 71130, USA
* Corresponding author.
E-mail address: bguthi@lsuhsc.edu

Neurol Clin 32 (2014) 943–955
http://dx.doi.org/10.1016/j.ncl.2014.07.010   **neurologic.theclinics.com**

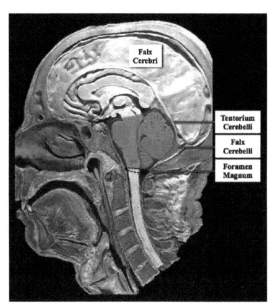

Fig. 1. Midsagittal view of human brain. The approximate location of posterior cranial fossa is shaded. The ring represents the location of foramen magnum. (*Courtesy of* John Beal, PhD, Department of Cellular Biology and Anatomy, Louisiana State University Health Sciences Center.)

a lower rate of occurrence, trauma to this area is associated with a higher rate of morbidity compared with supratentorial trauma.

By definition, TBI is the result of an external force impacting the head and causing a sudden change in acceleration of the brain. Anatomically, the posterior fossa is the largest of the three fossa (anterior, middle, and posterior), located along the floor of the cranial cavity. Its boundaries are marked by aspects of the sphenoid, occipital, parietal, and temporal bones, with a roof formed from reflections of the dura mater called the tentorium cerebelli that houses the clinically important transverse venous sinuses.[4] Although it is the largest fossa, the amount of space that is allowed for expansion is the smallest of the three fossa. Thus, the presence of critical structures that are contained within the posterior fossa combined with minimal compliance leads to significant morbidity from any mass-occupying lesions.[5]

Trauma to the posterior fossa may impair the function of cerebellum and/or the brainstem. When trauma affects the structures of the posterior fossa, the supratentorial region also may be affected. Studies have shown that more favorable outcomes were achieved when the supratentorial region was spared.[6] Skull fractures could further complicate the management of patients with TBI, especially if a fracture is open.

TBI is divided into primary and secondary brain injury. Primary brain injury refers to damage suffered as a direct result of the initial event, whereas secondary brain injury refers to the indirect insult to the brain as a result of the sequelae of the traumatic event. Primary traumatic injuries are commonly subdivided into blunt and penetrating injuries. Mass lesions from TBI are usually categorized as either intra- or extra-axial lesions. Intra-axial brain lesions are defined by intraparenchymal cerebellar or brainstem damage caused by hematoma, diffuse axonal injury from shearing forces, or delayed posttraumatic intracerebellar hematomas. Extra-axial injuries include epidural hematomas (EDH), subdural hematoma (SDH), and subarachnoid hemorrhage (SAH).[7]

INTRA-AXIAL LESIONS

Intraparenchymal cerebellar hemorrhage secondary to trauma constitutes about 3% of all the traumatic head injuries and about 25% of all the traumatic injuries to the posterior fossa.[3,8,9] Liu[10] reported the incidence of traumatic cerebellar hemorrhage to be 3.7% among all head injuries. Cerebellar hemorrhage may occur in patients of all age groups, although it may more commonly be observed in young patients because this age group is more commonly involved in motor vehicle accidents.

Pathophysiology

The exact mechanism of cerebellar contusion is unclear. They may be caused by blunt or penetrating trauma. Takeuchi and colleagues[11] proposed three mechanisms of injury in the pathogenesis of cerebellar hematoma. The first is coup injury, where the posterior fossa is the first site of impact. This type of injury typically results in contusion of one of the cerebellar hemispheres with a concomitant contusion of the frontal or temporal lobes. Typically, in a coup injury of the cerebellum, there is evidence of an overlying injury, such as an epidural or a SDH or a fracture of the occipital bone.

The second is contrecoup injury, where the site of first impact is other than the posterior fossa. Commonly, frontal or the temporal region is the first site of impact in this mechanism of injury. Again, in this type of injury, the cerebellar hemispheres are more commonly involved than the midline structures. However, in a contrecoup injury of the cerebellum, other traumatic lesions of the posterior fossa are rarely present.

The third is shear-related injury, caused by acceleration-deceleration forces. This type of injury is frequently associated with diffuse axonal injury. Differential movements of one portion of the brain with respect to the other lead to the development of shear-strain forces. The most common locations where these forces develop are the gray-white matter junction, brain-pia mater interface, cerebrospinal fluid–brain interface, and skull-dura interface. In the posterior fossa, these lesions are usually seen in the dorsolateral brainstem and in the cerebellar hemispheres.

In addition to the previously mentioned three mechanisms of injury, a fourth type of injury is also commonly observed. This is the delayed cerebellar hematoma, which develops secondary to cerebellar contusion as a result of secondary insult. The exact mechanism of this injury is unknown; however, this occurs more commonly in elderly people with underlying coagulopathy or hypertension.[12] Delayed intracerebellar hemorrhage develops a few hours to days after trauma. It may progress rapidly and lead to brainstem compression. Various mechanisms, such as increased endothelial permeability of small vessels in the posterior fossa and hyperoxidation within the endothelial cells, have been hypothesized in its development.[13,14] Therefore, it is essential to monitor the patients with posterior fossa trauma with serial imaging.

As the size of the hematoma grows, the cerebellar parenchyma is destroyed and the hematoma causes mass effect. This may result in fourth ventricular compression leading to obstructive hydrocephalus. Edema of the cerebellar parenchyma around the hematoma adds to the mass effect. In later stages, there may be direct compression of the brainstem resulting in alteration of mental status, stupor, coma, and ultimately death. This sequence of events corresponds to the medullary stage of transtentorial herniation as described by Plum and Posner.[15]

Herniation may occur when the cerebellar tonsils are forced through the foramen magnum (tonsillar herniation) or when the vermis is forced upward through the tentorial incisura (upward or reverse transtentorial herniation). The latter condition may occur when the supratentorial compartment is suddenly decompressed in the presence of a large posterior fossa lesion. It is fortunately a rare condition. There is up-ward displacement of the vermis through the tentorial incisura causing compression of brainstem and death.

Clinical Presentation

Traumatic parenchymal lesions of the cerebellum range from completely asymptom-atic to coma and death. The variety and extent of signs and symptoms depend on the site of hemorrhage, size of the hemorrhage, presence of perilesional edema, and mass effect on surrounding structures. Clinical features may be classified into the following stages and usually correlate with the progression of the underlying pathophysiologic process (secondary injury).

- Stage I: asymptomatic or mild symptoms (dizziness, headache, vertigo); no cere-bellar signs, no mass effect, no hydrocephalus, no brainstem compression; de-tected on imaging; the lesion is usually small, less than 2 cm; usually involving the cerebellar hemispheres
- Stage II: symptomatic; cerebellar signs present (axial or appendicular or both); mild mass effect over fourth ventricle, no hydrocephalus, no brainstem compres-sion; the lesion is usually greater than 2 cm
- Stage III: symptomatic; cerebellar signs present, moderate mass effect on fourth ventricle, mild hydrocephalus, mild brainstem compression; the lesion is about 3 to 4 cm
- Stage IV: symptomatic; cerebellar signs present, severe mass effect over fourth ventricle, severe hydrocephalus, brainstem compression, and altered mental status; the lesion is usually greater than 4 cm
- Stage V: symptomatic; severe brainstem compression; coma and death; lesion over 4 cm

Imaging Studies

As with other acute traumatic hemorrhagic lesions, acute cerebellar hemorrhage ap-pears hyperdense on computed tomography (CT) scan (**Fig. 2**) and isointense on T1-weighted and hypointense on T2-weighted magnetic resonance images. The following features should be observed on imaging while assessing a patient with cerebellar hemorrhage following trauma.

1. Location of hemorrhage (hemispheric, vermis, both)
2. Presence of perilesional edema
3. Associated posterior fossa traumatic lesions (EDH, SDH, fracture)
4. Mass effect over fourth ventricle
5. Ventricle size to assess for hydrocephalus
6. Compression of brainstem
7. Tonsillar herniation
8. Effacement of basal cisterns
9. Configuration of basal cisterns ("inverted smile" sign seen in upward herniation)
10. Presence of associated diffuse axonal injury or supratentorial traumatic lesions
11. Dissection of the hematoma into the brainstem through the fourth ventricle

Management Goals

The general management algorithm of a patient with TBI is beyond the scope of this article and is well described in the literature. In this section we discuss the specific management of focal cerebellar parenchymal hemorrhage. Conservative manage-ment of cerebellar contusion and hematoma may be considered in a fully alert patient

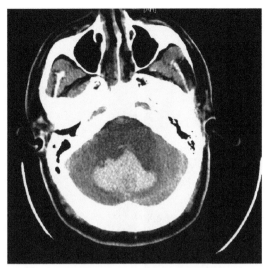

Fig. 2. Cerebellar hematoma. Traumatic vermian hematoma in a patient. The hematoma has extended into the fourth ventricle and compressed it. There is also edema around the hematoma.

with a small lesion. Close monitoring is required to detect early signs of deterioration, which mandates surgical evacuation. Surgical evacuation for intraparenchymal cerebellar hemorrhage is usually indicated in the following situations: (1) contusion or hematoma greater than 3 cm in maximum dimension, (2) effacement of the basal cisterns, (3) moderate to severe mass effect over fourth ventricle causing hydrocephalus, (4) signs of tonsillar or upward herniation, and (5) moderate to severe brainstem compression.

EXTRA-AXIAL LESIONS

External forces that give rise to TBI first stop at the skull and are then transmitted to the underlying structures in a linear fashion. This causes a vertical force on the brain tissue adjacent to the inner table of the skull at the site of the impact.[16] As a result, the formation of intracranial, extra-axial hematomas after head injury is a common occurrence.[17]

Pathophysiology

EDH occurs in 2% to 5% of head-injured patients and posterior fossa EDH constitutes 4% to 13% of all EDH.[18] EDHs are located between the outer (periosteal) layer of the dura mater and the inner table of the skull (**Fig. 3**). They typically develop at the moment of impact at the coup site. They are often associated with overlying occipital fractures.[7] In comparison with the supratentorium EDH, posterior fossa EDHs are more frequently of venous rather than arterial origin. They are most often caused by transverse sinus injury from direct occipital trauma. Clival EDHs are an even rarer variant of posterior fossa EDHs and may occur by hyperflexion or extension cervical injuries or basilar clival fractures.[19]

SDHs are located between the inner (meningeal) layer of the dura mater and the arachnoid. SDHs are not always a result of the direct impact in head trauma but can result from shearing of bridging veins and venous sinuses. They occur in approximately 11% of head-injured patients. SDHs are associated with the highest mortality rate of all traumatic intracranial injuries. The rate is more than four times higher in

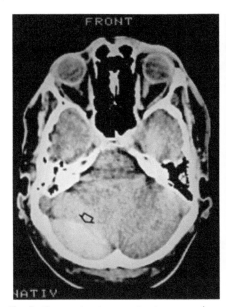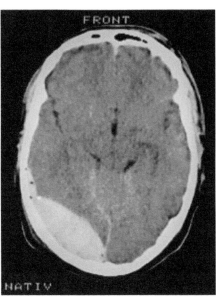

Fig. 3. Noncontrast computer tomography scan of a 23-year-old man with an epidural hematoma of the posterior fossa located between the outer layer of the dura mater and the inner table of the skull. Note the characteristic hyperdense, biconvex appearance of the lesion. *Arrowhead* showing biconvex hyperdense collection consistent with an epidural hematoma. (*From* Maschke M, Morsdorf MM, Timman D, et al. Posterior fossa trauma. In: Manto M, Gruol D, Schmahmann J, et al, editors. Handbook of cerebellum and cerebellar disorders. New York: Springer Science+Business Media, 2013; with permission.)

patients older than 65 years. SDHs are more likely to be associated with moderate to severe underlying parenchymal injury, which is considered to be a contributor to the overall poor outcome of patients with SDHs.[20]

Traumatic SAH, like EDH of the posterior fossa, usually occurs because of rupture of venous structures. Despite its venous origin, traumatic SAH of the posterior fossa can occasionally lead to vasospasm of intracerebral arteries.

The two most common types of fractures to the skull are linear and depressed fractures. Linear fractures are more common and have better patient outcomes compared with depressed fractures.[10] Fractures to the occipital bone are of special concern because it is the major bone of the posterior cranial fossa and transmits many important anatomic structures including the vertebral arteries, hypoglossal nerves (cranial nerve XII), meningeal branches of ascending pharyngeal artery, transverse sinus, sigmoid sinus, and vagus nerves (**Fig. 4**).

Clinical Findings

The classic "lucid" interval described in EDH occurs in 15% to 30% of patients and even less commonly in EDHs occurring in the posterior fossa. It consists of a brief loss of consciousness, caused by impact, followed by an awake period and late deterioration caused by mass effect and increasing intracranial pressure (ICP). With compressive lesions of the posterior fossa, including EDHs and SDHs, patients usually present with headache, nausea, and vomiting followed by loss of consciousness. Because of the limited size of the posterior fossa, early detection is imperative to avoid rapid and life-threatening neurologic deterioration.

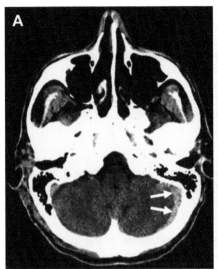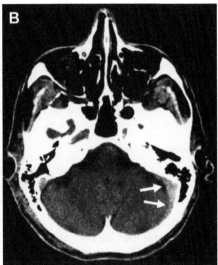

Fig. 4. Both (*A*) and (*B*) are noncontrast computed tomography scans of the head showing the crescentic or concave shape of an acute subdural hematoma. (*A*) shows the lower compartment of the the posterior fossa whereas (*B*) shows a higher cut at the the superior poles of the cerebellum depicting the crescentic nature of an acute subdural hematoma. (*From* Maschke M, Morsdorf MM, Timman D, et al. Posterior fossa trauma. In: Manto M, Gruol D, Schmahmann J, et al, editors. Handbook of cerebellum and cerebellar disorders. New York: Springer Science+Business Media, 2013; with permission.)

Clinical Examination

Pupillary examination by assessment of pupil size and reactivity to light is imperative in posterior fossa trauma, especially in patients with suspected mass lesions (eg, EDH, SDH). Sluggish or no pupillary reactivity may indicate compression of the fourth ventricle or brainstem and/or hydrocephalus. Downward deviation of the eyes may also be associated with unreactive pupils and possible hydrocephalus.

The Glasgow Coma Scale (GCS) is used to assess level of consciousness. Consciousness has two components: arousal and content. Impairment of arousal can vary from drowsiness to obtundation to coma. Coma is the most severe form of arousal impairment, and is defined as the inability to follow commands, speak, or open eyes to pain.[21]

Cranial nerve III and VI palsies may indicate impending herniation or increased ICP, respectively.

Motor examination should evaluate muscle tone, reflexes, coordination, and motor strength.

Imaging Studies

CT scanning is the imaging modality of choice for evaluation of head-injured patients. It allows rapid assessment of the location, extent, and type of intracranial lesions caused by the head injury.[19] According to Pascual and Prieto[22] three major findings should be evaluated on a head-injured patient's CT: (1) presence of intracranial hematomas, (2) appearance of basal cisterns, and (3) presence of traumatic SAH. Studies have indicated a relationship between status of basal cisterns and outcome. Compressed or absent basal cisterns indicate a threefold risk of increased ICP.[19]

The characteristic CT appearance of acute EDH is hyperdense, biconvex lesions adjacent to the skull. Mass effect is common.[23] Occasionally, EDHs may appear heterogeneous with hyperdense and isodense areas, which may indicate active bleeding.

Acute SDH appears as hyperdense, crescentic collections between the dura and brain parenchyma on CT (**Fig. 5**). In contrast with acute EDHs, acute SDHs are more diffuse, less uniform, and concave over the brain surface.[24]

CT scan is more sensitive than magnetic resonance imaging to disclose SAH at the acute stage, showing hyperdense fluid within the cisterns and sulci, around the falx of cerebellum, or in ventricles (**Fig. 6**).[7]

Management Goals

There are no class I or II guidelines for specific management of posterior fossa traumatic injuries. Factors that determine surgical versus nonsurgical management of injuries to the posterior fossa are discussed next.[24,25]

Acute epidural hematomas

Volume greater than 30 cm³ and compression or obliteration of the fourth ventricle regardless of GCS score should undergo surgical evacuation as soon as possible.

Volume less than 30 cm³, thickness less than 15 mm, no compression or mild compression of the fourth ventricle, GCS greater than 8, and no focal deficit can be managed with serial CT scans and close neurologic examinations.

Acute subdural hematoma

Thickness greater than 10 mm and/or compression of the fourth ventricle regardless of GCS score should undergo surgical decompression as soon as possible.

Thickness less than 10 mm, GCS score less than 9 with decrease in greater than 2 points between injury and hospital admission, and asymmetric or fixed pupils should undergo surgical decompression. GCS score less than 9 should undergo ICP monitoring.

Skull fractures

Open skull fractures, closed depressed skull fracture greater than 1 cm, and fractures with significant underlying intracranial hematoma should undergo surgical intervention.

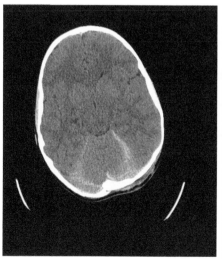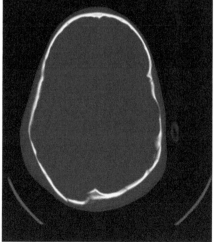

Fig. 5. Noncontrast computer tomography scan depicting a depressed occipital bone fracture abutting the right transverse sinus.

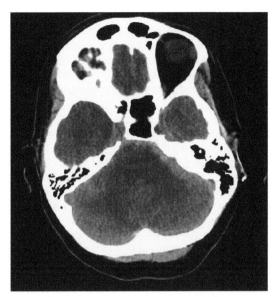

Fig. 6. Noncontrast computed tomography scan of a 43-year-old woman with sudden-onset severe headache following trauma. There is subarachnoid hemorrhage in the basal cisterns.

Open skull fractures depressed greater than the thickness of the cranium should undergo surgical debridement to prevent infection.

Nondepressed cranial fractures, fractures without clinical or radiographic evidence of violation of the dura, depression less than 1 cm, and fractures without significant intracranial hematomas do not require surgical intervention. Simple linear skull fractures do not require surgical intervention.

Surgical Intervention

The general principles of craniotomy and craniectomy in the posterior fossa apply. In general, a large craniectomy is preferred to provide adequate decompression. The foramen magnum rim should be removed to provide adequate room for the tonsils and prevent tonsillar herniation. Placement of an external ventricular drain before performing posterior fossa decompression is recommended in light of the risk of obstructive hydrocephalus. Earlier literature warned against such intervention to avoid the possibility of upward herniation; however, to circumvent this occurrence, care should be taken to allow for minimal drainage of cerebrospinal fluid on placement of the ventricular drain. It is also important not to chase the hematoma beyond the fourth ventricle and into the brainstem because the risk of causing inadvertent injury to the surrounding normal brainstem parenchyma is very high. The goal of surgery in posterior fossa traumatic lesions is to reduce the intracranial tension and the mass effect on the fourth ventricle. Meticulous hemostasis is of great importance as in any neurosurgery. The dura should not be closed under tension and if there is any difficulty, a dural graft should be used.

VASCULAR INJURIES

Arterial dissections are possible but rare in trauma to the posterior fossa. Damage to the arteries of the posterior fossa are usually associated with fractures but can occur without bony injury. Studies suggest that the vertebral artery (VA) is less commonly injured in all traumatic events compared with the carotid arteries (internal, external, and common carotid). The exception to this is when there is cervical spinal trauma affecting the foramen transversarium.[26] Transverse fracture of the petrous bone can extend into the occipital bone leading to laceration of major venous sinuses, such as the sigmoid sinus.[27] These venous sinus injuries could lead to venous EDH. Other vascular injuries usually involve the posteroinferior cerebellar artery (PICA).

Pathophysiology

Rapid acceleration-deceleration causing rotation and hyperextension of the neck is a mechanism causing VA injuries (VAI).[28] This injury has the potential to cause posterior circulation or cerebellar/brainstem stroke. Degree of VAI is classified into five grades. Grade I injury is described as arterial dissections with less than 25% luminal narrowing. Grade II injury is arterial dissection with more than 25% luminal narrowing. Grade III injury is when there is pseudoaneurysm of the VA. Grade IV injury occurs when there is occlusion of the VA. Grade V injury is a VA transsection.[29]

The most common cause of SAH is trauma. Traumatic SAH in the posterior fossa has been associated with rupture or dissection of VA or its branches, and formation of true or pseudoaneurysms.[30]

Clinical Findings

Most patients that suffer VAI are asymptomatic initially after trauma. The symptom-free period can range from 10 to 72 hours, which makes early diagnosis difficult.[28] CT angiography (CTA) is recommended as the screening tool in patients after blunt trauma for suspected VAI.[29] VAI may cause neurologic deterioration from distal thromboembolic events causing ischemic stroke in the posterior fossa.

The gold standard for diagnosis of VAI is digital subtraction angiography (DSA).[31] However, CTA can be incorporated into the trauma CT scan of the entire body. Current CT scans can effectively image large segments of the body in a short period of time.[32] CTA with three-dimensional reconstruction has quality that matches the imaging of DSA. On CTA, double-lumen appearance with eccentric round-shaped hyperdensity of the true lumen and a surrounding crescentic hypodensity corresponding to the false lumen is an indication of VA dissection. Another radiographic feature suggesting VA dissection is seen when the vessel has an increased overall diameter but poor visualization of the lumen.[31] CTA excels in identifying occlusion of vessel lumen, intimal flap, and pseudoaneuysms. VAI is a dynamic process, with gradual progression, spontaneous improvement, or immediate deterioration. No single imaging modality is definite for diagnosis because of this fact. If CTA is not conclusive on diagnosis, DSA is performed. Classic findings on angiogram include pearl and string sign, a double lumen, or a fusiform dilatation of the dissected segment (**Fig. 7**). False lumen of the dissected vessel is seen when there is delayed contrast clearance.[32] Definite diagnosis is often made by combination of clinical findings, CTA, and/or DSA.

Traumatic intradural VA and PICA aneurysm may result from blunt or penetrating head trauma. Direct trauma with compression of the artery against the fixed edges of the falx or tentorium may cause vascular injury leading to the formation of dissection or pseudoaneurysm.[33] Rupture of these aneurysms causes severe morbidity and mortality. Patients after head trauma with posterior fossa SAH or fourth ventricular intraventricular hemorrhage should be fully evaluated for vascular lesions.

Management and Treatment

Traumatic VAI may cause ischemic stroke in the posterior fossa. Anticoagulation or antiplatelet therapy is used to reduce the risk of stroke. VAI usually occurs in the

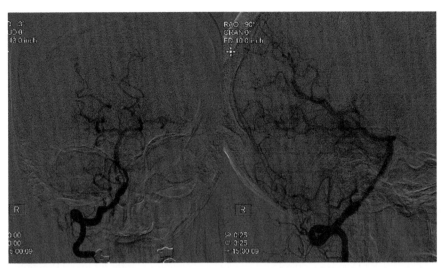

Fig. 7. (*Left image*) Right vertebral injection anteroposterior view showing fusiform enlargement of the V4 segment of the vertebral artery followed by abrupt narrowing. This string sign is characteristic of subarachnoid hemorrhage. (*Right image*) Right vertebral injection lateral view showing enlargement of the V4 segment of the vertebral artery with abrupt narrowing. The posterior inferior cerebellar artery arises from the segment that has dissection.

setting of patients with severe traumatic brain, spine, or intra-abdominal injury. In those patients, anticoagulation or antiplatelet therapy could be contraindicated because of increased risk of bleeding.[29] Surgical options involve proximal ligation of the dissected vessels, clipping or wrapping of associated pseudoaneuysms, and extracranial to intracranial bypass.[32] Open surgery has been shown to have high rates of morbidity and mortality. More recently, advances in endovascular intervention have provided alternative management strategies often with lower associated morbidity. Endovascular therapy offers minimal invasive technique, decreased operative time, and eliminates the need for donor vessel for bypass procedure. Also, when angiogram is performed for diagnosis, intervention could immediately be performed. In the setting of multisystem trauma, the diseased vessel could be accessed from a distal site away from patient injuries. Treatments include use of detachable balloons, coils, and liquid embolic agents to completely eliminate the blood flow over the diseased vessel or obliterate dissecting aneurysms.[32] The choice of therapy for patients with VAI should be determined on an individual basis, taking into account the type and severity of vascular injury, associated traumatic injuries, and the risk of bleeding associated with anticoagulation or antiplatelet therapy.[29]

Treatment of traumatic PICA aneurysm is usually by surgical clipping or endovascular obliteration when the patient is stable for such a procedure. Although traumatic PICA aneurysms are uncommon, they can cause significant morbidity because of risk of hemorrhage. Surgical approaches to PICA aneurysm depend on the specific location of the aneurysm. Combined subtemporal presigmoid transtentorial, far lateral suboccipital, midline suboccipital, and combined lateral and medial suboccipital are some of the approaches for clipping of PICA aneurysm. Endovascular treatment of PICA aneurysms can be achieved with good success rate and low morbidity.[34] However, the best treatment option is determined on a case-by-case basis depending on the location and type of pathology and the patient's associated comorbidities.

SUMMARY

Traumatic injury to the posterior fossa is a complex pathologic condition because of the great heterogeneity of lesions present. As with all TBI, treatment of primary brain injuries and prevention of secondary brain injuries is the mainstay of management. It is imperative to recognize traumatic lesions of the posterior fossa early because of the occurrence of rapid neurologic decline. Overall, the decision regarding whether or not to proceed with surgical intervention depends on the patient's clinical condition, neurologic status, and imaging findings. In general, nonoperative management should be considered only if the patient is fully conscious and the associated posterior fossa lesions are small with little or no mass effect. Posterior fossa traumatic vascular injuries should also be managed either by an open surgical or endovascular approach.[19]

REFERENCES

1. Faul M, Xu L, Wald MM, et al. Traumatic brain injury in the United States: emergency department visits, hospitalizations and deaths 2002–2006. Atlanta (GA): Centers for Disease Control and Prevention, National Center for Injury Prevention and Control; 2010.
2. Snell RS. Clinical neuroanatomy. 7th edition. Philadelphia: Wolters Kluwer Health/Lippincott Williams & Wilkins; 2010.
3. Tsai FY, Teal JS, Itabashi HH, et al. Computed tomography of posterior fossa trauma. J Comput Assist Tomogr 1980;4:291–305.
4. (editor-in-chief). In: Standring S, editor. Gray's anatomy: the anatomical basis of clinical practice. 39th edition. Spain: Elsevier Publishing; 2005. p. 1549.
5. Atkinson JL. Acute epidural hematoma. In: Batjer HH, Loftus CM, editors. Textbook of neurological surgery: principles and practice. Philadelphia: Lippincott Williams and Wilkins; 2005. p. 2843.
6. Hashimoto T, Nakamura N, Richard KE, et al. Primary brain stem lesions caused by closed head injuries. Neurosurg Rev 1993;16:291–8.
7. Maschke M, Morsdorf M, Timmann D, et al. Posterior fossa trauma. In: Manto M, Schmahmann DJ, Rossi F, et al, editors. Handbook of cerebellum and cerebellar disorders. New York: Springer Science; 2013. p. 2055–78.
8. Karasawa H, Furuya H, Naito H, et al. Acute hydrocephalus in posterior fossa injury. J Neurosurg 1997;86:629–32.
9. Wright RL. Traumatic hematomas of the posterior cranial fossa. J Neurosurg 1966;25:402–9.
10. Liu K. Characteristics of diagnosis and treatment of traumatic intracerebellar hemorrhage. Zhonghua Wai Ke Za Zhi 1997;35:166–7 [in Chinese].
11. Takeuchi S, Takasato Y, Masaoka H, et al. Traumatic intra-cerebellar haematoma: study of 17 cases. Br J Neurosurg 2011;25:62–7.
12. d'Avella D, Servadei F, Scerrati M, et al. Traumatic intracerebellar hemorrhage: clinicoradiological analysis of 81 patients. Neurosurgery 2002;50:16–25.
13. Evans JP, Scheinker IM. Histologic studies of the brain following head trauma; post-traumatic petechial and massive intracerebral hemorrhage. J Neurosurg 1946;3:101–13.
14. Tsubokawa T, Yamada J, Tomizawa N, et al. Classification of traumatic intracerebral hematoma by repeated CT-scan and clinical course (author's transl). Neurol Med Chir (Tokyo) 1979;19:1127–37 [in Japanese].
15. Posner J, Saper C, Schiff N, et al. Plum and Posner's Diagnosis of Stupor and Coma. New York: Oxford University Press; 2007.

16. Denny-Brown D, Russell WR. Experimental cerebral concussion. J Physiol 1940; 99:153.
17. Saatman KE, Duhaime AC, Bullock R, et al. Classification of traumatic brain injury for targeted therapies. J Neurotrauma 2008;25(7):719–38.
18. Balik V, Lehto H, Sulla I, et al. Posterior fossa extradural haematomas. Cent Eur Neurosurg 2010;71(4):167–72.
19. Quinones-Hinojosa A, editor. Schmidek and sweet operative neurosurgical techniques. 6th edition. Philadelphia: Elsevier; 2012.
20. Gulsen S, Sonmez E, Yilmaz C, et al. Traumatic acute subdural hematoma extending from the posterior cranial fossa to the cerebellopontine angle. J Korean Neurosurg Soc 2009;46(3):277–80.
21. Greenberg M. Handbook of neurosurgery. 7th edition. New York: Thieme; 2010.
22. Pascual JM, Prieto R. Surgical management of severe closed head injury in adults. In: Quinones-Hinojosa A, editor. Schmidek and sweet operative neurosurgical techniques. 6th edition. Philadelphia: Elsevier; 2012. p. 1513–38.
23. Servadei F, Compagnone C, Sahuquillo J. The role of surgery in traumatic brain injury. Curr Opin Crit Care 2007;13:163–8.
24. Bullock MR, Chesnut R, Ghajar J, et al. Guidelines for the surgical management of traumatic brain injury. Neurosurgery 2006;58(S2):1–62.
25. Brain Trauma Foundation, American Association of Neurological Surgeons, Congress of Neurological Surgeons. Guidelines for the management of severe traumatic brain injury. J Neurotrauma 2007;24:S1–106.
26. Desouza RM, Crocker MJ, Haliasos N, et al. Blunt traumatic vertebral artery injury: a clinical review. Eur Spine J 2011;20(9):1405–16.
27. Samii M, Tatagiba M. Skull base trauma: diagnosis and management. Neurol Res 2002;24:147–56.
28. Majidi S, Hassan A, Adil M, et al. Incidence and outcome of vertebral artery dissection in trauma setting: analysis of national trauma data base. Neurocrit Care 2014. [Epub ahead of print].
29. Harrigan M, Hadley M, Dhall S, et al. Management of vertebral artery injuries following non-penetrating cervical trauma. Neurosurgery 2013;72:234–43.
30. Schuster J, Santiago P, Elliott J, et al. Acute traumatic posteroinferior cerebellar artery aneurysms: report of three cases. Neurosurgery 1999;45:1465–7.
31. Soper J, Parker G, Hallinan J. Vertebral artery dissection diagnosed with CT. AJNR Am J Neuroradiol 1995;16:952–4.
32. Ali M, Amenta P, Starke R, et al. Intracranial vertebral artery dissections: evolving perspectives. Interv Neuroradiol 2012;18:469–83.
33. Nishioka T, Maeda Y, Tomogane Y, et al. Unexpected delayed rupture of the vertebral-posterior inferior cerebellar artery aneurysms following closed head injury. Acta Neurochir (Wien) 2002;144:839–45.
34. Chalouhi N, Jabbour P, Starke R, et al. Endovascular treatment of proximal and distal posterior inferior cerebellar artery aneurysms. J Neurosurg 2013;118: 991–9.

Multiple Sclerosis and the Cerebellum

Leticia Tornes, MD[a,b], Brittani Conway, MD[c], William Sheremata, MD, FRCP(C)[a,b,*]

KEYWORDS

- Multiple sclerosis • Tremor • Nystagmus • Clinically isolated syndrome • Cerebellar
- MRI • Disability

KEY POINTS

- Tremor is the most common cerebellar manifestation in multiple sclerosis (MS).
- Cerebellar manifestations in MS are predictors of progression and disability.
- The clinical examination is often superior to magnetic resonance imaging in detecting cerebellar dysfunction in MS.
- Patients with progressive forms of MS often have cerebellar disease, which is often a major cause of their disability.

INTRODUCTION

Multiple sclerosis (MS) is an inflammatory, demyelinating, degenerative disorder of the central nervous system that is most prevalent in young adults of European descent. Illness is characterized by relapses of disease affecting various areas of the brain, optic nerves, and spinal cord over time. It is the most common cause of disability in young adults.[1] The clinical manifestations of disease are disseminated in both time and space and its protean manifestations prominently include signs of cerebellar dysfunction. In patients with MS, the appearance of cerebellar manifestations portends a poor prognosis and greater disability. Weinshenker and colleagues,[2] in a population study, noted that cerebellar involvement was the most significant predictor in determining time to disability, that is, the need to use a cane.

Tremor is the most clinically evident cerebellar manifestation seen in MS.[3] Charcot, the world's first professor of neurology and the first to characterize MS, was also the first to recognize intention tremor in a living MS patient at the Salpetrier (in Paris) in 1878. It was Charcot who first distinguished intention tremor from the tremor associated with paralysis agitans, described by Parkinson in 1817.

[a] Clinical Neurology, University of Miami, MS Center of Excellence, 1150 Northwest 14th Street, Miami, FL 33136, USA; [b] Department of Neurology, Multiple Sclerosis Center of Excellence, Miller School of Medicine, Clinical Research Building, 13th Floor, 1120 Northwest 14th Street, Miami, FL 33136, USA; [c] Department of Neurology, Jackson Memorial Hospital, 1611 Northwest 12th Avenue, Miami, FL 33136, USA
* Corresponding author. 1120 Northwest 14th Street, 13th Floor, Miami, FL 33136.
E-mail address: WSherema@med.miami.edu

Neurol Clin 32 (2014) 957–977
http://dx.doi.org/10.1016/j.ncl.2014.08.001
0733-8619/14/$ – see front matter © 2014 Elsevier Inc. All rights reserved.

Charcot in a remarkably modern sounding admonition said, "Now, it is especially, when the disease is in its earliest stage ... that it is important to know how to recognize it by the slightest indicia." He described a 21-year-old woman "Vauthier" with a history of (recurrent) vertigo from the age of 14 that disappeared with pregnancy at age 21. However, on her admission to the Salpetrier she demonstrated nystagmus, weakness, and tremor of her upper extremities. After 1 year, her right-sided weakness and tremor had increased and she could no longer stand. She died 4 years after her admission and at necropsy the findings included plaques in both middle cerebellar peduncles (**Fig. 1**).

EPIDEMIOLOGY

Onset typically occurs between the ages of 20 and 40 with a mean age of 30. MS can occur in children and the elderly, but it is uncommon. Relapsing-remitting MS (RRMS) typically presents at an earlier age than primary progressive MS (PPMS). MS is at least twice as common in women as in men, with the number of women diagnosed with MS increasing with passing time.[4] The incidence and prevalence of MS varies geographically, with higher frequency in northern latitudes. However, this North–South gradient has disappeared in the United States. Those from Northern Europe seem to be the most susceptible with Asians, Africans, and American Indians with the lowest risk. Weinshenker and associates[2] found that in Southern Ontario the proportion of MS patients at presentation had (shown as percent) pyramidal tract dysfunction 57%, sensory abnormalities 35%, and cerebellar involvement 33%.

ETIOLOGY AND PATHOPHYSIOLOGY

MS was initially described as a disease of the white matter, but recent studies have revealed evidence of inflammation and demyelination of both white and gray matter, as well as axonal injury.[5] Although the etiology of MS is unknown, evidence points to the likely interaction of multiple factors, predominantly genetic and environmental, that trigger an immune response leading to central nervous system injury. Contributing environmental factors that have been implicated in increasing the risk of MS include vitamin D and smoking. There seems to be a central role for Epstein-Barr virus and

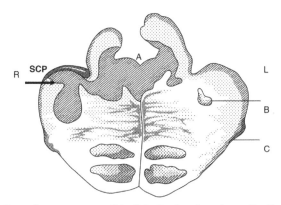

Fig. 1. Cross-section of upper pons, "Vauthier", showing demyelinating plaques (A–C) involving the superior cerebellar peduncle (SCP) and the tegmentum. (*From* Charcot JM. Lectures on the disease of the nervous system delivered the Salpetriere. London: The Sydenham Society; 1877.)

perhaps a role for other viruses.[6,7] Recently, salt intake has also been shown to be associated with an increased the risk of developing MS, apparently through mechanisms involving induction of T helper 17 cells.[8]

CLINICAL COURSE AND DIAGNOSIS

The clinical course of the disease is unpredictable and varies greatly in its symptomatology and its severity. Four disease courses have been defined: RRMS, secondary progressive MS (SPMS), PPMS, and progressive relapsing MS (**Table 1**). The most common form is RRMS, seen in approximately 80% to 85% of patients at presentation.[9] These patients present with attacks of new or recurrent neurologic deficits followed by periods of remission of symptoms and, by definition, without progression of disability between attacks. It is estimated that 50% of patients with RRMS go on to develop SPMS.[10] Of the MS population, 10% to 15% presents with PPMS. The typical clinical course of these patients is an insidious, progressive myelopathy[11] and, unlike RRMS, the female to male ratio is 1:1. The Kurtzke Extended Disability Status Scale is used universally in assessing the MS patients' impairment and disability.[12] A score of zero indicates no disability, 6 the use of unilateral assistance in ambulation (ie, 1 cane), and 10 is death from MS.

To establish a diagnosis of MS, lesions in the central nervous system must be separated both in time and space. The 2010 revised McDonald criteria include a simplified iteration of magnetic resonance imaging (MRI) requirements to establish the diagnosis of MS or clinically isolated syndrome (CIS), allowing identification of MS with high probability at its first clinical manifestation.[13] Importantly, the diagnosis of MS rests on ruling out other disorders that may have similar clinical presentations.

Differential Diagnosis

The differential diagnosis of MS is extensive. The patient's clinical history and neurologic findings as well as concomitant systemic findings are crucial in distinguishing between MS from other diseases (**Box 1**). When MS presents with signs and symptoms of cerebellar disease, the differential diagnosis of the adult-onset sporadic ataxias must be entertained. A history of toxic or metabolic exposures should be explored because alcohol, hypoglycemia, or toxic exposure may point to an alternative diagnosis. Another clue may be a history of diarrhea, because this may be seen in both vitamin E deficiency and Whipple disease.[14] Patients with Friedreich ataxia, an autosomal-recessive disorder, likely do not have family history. The Cajun form of illness presents later in life and its presentation in young adults with spinal cord atrophy, dysarthria, dorsal column dysfunction, and ataxia may be mistaken for MS.[15]

Table 1 Multiple sclerosis disease courses		
Course	Percent at Presentation	Characteristics and Definitions
Relapsing remitting	85	Relapse with recovery or recovery with some residual deficits. No progression between "attacks"
Secondary progressive		Follows relapsing-remitting course, continuous progression
Primary progressive	10–15	Progression from onset, occasionally plateaus
Progressive relapsing		Progressive from onset with superimposed relapses (may or may not remit)

Box 1
Differential diagnosis of multiple sclerosis

Infectious

  Lyme disease

  Syphilis

  Progressive multifocal leukodystrophy (PML)

  Human immunodeficiency virus (HIV)

  Human T-cell lymphotrophic virus (HTLV-1)

  Hepatitis C

  Whipple's disease

Inflammatory

  Acute disseminated encephalomyelitis (ADEM)

  Neuromyelitis optica (NMO)

  Sarcoidosis

  Systemic lupus erythematosus (SLE)

  Sjögren syndrome

Vascular

  Small vessel disease

  Neurologic vasculitis

  Anti-phospholipid antibody syndrome

  Cerebral autosomal dominant arteriopathy with subcortical infarcts and leukoencephalopathy (CADASIL)

Hereditary/degenerative

  Spinocerebellar ataxia (SCA)

  Adrenoleukodystrophy

  Metachromatic leukodystrophy

  Mitochondrial disease

  Leber's hereditary optic neuropathy

  Multiple system atrophy (MSA)

Nutritional/metabolic

  Vitamin B_{12} deficiency

  Copper deficiency

  Alcohol

  Hyperglycemia

Neoplastic

  Neurologic lymphoma

  Paraneoplastic syndromes

Other

  Complicated migraine

  Psychogenic

Vitamin B_{12} deficiency may mimic MS in that both present with myelopathy, ataxia and cognitive effects. Vitamin B_{12} deficiency may also present with T2 hyperintensities in the spinal cord like those seen in MS. However, vitamin B_{12} deficiency is more common in elderly patients, although it may present in young adults who are vegan, post gastrointestinal surgery, or in those with malabsorption.[16]

The spinocerebellar ataxias (SCA) are a group pf 31 autosomal-dominant ataxias that have multiple, underlying mutations.[17] In most cases, a family history is present; however, sporadic cases can occur such as SCA 6 and SCA 17.[18] In SCA 6, the onset is in adulthood, followed by a slowly progressive cerebellar ataxia, dysarthria, and nystagmus. Patients may present similarly to those with PPMS, presenting with gait instability and imbalance. In addition, there may be visual disturbances (such as diplopia and nystagmus), hyperreflexia, and extensor plantar responses.[14,17,19] These symptoms are commonly seen in MS, especially in patients with secondary progressive illness.

Multiple systems atrophy (MSA), is a late-onset (mean age about 54), sporadic, neurodegenerative disorder that is characterized by a presentation with features of either parkinsonism or cerebellar ataxia plus autonomic failure and pyramidal tract dysfunction. There are 2 main types, MSA–parkinsonian variant and MSA-cerebellar variant. The cerebellar variant is less common, but shares many symptoms with MS. It presents with gait ataxia, limb ataxia, scanning dysarthria, and oculomotor disturbances.[20] In most instances, the patients develop other signs of MSA, such as autonomic instability, but in cases where cerebellar signs are predominant, it may be virtually indistinguishable from MS. Patients with PPMS and MSA both present later in life and exhibit a progressive course. One can differentiate between the 2 with imaging and cerebrospinal fluid analysis. Rarely, the 2 diseases can present concomitantly.[21]

TREATMENT

The pharmacologic treatment of MS is 3-fold and involves treatment of acute attacks, disease-modifying drugs, and the use of symptomatic therapies. MS attacks or exacerbations typically abate spontaneously without pharmacologic intervention; nonetheless, one can abbreviate the more severe MS flares with medications. In the acute attack, intravenous steroids, high-dose oral steroids, or adrenocorticotrophic hormone may be used. In cases when the attack is severe and refractory to steroid, or adrenocorticotrophic hormone therapy, or both, it has been shown that plasma exchange statistically improved outcomes when compared with placebo (42.1% vs 5.9%).[22]

In the last 2 decades, a number of drugs have been approved for the management of MS (**Table 2**). The interferons and glatiramer acetate result in a similar reduction in relapse rate of approximately 30%. The most attractive aspect of these medications is their long-term safety profile, established over the last 2 decades. In addition, these medications have been studied in CIS. Such presentations (CIS) may be the first clinical presentation of RRMS, usually presenting as unilateral optic neuritis, transverse myelitis, or a brain stem attack.[23] Patients with CIS with an abnormal brain MRI are highly likely, close to 90%, to develop clinically definite MS.[24–26] All CIS trials showed that treatment significantly delayed both a second attack and MRI lesion activity.[27]

In addition to the injectable therapies described, 1 drug infused intravenously, natalizumab (Tysabri, Biogen Idec, Cambridge, MA, USA) and 3 oral medications have been approved by the food and drug administration for the treatment of MS. Fingolimod (Gilenya, Novartis, Basel, Switzerland) is a sphingosine-1-phosphate receptor

Table 2
Food and drug administration-approved immunomodulating medications for multiple sclerosis

Generic Name	Brand Name	Route and Frequency	Adverse Effects
Interferon β-1b	Betaseron, Extavia	SQ every other day	Flulike symptoms
Interferon β1-a	Avonex, Rebif	Intramuscular weekly SQ 3 times weekly	Flulike symptoms
Glatiramer acetate	Copaxone	SQ 20 mg daily or SQ 40 mg 3 times weekly	Idiosyncratic chest pain
Natalizumab	Tysabri	Infusion every 4 wk	PML
Fingolimod	Gilenya	Oral once a day	Bradycardia, AV block, macular edema, reductions in lymphocyte counts
Teriflunomide	Aubagio	Oral once a day	Hair loss, hepatotoxicity, teratogenesis
Dimethyl fumarate	Tecfidera	Oral twice a day	Nausea, flushing

Abbreviations: AV, atrioventricular; PML, progressive multifocal leukoencephalopathy; SQ, subcutaneously.

agonist that was the first oral agent approved for the treatment of RRMS based on its clinical and MRI efficacy demonstrated in clinical trials.[28,29] Teriflunomide (Aubagio, Sanofi Aventis, Bridgewater, NJ, USA) a pyrimidine synthesis inhibitor is the second oral drug approved for MS. It has a black box warning for tetratogenesis and hepatotoxicity.[30] Dimethyl fumerate (Tecfidera, Biogen Idec, Cambridge, MA, USA) is the third oral agent available. In clinical trials, it decreased the annualized relapse rate and the number of new or enhancing MRI lesions.[31,32] Natalizumab is a monoclonal antibody that in clinical trials is the most potent approved drug, showing a 67% reduction in relapse rates over 2 years compared with placebo.[33] Unfortunately, natalizumab is associated with a risk of progressive multifocal leukoencephalopathy and in risk management the patient must be counseled regarding this risk. The risk to the patient is increased by previous exposure to immunosuppressive therapy (particularly mitoxantrone and methotrexate), duration of therapy, and John Cunningham Virus (JCV) antibody status.[34]

CLINICAL MANIFESTATIONS OF CEREBELLAR DYSFUNCTION IN MULTIPLE SCLEROSIS

MS patients commonly exhibit cerebellar manifestations that may include tremor, ataxia, imbalance, and speech disturbance. The physical examination may reveal intention tremor in the extremities (dysmetria), ataxia, head titubation, and truncal ataxia. Ocular findings of nystagmus, ocular dysmetria, and failure of fixation suppression (square wave jerks) suggest cerebellar or cerebellovestibular connection dysfunction. Speech can be scanning in character or explosive. It is often difficult to distinguish pure cerebellar dysfunction on examination because there is overlap with motor, sensory, and cerebral dysfunction. For example, involvement of the vermis typically presents with a wide-based and unsteady gait. However, this truncal ataxia may not be from a pure cerebellar lesion in an MS patient, and is more likely to be the consequence of multiple lesions. Proprioceptive loss owing to posterior column involvement is often a contributing factor to the gait abnormality. If a patient has a lesion of the intermediate cerebellar hemisphere, there may be ataxia on examination. If there is motor involvement, it may be difficult to assess cerebellar lesions.

Cerebellar manifestations are rare in CIS. Miller and colleagues[23] reviewed CIS cases and found that 21% presented with optic neuritis, 46% with long tract symptoms and signs, 10% with a brain stem dysfunction, and 23% with multifocal abnormalities. The initial presentation of MS may affect the disease course and prognosis Interestingly, patients with early onset MS (age of onset before 16) have clinical features mainly of relapsing remitting disease, but more frequently present with brain stem–cerebellar dysfunction (28.6%), pyramidal symptoms (18.4%), and optic neuritis (14.3%).[35]

In MS, infratentorial lesions detectable with gadolinium-enhanced MRI are less prevalent than lesions of the cerebrum. Importantly, the clinical examination may be more sensitive in detecting evidence of cerebellar disease than imaging. In 2007, Kutzelnigg and colleagues[36] reported extensive demyelination in the cerebellar cortex that was equivalent to or worse than that seen in the cerebral cortex. Interestingly, these patients did not have apparent lesions on MRI. In their series, the cerebellar cortex had large areas of demyelination. The SPMS patients had 38.8% of the cerebellar area affected and in PPMS 36.9% was affected.

Case 1: Cerebellar Findings Without MRI Changes

A 46-year-old, right-handed woman was diagnosed with RRMS at age 17 has now entered a secondary-progressive phase (**Figs. 2** and **3**). Examination is remarkable for chronic left hemiparesis and the new onset of marked truncal ataxia, bilateral intention tremor, and dysdiadochokinesia. MRI does not reveal any hyperintense lesions in the cerebellum on fluid-attenuated inversion recovery MRI sequence, and there are no new gadolinium-enhancing lesions.

Lesions within the brain stem often affect the cerebellum and its afferent and efferent tracts, resulting in symptoms such as tremor, nystagmus, vertigo, cognitive impairment, and dysarthria. This section focuses on each of these symptoms with emphasis on clinical presentation, MRI findings, and treatment.

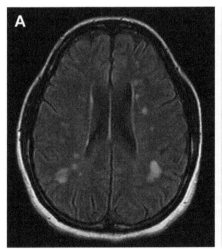 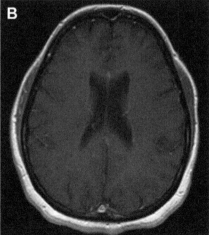

Fig. 2. (*A*) Brain MRI, axial fluid-attenuated inversion recovery MRI with T2 hyperintensities. (*B*) Brain MRI, axial T1 post contrast with no acute lesions.

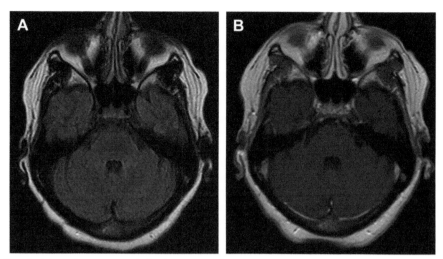

Fig. 3. (*A*) Brain MRI, axial fluid-attenuated inversion recovery MRI with no cerebellar lesions. (*B*) Brain MRI, axial T1 post contrast with no cerebellar lesions.

Occurrence of Tremor in Multiple Sclerosis

McAlpine and Compston,[37] in a prospective study of the natural history of MS, recognized tremor as relatively uncommon. Of 146 patients with RRMS, only 1 patient had "motor and cerebellar" manifestations compared with 8 of 146 with progressive disease. Since then, there have been 3 major studies with prevalence data on tremor in MS that reported higher prevalence of tremor occurring in MS than McAlpine and Compston. Weinshenker and colleagues'[2] series from a Southern Ontario MS clinic found clinically relevant tremor present in one third of 259 patients followed for 3 years. In contrast, Alusi and coworkers,[3] in their prospective study of tremor in 100 randomly selected MS patients in London, tremor was found in 58 patients; however, it was asymptomatic in only 20 patients. The tremor affected the arms (58%), legs (10%), head (9%), and trunk (7%).[3] Severity of the tremor correlated with other cerebellar deficits, including dysarthria, dysmetria, and dysdiadochokinesia. Of these, 27% were reported to have disability related to their tremor.[3] The tremor began approximately 13 years after the first MS symptoms and was progressive. No patient had resolution or remission of the tremors.[3] Last, Pittock and associates'[38] 200 patients from a community-based clinic in Minnesota had the lowest (25.5%) prevalence of tremor. The discrepancy in prevalence is derived from 2 population studies that differed significantly in patient selection. The higher prevalence rate was reported in a study published by Alusi and colleagues,[3] who evaluated randomly selected patients from an MS clinic registry. The study group included a disproportionately large representation of patients with progressive forms of MS (63% SPMS, 22% PPMS, 15% RRMS) and a relatively high median Kurtzke Extended Disability Status Scale score of 6.0. In contrast, our clinic has 50% of patients with RRMS. Conversely, a study published by Pittock and colleagues[38] was performed on a community-based population of patients diagnosed with MS and reported a 25% prevalence of tremor. This study included a more representative distribution of MS forms (65% RRMS, 30% SPMS, 5% PPMS) and median Kurtzke Extended Disability Status Scale score of 3.0. Twenty-five percent may be a more accurate estimation of tremor prevalence in MS, but the prevalence among patients with progressive forms of MS and with more advanced disability is likely to be higher.

The tremor observed in MS has a characteristic presentation described as an action tremor of the upper extremities.[3,38] Action tremor can range from being postural, kinetic, or intentional in nature. Onset of tremor in MS correlates with earlier retirement and probability of unemployment, demonstrating that tremor is an important predictor of morbidity associated with MS that must be managed appropriately.[38]

A correlation of tremor and cerebellar examination findings has been reported; thus, the most likely location of tremor-causing lesions is the cerebellum and its afferent and efferent tracts.[3,38] Although lesions in the cerebellar hemispheres are often implicated in tremor and ataxia, a cohort study of Japanese MS patients with brain stem and/or cerebellar examination findings demonstrated that those with cerebellar hemisphere lesions (6%) were the minority, whereas lesions within the middle cerebellar peduncle and pons were up to 8 times more common.[39] In a separate study, the severity of tremor correlated with lesion load in the contralateral pons rather than the cerebellar hemispheres, further suggesting that lesions of the cerebellar afferent or efferent pathways are more likely to produce ataxia or tremor.[40] In summary, it may be concluded that the incidence of cerebellar hemispheric lesions evidence by MRI is relatively low, and patients with severe ataxia and tremor often have lesions within the cerebellar peduncle or brain stem.[39]

Case 2: Upper Extremity Tremor

A 25-year-old right-handed man with RRMS diagnosed at age 12 presents with a new right upper extremity tremor (**Fig. 4**). Examination is remarkable for an intention and postural tremor in the right upper extremity, marked ataxia, and dysmetria on finger-to-nose and heel-to-shin testing of the right side. MRI revealed a hyperintense lesion in the right middle cerebellar peduncle (see **Fig. 4**). He was started on propranolol and in follow-up 1 month later, there was moderate improvement in the tremor.

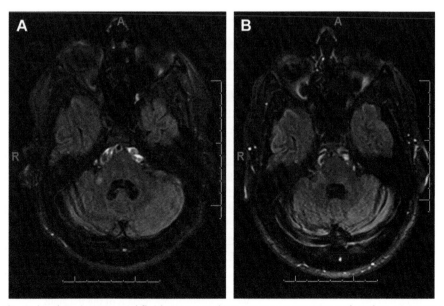

Fig. 4. (*A, B*) Brain MRI, axial fluid-attenuated inversion recovery MRI with T2 hyperintensity in right middle cerebellar peduncle.

Management of tremor in MS patients ordinarily begins with pharmacotherapy to attenuate the severity of the tremor and to improve functional status. Numerous medications have been investigated for the treatment of tremor and ataxia (**Table 3**), but evidence is limited owing to small study group size. Koch and colleagues[52] performed a thorough review of oral medications tested for tremor in MS. Medications, including primidone, carbamazepine, glutethimide, ondansetron, and propranolol, were shown to have modest effects, but all studies were either open label or performed on small cohorts. Similarly, topiramate and clonazepam have been demonstrated to reduce tremor, but evidence is limited to isolated case reports.[53,54] Levetiracetam was an appealing treatment option because of its limited side effect and limited drug–drug interaction profile. Unfortunately, a well-designed investigation of oral doses ranging from 1000 to 2000 mg daily demonstrated no effect on tremor in a cohort of 18 patients.[48,55] Oral isoniazid is perhaps the most investigated treatment for tremor in MS. Multiple evaluations of oral isoniazid in doses up to 20 mg/kg have been performed, including well-designed double-blind, placebo-controlled studies that demonstrated improvement in tremor but no improvement in functional status.[52,56]

Cannabis and cannabis extract are becoming more readily available in the United States and have been postulated to alleviate tremor symptoms. Three randomized, double-blind, placebo-controlled studies have demonstrated no reduction in tremor or improvement in functional outcome despite patient surveys indicating improvement in tremor.[50,52] Fox and colleagues[50] performed the largest, most objective evaluation of cannabis extract attenuation of tremor, but no improvement was observed. Regardless of the absence of well-designed investigations demonstrating improvement in tremor severity or function, a trial of at least 2 or 3 of the medications listed in **Table 3** is warranted before consideration of other treatment options. In our experience, patients with low-frequency tremors (3–5 Hz/s) seem to benefit from doses of propranolol ranging from 40 to 240 mg daily. It is important to escalate the dosage

Table 3	
Therapeutic options for tremor in multiple sclerosis	
Treatment	**Dose**
Pharmacologic	
Primidone	Maximum 750 mg orally daily[41]
Propranolol	100 mg orally daily[42]
Clonazepam	Maximum 15 mg orally daily[43]
Isoniazid	Maximum 20 mg/kg orally daily[44]
Glutethimide	750–1250 mg orally daily[45]
Ondansetron	8 mg intravenously one-time dose[46]
Carbamazepine	600 mg orally daily dose[47]
Levetiracetam	1000–2000 mg orally daily[48]
Topiramate	Titration to 150 mg orally daily[49]
Cannabis and extracts	Maximum 0.125 mg/kg orally daily[50]
Botulinum toxin type A	Maximum 100 IU injected intramuscularly per limb[51]
Surgical	
Vagal nerve stimulator	Vagus nerve
Thalamotomy	Ventral intermediate nucleus of the thalamus
Deep brain stimulation	Ventral intermediate nucleus of the thalamus

slowly to avoid hypotension. Other drugs in our armamentarium have not impressed either patients or the attending neurologists.

Botulinum toxin A is an injectable pharmacotherapy that is increasing in popularity. When evaluated in the management of cerebellar tremor in MS patients, the first randomized, placebo-controlled, crossover trial demonstrated promising results. Patients with either RRMS or SPMS and a cerebellar tremor were randomized to either botulinum toxin type A or saline injections into agonist and antagonist muscle groups of the upper extremity. Reevaluation of tremor at 3 months after intramuscular botulinum toxin injections revealed that the median tremor severity score was significantly reduced from moderate to mild severity when compared with saline injections.[51] Similarly, functional improvement was noted in the ability to perform tasks such as writing and drinking from a cup.[51] The only reported adverse reaction was weakness, which typically improved after 2 weeks duration. At present, a phase III trial is needed to further validate the findings demonstrated in this crossover study.

When tremor is disabling and no improvement is achieved with oral medications, surgical therapy is considered. Current surgical options range from the placement of a vagal nerve stimulator to more invasive intracranial operations. The vagal nerve stimulator was initially postulated by Marrosu and colleagues[57] to reduce the severity of cerebellar tremor in MS patients via a feedback mechanism to the inferior olivary nucleus. In the original case report published in 2005,[57] no improvement in tremor of the limbs or head was appreciated after 1 year. However, when the stimulation current and frequency were reduced, there was a 20% reduction in the tremor scale within 6 months. The success of this therapy was further demonstrated in a case series performed on 3 MS patients with a cerebellar tremor and reported 67% improvement in the tremor scale at 3 months.[58] These results have not been confirmed with a randomized, controlled trial; nonetheless, early results are encouraging.

Two intracranial procedures are currently used to alleviate disabling tremor in MS: Thalamotomy and deep brain stimulation. Both procedures commonly target the ventral intermediate nucleus of the thalamus, which lies between the ventral lateral and ventral posterior thalamic nuclei. A metaanalysis performed by Yap and colleagues[59] comparing thalamotomy and deep brain stimulation revealed that both procedures are effective at reducing tremor with rates of tremor suppression ranging from 70% to 100%, but favoring deep brain stimulation. An early study performed by Matsumoto and colleagues[60] recognized the need to select patients who will benefit from surgical therapy. They identified that patients with a greater severity of tremor at baseline, as measured with a dedicated instrument, were more likely to improve postoperatively from either procedure than those with a mild or moderate tremor.[60] Adverse outcomes for each procedure are relatively similar and include hemiparesis, dysarthria, dysphagia, and cognitive changes that are predominately related to instrumentation-provoked hemorrhage. Unfortunately, the challenge remains in choosing the optimal procedure. As Yap and colleagues[59] recognize, deep brain stimulation allows for titration of effect as the disease progresses, but data from long-term follow-up are still needed. In our experience, thalamotomy in 7 patients resulted in effective resolution of tremor but failure of functional improvement, but was a disappointment to the patients. However, the patient's families were pleased with the resolution of the severe tremor.

Nystagmus

Nystagmus is an abnormal, involuntary eye movement produced in response to the inability to fix gaze on a target. It is typically composed of an initial slow phase followed by a fast, corrective phase.[61] Fixation of gaze is complex task that is mediated by neural integrators within the midbrain, pons, and cerebellum, placing it vulnerable to MS plaques. Nystagmus is observed in 40% to 60% of patients with MS and is often poorly recognized on clinical examination.[62,63] The most common forms of nystagmus observed in MS are pendular nystagmus and gaze-evoked upbeat nystagmus.[64,65]

Case 3: Nystagmus, Tremor, Dysmetria, Truncal Ataxia, and Dysdiadochokinesia

A 22-year-old right-handed woman has had an aggressive course of RRMS for 9 years. Her clinical course was stabilized after starting monthly natalizumab infusions (**Figs. 5** and **6**). Treatment was discontinued in anticipation of a planned pregnancy and 2 months later she presents with right-sided weakness, numbness, and impaired balance. Examination was remarkable for gaze-evoked nystagmus to the right, intact strength in all 4 extremities, bilateral upper extremity intention tremor, truncal ataxia, dysmetria bilaterally on finger-to-nose and heel-to-shin testing, and bilateral dysdiadochokinesia in the upper extremities. MRI revealed multiple new gadolinium-enhancing lesions within the bilateral periventricular region, right cerebellar hemisphere, right cerebral peduncle, and the left cerebellopontine junction. The monthly natalizumab infusions were resumed and within 2 months her examination stabilized.

Pendular nystagmus is an involuntary sinusoidal ocular movement with a frequency of 2.5 to 6 Hz that can occur in any plane and can be monocular or binocular.[66–68] Pendular nystagmus is unique because there is no differentiation between the slow and fast phases. Lesions within the dentate–rubro–olivary triangle are most commonly associated with pendular nystagmus.[61] Before the convenience of MRI, 1 study identified 25 patients with acquired pendular nystagmus in a cohort of 644 patients with MS. The prevalence of cerebellar signs (truncal ataxia, head tremor, intention tremor, and ataxic dysarthria) was significantly higher among the 25 patients with acquired pendular nystagmus compared with patients without pendular nystagmus. Necropsy evaluation of these patients demonstrated extensive cerebellar lesions compared with controls.[68] A more recent study utilizing MRI has demonstrated that the majority of

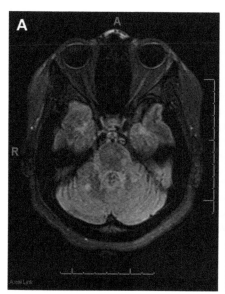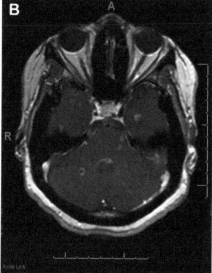

Fig. 5. (A) Brain MRI, fluid-attenuated inversion recovery MRI with right cerebellar and left brain stem lesions. (B) Brain MRI T1 post contrast with corresponding enhancing lesions.

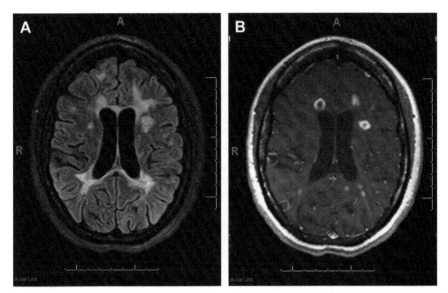

Fig. 6. (*A*) Brain MRI, axial fluid-attenuated inversion recovery MRI. (*B*) T1 post contrast with periventricular disease with multiple enhancing lesions, some with open ring pattern of enhancement.

patients with pendular nystagmus have lesions within the pontomedullary region rather than the cerebellum. This study corroborated the high prevalence of cerebellar signs in patients with pendular nystagmus, indicating that these signs are likely related to lesions of cerebellar pathways.[67]

Primary position upbeat nystagmus can also be seen in MS patients with cerebellar lesions.[65] This clinical finding is characterized by a slow downward movement of the eyes followed by upbeating, correctional saccades in primary gaze that increase in amplitude with upward gaze, decrease in amplitude with downward gaze, and are unaffected by horizontal gaze.[65] Primary position upbeat nystagmus is observed in patients with lesions in the pontomesencephalic junction, pontomedullary junction, and occasionally within the cerebellum.[65,69]

Downbeat nystagmus is most commonly observed in patients with Arnold–Chiari malformation or cerebellar degenerative disorders, but a few cases have been reported in association with MS.[66,70,71] A slow, upward drift of the eyes followed by a fast, downward correctional saccade characterizes this form of nystagmus. Downbeat nystagmus is often associated with lesions of the flocculus and surrounding regions.[61,66] One study corroborated this association in MS and identified 2 MS patients with downbeat nystagmus who had extensive parafloccular and middle cerebellar peduncle lesions.[70]

Periodic alternating nystagmus is more common in primary cerebellar disorders, but has been reported in MS.[66,72] It is a unique form of nystagmus that can occur in any plane and has a very predictable cycle: Fast-phase corrective saccades with increasing amplitude followed by decreasing amplitude and eventually a brief period of inactivity, then the cycle continues in the opposite direction. Periodic alternating nystagmus is most commonly seen in lesions of the nodulus, a central cerebellar structure that provides inhibitory input to the vestibular nuclei.[61]

Optimal treatment of nystagmus is specific for the type of nystagmus (**Table 4**). Pendular nystagmus can be treated with gabapentin or memantine.[73] The mechanism

Table 4	
Treatment of nystagmus	
Condition	Treatment
Pendular nystagmus	Gabapentin, memantine
Primary position upbeat nystagmus	4-Aminopyridine
Downbeat nystagmus	4-Aminopyridine
Periodic alternating nystagmus	Baclofen

leading to reduction of pendular nystagmus is poorly understood, but is potentially related to N-methyl-D-aspartate receptor modulation. One examiner-blinded, cross-over treatment study compared memantine and gabapentin in 11 patients with acquired pendular nystagmus. Reduction in amplitude of nystagmus was noted with each treatment, and in some cases cessation of nystagmus was achieved after 1 week of therapy.[74] In this study, memantine was more efficacious, but larger studies are necessary for confirmation. Upbeat and downbeat nystagmus have both been demonstrated to respond to 4-aminopyridine, but the evidence for efficacy in upbeat nystagmus is limited to a case report.[75–77] Baclofen is an efficacious therapy for both upbeat and periodic alternating nystagmus.[73]

Dysarthria

Dysarthria has been recognized as a common sign of MS and is hallmark of Charcot's triad. In the late 1800s, Charcot identified 3 clinical signs—nystagmus, intention tremor, and scanning speech—that were shared in patients who suffered from the disease for years.[78] Dysarthria associated with MS was initially described as scanning speech where words are spoken in distinct syllables separated by pauses. Further studies revealed that the more common presentation of dysarthria is a mixture of ataxic and spastic speech qualities.[79] Often, the speech is described as harsh in quality with irregularity in volume and occasional errors in articulation[78,79]; the ataxic nature of the dysarthria led many to believe that it correlated with cerebellar signs on examination. A large observational study by Darley and colleagues[78] demonstrated that cerebellar findings are common in MS patients with dysarthria. Although cerebellar signs are frequently observed, the severity of dysarthria is more intimately correlated with overall neurologic impairment rather than the degree of cerebellar dysfunction.[78,79] The effectiveness of speech therapy for the treatment of dysarthria is not proven; nonetheless, patients with MS who are severely affected by dysarthria should be referred to speech therapy for evaluation and subsequent treatment.

Case 4: Dysarthria, Nystagmus, and Ataxia

A 35-year-old right-handed woman was diagnosed with RRMS 12 years prior. The patient had prior episodes of optic neuritis and transverse myelitis, and recurrent relapses despite the use of immunomodulating therapy with interferons (**Figs. 7** and **8**). She presented for first evaluation and was found to have decreased visual acuity, decreased vibration in the lower extremities, and a positive Romberg sign. There was dysmetria on the left upper extremity and ataxia on the left lower extremity. She also had significant spasticity with hyperreflexia in the lower extremities. She was unable to perform tandem gait, and exhibited a spastic gait. She required a cane to ambulate. MRI of the brain revealed extensive supratentorial T2 and fluid-attenuated inversion recovery hyperintensies. There were also cerebral peduncles,

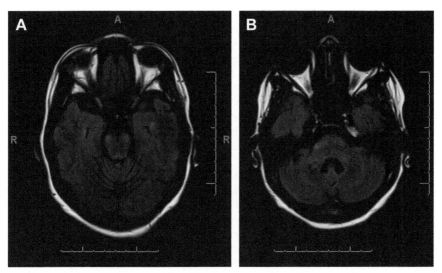

Fig. 7. (*A*, *B*) Brain MRI, axial fluid-attenuated inversion recovery MRI with cerebellar peduncle lesions.

and pons and middle cerebellar peduncles lesions. The patient was started on natalizumab and stabilized.

Vertigo

Although vertigo is not a manifestation of cerebellar disease, we include a discussion of this topic because it commonly presents in the company of cerebellar findings

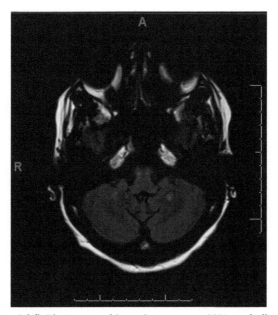

Fig. 8. Brain MRI, axial fluid-attenuated inversion recovery MRI cerebellar lesion.

owing to plaques disturbing connections to and from the cerebellum. The most challenging aspect of managing patients with MS is the determination whether a new symptom is secondary to a demyelinating plaque or some other neurologic disorder. This is particularly true when investigating the acute onset of vertigo. Vertigo related to the presence of an acute plaque, rather than benign paroxysmal positional vertigo or other vestibulopathies, can be challenging to differentiate before obtaining imaging. In 1 retrospective study, 25 patients with MS had presented with acute onset of vertigo and had undergone extensive neurootologic examination, ultimately revealing that 13 of the 25 patients had vertigo related to benign paroxysmal positional vertigo, 8 of the 25 were related to a new MS plaque, and the remaining 4 of the 25 were found to have other causes of vertigo.[80]

Acute vertigo related to an MS plaque may be constant or intermittent, but is regularly associated with spontaneous nystagmus. Benign positional vertigo is always positional and is not associated with spontaneous nystagmus.[80] When it is still unclear whether the vertigo is central rather than peripheral in origin, the HINTS examination can be useful. HINTS is an acronym for *head impulse test, nystagmus, and test of skew*. Signs on this examination that suggest central origin of vertigo include a negative head impulse test, direction-changing nystagmus, and presence of skew gaze deviation. MS plaques causing vertigo are often localized to the root of the vestibulocochlear nerve, medial vestibular nucleus, or the cerebellar peduncles.[80,81]

Treating vertigo in MS can be challenging. If the patient presents with acute vertigo that is related to an MS plaque, as previously described, then treatment should be aimed at the acute attack, including intravenous steroids or high-dose oral steroids. There is no established therapy for chronic vertigo secondary to a prior plaque, but some physicians find that low-dose, long-acting benzodiazepines offer some relief.[82]

Case 5: Vertigo and Truncal and Appendicular Ataxia

A 48-year-old right-handed man presented with subacute imbalance and vertigo (**Figs. 9–11**). Symptoms worsened and he then developed incoordination of the right

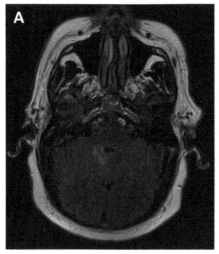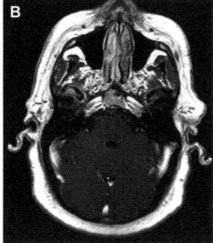

Fig. 9. (*A*) Brain MRI, axial fluid-attenuated inversion recovery MRI. (*B*) T1 post contrast with active lesion of vermis.

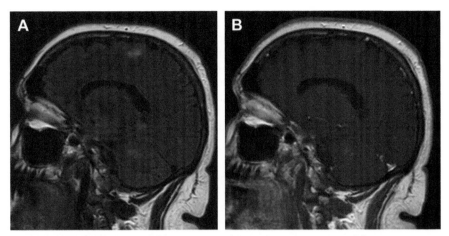

Fig. 10. (A) Brain MRI, sagittal fluid-attenuated inversion recovery MRI. (B) T1 post contrast with lesions of cerebral cortex and cerebellum.

arm and leg to the point where he needed to use his left arm to shave and was having trouble ambulating. His examination revealed dysarthria, loss of smooth pursuit, slight horizontal nystagmus, and a positive Romberg sign. Ataxia of the right upper and lower extremities and right-sided dysdiadochokinesia were noted. Reflexes were brisk in the lower extremities, right more than left. He was unable to tandem and had truncal ataxia. MRI scan of the brain showed multiple T2 hyperintensities both supratentorial and infratentorial in location with contrast enhancement. Cerebellar lesion was involving the right hemisphere and vermis. The patient was treated with intravenous steroids with some improvement of symptoms and then started on dimethyl fumerate with good response thus far.

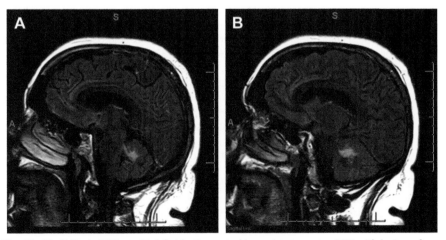

Fig. 11. (A, B) Brain MRI, sagittal fluid-attenuated inversion recovery MRI with lesion of cerebellum midline and lateral views.

SUMMARY

Cerebellar manifestations in MS are common, especially once the disease becomes progressive. Patients who have cerebellar manifestations early in the disease course tend to have a more aggressive course with higher disability and more disease burden as evidenced in some of the cases presented. When treating patients such as these, is important to keep in mind their disease course and treat it aggressively when appropriate. Of all the cerebellar manifestations, tremor is the most common. There are a myriad of treatment options available for patients with tremor.

REFERENCES

1. Noseworthy JH, Lucchinetti C, Rodriguez M, et al. Multiple sclerosis. N Engl J Med 2000;343(13):938–52.
2. Weinshenker BG, Issa MF, Baskerville J. Long-term and short-term outcome of multiple sclerosis: a 3-year follow-up study. Arch Neurol 1996;53(4):353–8.
3. Alusi SH, Worthington JF, Glickman S, et al. A study of tremor in multiple sclerosis. Brain 2001;124(Pt 4):720–30.
4. Koch-Henriksen N, Sorensen PS. The changing demographic pattern of multiple sclerosis epidemiology. Lancet Neurol 2010;9(5):520–32.
5. Trapp BD, Peterson J, Ransohoff RM, et al. Axonal transection in the lesions of multiple sclerosis. N Engl J Med 1998;338(5):278–85.
6. Ebers GC. Environmental factors and multiple sclerosis. Lancet Neurol 2008; 7(3):268–77.
7. Wingerchuk DM. Environmental factors in multiple sclerosis: Epstein-Barr virus, vitamin D, and cigarette smoking. Mt Sinai J Med 2011;78(2):221–30.
8. Kleinewietfeld M, Manzel AF, Titze JF, et al. Sodium chloride drives autoimmune disease by the induction of pathogenic TH17 cells. Nature 2013;496(7446): 518–22.
9. Compston A, Confavreux C, Lassmann H, et al. McAlpine's multiple sclerosis. 4th edition. London: Elsevier; 2006.
10. Weinshenker BG, Bass B, Rice GP, et al. The natural history of multiple sclerosis: a geographically based study: 2 predictive value of the early clinical course. Brain 1989;112(6):1419–28.
11. Thompson AJ, Polman CH, Miller DH, et al. Primary progressive multiple sclerosis. Brain 1997;120(Pt 6):1085–96.
12. Kurtzke JF. Rating neurologic impairment in multiple sclerosis: an expanded disability status scale (EDSS). Neurology 1983;33(11):1444–52.
13. Polman CH, Reingold SC, Banwell B, et al. Diagnostic criteria for multiple sclerosis: 2010 revisions to the McDonald criteria. Ann Neurol 2011;69(2):292–302.
14. Klockgether T. Sporadic ataxia with adult onset: classification and diagnostic criteria. Lancet Neurol 2010;9(1):94–104.
15. Marmolino D. Friedreich's ataxia: past, present and future. Brain Res Rev 2011; 67(1–2):311–30.
16. Oh R, Brown DL. Vitamin B_{12} deficiency. Am Fam Physician 1990;42(5): 1217–20.
17. Seidel K, Siswanto S, Brunt ER, et al. Brain pathology of spinocerebellar ataxias. Acta Neuropathol 2012;124(1):1–21.
18. Lin DJ, Hermann KL, Schmahmann JD. Multiple system atrophy of the cerebellar type: clinical state of the art. Mov Disord 2014;29(3):294–304.
19. Abele M, Bürk K, Schöls L, et al. The aetiology of sporadic adult-onset ataxia. Brain 2002;125(5):961–8.

20. Wenning GK, Colosimo CF, Geser FF, et al. Multiple system atrophy. Lancet Neurol 2004;3(2):93–103.
21. Finke C, Siebert EF, Plotkin M, et al. Multiple system atrophy masking multiple sclerosis. Clin Neurol Neurosurg 2010;112(1):59–61.
22. Weinshenker BG, O'Brien PC, Petterson TM, et al. A randomized trial of plasma exchange in acute central nervous system inflammatory demyelinating disease. Ann Neurol 1999;46(6):878–86.
23. Miller D, Barkhof F, Montalban X, et al. Clinically isolated syndromes suggestive of multiple sclerosis, part I: natural history, pathogenesis, diagnosis, and prognosis. Lancet Neurol 2005;4(5):281–8.
24. Brex PA, Ciccarelli O, O'Riordan JI, et al. A longitudinal study of abnormalities on MRI and disability from multiple sclerosis. N Engl J Med 2002;346(3):158–64.
25. O'Riordan JI, Thompson AJ, Kingsley DP, et al. The prognostic value of brain MRI in clinically isolated syndromes of the CNS. A 10-year follow-up. Brain 1998;121(Pt 3):495–503.
26. Fisniku LK, Brex PA, Altmann DR, et al. Disability and T2 MRI lesions: a 20-year follow-up of patients with relapse onset of multiple sclerosis. Brain 2008;131(Pt 3):808–17.
27. Coyle PK. Early treatment of multiple sclerosis to prevent neurologic damage. Neurology 2008;71(24 Suppl 3):S3–7.
28. Cohen JA, Barkhof F, Comi G, et al. Oral fingolimod or intramuscular interferon for relapsing multiple sclerosis. N Engl J Med 2010;362(5):402–15.
29. Kappos L, Radue EW, O'Connor P, et al. A placebo-controlled trial of oral fingolimod in relapsing multiple sclerosis. N Engl J Med 2010;362(5):387–401.
30. O'Connor P, Wolinsky JS, Confavreux C, et al. Randomized trial of oral teriflunomide for relapsing multiple sclerosis. N Engl J Med 2011;365(14):1293–303.
31. Fox RJ, Miller DH, Phillips JT, et al. Placebo-controlled phase 3 study of oral BG-12 or glatiramer in multiple sclerosis. N Engl J Med 2012;367(12):1087–97.
32. Gold R, Kappos L, Arnold DL, et al. Placebo-controlled phase 3 study of oral BG-12 for relapsing multiple sclerosis. N Engl J Med 2012;367(12):1098–107.
33. Polman CH, O'Connor PW, Havrdova E, et al. A randomized, placebo-controlled trial of natalizumab for relapsing multiple sclerosis. N Engl J Med 2006;354(9):899–910.
34. Fox RJ, Rudick RA. Risk stratification and patient counseling for natalizumab in multiple sclerosis. Neurology 2012;78(6):436–7.
35. Deryck O, Ketelaer PF, Dubois B. Clinical characteristics and long term prognosis in early onset multiple sclerosis. J Neurol 2006;253(6):720–3.
36. Kutzelnigg A, Faber-Rod JC, Bauer J, et al. Widespread demyelination in the cerebellar cortex in multiple sclerosis. Brain Pathol 2007;17(1):38–44.
37. McAlpine DF, Compston N. Some aspects of the natural history of disseminated sclerosis. Q J Med 1952;21(82):135–67.
38. Pittock SJ, McClelland RL, Mayr WT, et al. Prevalence of tremor in multiple sclerosis and associated disability in the Olmsted county population. Mov Disord 2004;19(12):1482–5.
39. Nakashima I, Fujihara K, Okita N, et al. Clinical and MRI study of brain stem and cerebellar involvement in Japanese patients with multiple sclerosis. J Neurol Neurosurg Psychiatry 1999;67(2):153–7.
40. Feys P, Maes F, Nuttin B, et al. Relationship between multiple sclerosis intention tremor severity and lesion load in the brainstem. Neuroreport 2005;16(12):1379–82.

41. Naderi F, Javadi SA, Motamedi M, et al. The efficacy of primidone in reducing severe cerebellar tremors in patients with multiple sclerosis. Clinical Neuropharmacology 2012;35(5):224–6.

42. Koller WC. Pharmacologic trials in the treatment of cerebellar tremor. Archives of Neurology 1984;41(3):280–1.

43. Trelles L, Trelles JO, Castro C, et al. Successful treatment of two cases of intention tremor with clonazepam. Ann Neurol 1984;16(5):621–621.

44. Bozek CB, Kastrukoff LF, Wright JM, et al. A controlled trial of isoniazid therapy for action tremor in multiple sclerosis. Journal of Neurology 1987;234(1):36–9.

45. Aisen ML, Holzer M, Rosen M, et al. Glutethimide treatment of disabling action tremor in patients with multiple sclerosis and traumatic brain injury. Archives of Neurology 1991;48(5):513–5.

46. Rice GP, Lesaux J, Vandervoort P, et al. Ondansetron, a 5-HT3 antagonist, improves cerebellar tremor. Journal of Neurology. Neurosurgery & Psychiatry 1997;62(3):282–4.

47. Sechi GP, Zuddas M, Piredda M, et al. Treatment of cerebellar tremors with carbamazepine: A controlled trial with long-term follow-up. Neurology 1989;39(8):1113.

48. Feys P, D'hooghe MB, Nagels G, et al. The effect of levetiracetam on tremor severity and functionality in patients with multiple sclerosis. Multiple Sclerosis 2009;15(3):371–8.

49. Schroeder A, Linker R, Lukas C, et al. Successful treatment of cerebellar ataxia and tremor in multiple scerlosis with topiramate: A case report. Clinical Neuropharmacology 2010;33(6):317–8.

50. Fox P, Bain PG, Glickman S, et al. The effect of cannabis on tremor in patients with multiple sclerosis. Neurology 2004;62(7):1105–9.

51. Van Der Walt A, Sung S, Spelman T, et al. A double-blind, randomized, controlled study of botulinum toxin type A in MS-related tremor. Neurology 2012;79(1):92–9.

52. Koch M, Mostert J, Heersema D, et al. Tremor in multiple sclerosis. J Neurol 2007;254(2):133–45.

53. Schroeder A, Linker R, Lukas C, et al. Successful treatment of cerebellar ataxia and tremor in multiple sclerosis with topiramate: a case report. Clin Neuropharmacol 2010;33(6):317–8.

54. Trelles L, Trelles JO, Castro C, et al. Successful treatment of two cases of intention tremor with clonazepam. Ann Neurol 1984;16(5):621.

55. Feys P, D'hooghe MB, Nagels G, et al. The effect of levetiracetam on tremor severity and functionality in patients with multiple sclerosis. Mult Scler 2009;15(3):371–8.

56. Bozek CB, Kastrukoff LF, Wright JM, et al. A controlled trial of isoniazid therapy for action tremor in multiple sclerosis. J Neurol 1987;234(1):36–9.

57. Marrosu F, Maleci A, Cocco E, et al. Vagal nerve stimulation effects on cerebellar tremor in multiple sclerosis. Neurology 2005;65(3):490.

58. Marrosu F, Maleci A, Cocco E, et al. Vagal nerve stimulation improves cerebellar tremor and dysphagia in multiple sclerosis. Multiple Sclerosis 2007;13(9):1200–2.

59. Yap L, Kouyialis A, Varma TRK. Stereotactic neurosurgery for disabling tremor in multiple sclerosis: Thalamotomy or deep brain stimulation? British Journal of Neurosurgery 2007;21(4):349–54.

60. Matsumoto J, Morrow D, Kaufman K, et al. Surgical therapy for tremor in multiple sclerosis. Neurology 2001;57:1876–82.

61. Lavin P. Neuro-ophthalmology: ocular motor system. In: Daroff RB, Fenichel GM, Jankovic J, et al, editors. Bradley's neurology in clinical practice. 6th edition. Philadelphia: Saunders; 2012. p. 587–633.
62. Solingen LD, Baloh RW, Myers L, et al. Subclinical eye movement disorders in patients with multiple sclerosis. Neurology 1977;27(7):614–9.
63. Aantaa E, Riekkinen PJ, Frey HJ. Electronystagmographic findings in multiple sclerosis. Acta Otolaryngol 1973;75(1):1–5.
64. Roodhooft J. Summary of eye examinations of 284 patients with multiple sclerosis. Int J MS Care 2012;14(1):31–8.
65. Kim J, Jeong I, Lim Y, et al. Primary position upbeat nystagmus during an acute attack of multiple sclerosis. J Clin Neurol 2014;10(1):37–41.
66. Barnes D, McDonald WI. The ocular manifestations of multiple sclerosis. 2. Abnormalities of eye movements. J Neurol Neurosurg Psychiatry 1992;55:863–8.
67. Lopez LI, Bronstein AM, Gresty MA, et al. Clinical and MRI correlates in 27 patients with acquired pendular nystagmus. Brain 1996;119(2):465–72.
68. Aschoff JC, Conrad B, Kornhuber HH. Acquired pendular nystagmus with oscillopsia in multiple sclerosis: A sign of cerebellar nuclei disease. Journal of Neurology,. Neurosurgery & Psychiatry 1974;37(5):570–7.
69. Fisher A, Gresty M, Chambers B, et al. Primary position upbeating nystagmus: A variety of central positional nystagmus. Brain 1983;106(4):949–64.
70. Bronstein AM, Miller DH, Rudge P, et al. Down beating nystagmus: magnetic resonance imaging and neuro-otological findings. J Neurol Sci 1987;81(2–3):173–84.
71. Baloh RW, Spooner JW. Downbeat nystagmus: a type of central vestibular nystagmus. Neurology 1981;31(3):304–10.
72. Matsumoto S, Ohyagi Y, Inoue I, et al. Periodic alternating nystagmus in a patient with MS. Neurology 2001;56(2):276–7.
73. Mehta A, Kennard C. The pharmacological treatment of acquired nystagmus. Practical Neurology 2012;12(3):147–53.
74. Starck M, Albrecht H, Pöllmann W, et al. Acquired pendular nystagmus in multiple sclerosis: An examiner-blind cross-over treatment study of memantine and gabapentin. Journal of Neurology 2010;257:322–7.
75. Kalla R, Glasauer SF, Buttner UF, et al. 4-aminopyridine restores vertical and horizontal neural integrator function in downbeat nystagmus. Brain 2007;130(Pt 9): 2441–51.
76. Glasauer S, Kalla R, Büttner U, et al. 4-aminopyridine restores visual ocular motor function in upbeat nystagmus. J Neurol Neurosurg Psychiatry 2005; 76(3):451–3.
77. Kalla R, Spiegel R, Claassen J, et al. Comparison of 10-mg doses of 4-aminopyridine and 3,4-diaminopyridine for the treatment of downbeat nystagmus. J Neuroophthalmol 2011;31(4):320–5.
78. Darley FL, Brown JR, Goldstein NP. Dysarthria in multiple sclerosis. Journal of Speech, Language, and Hearing Research 1972;15:229–45.
79. Hartelius L, Runmaker B, Andersen O. Prevalence and characteristics of dysarthria in a multiple-sclerosis incidence cohort: Relation to neurological data. Folia Phoniatrica et Logopaedica 2000;52(4):160–77.
80. Frohman EM, Zhang H, Dewey RB, et al. Vertigo in MS: utility of positional and particle repositioning maneuvers. Neurology 2000;55(10):1566–9.
81. Pula JH, Newman-Toker DE, Kattah JC. Multiple sclerosis as a cause of the acute vestibular syndrome. J Neurol 2013;260(6):1649–54.
82. Schapiro RT. Symptom management in multiple sclerosis. Ann Neurol 1994; 36(Suppl):S123–9.

Cerebellar Infarction

Sudhir Datar, MD*, Alejandro A. Rabinstein, MD

KEYWORDS

- Cerebellar stroke • Posterior circulation stroke • Cerebellar infarction • Vertigo
- Ataxia

KEY POINTS

- Cerebellar infarction often presents with nonspecific symptoms such as nausea, vomiting, headache, and dizziness. It can be difficult to recognize because it is a less common cause of these symptoms than other more benign diseases.
- Cardioembolism, large artery atherosclerosis, and basilar or vertebral artery dissection are important causes.
- Complications such as tissue swelling and mass effect can be life threatening because of brain stem compression and/or obstructive hydrocephalus.
- Close monitoring is essential in the acute phase for timely recognition and treatment of these complications.
- Patients can have a good outcome if managed appropriately. Decompressive suboccipital craniectomy is necessary in the most severe cases.

INTRODUCTION

Cerebellar stroke accounts for approximately 2% to 3% of all strokes.[1–3] Approximately 20,000 new cerebellar infarctions occur each year in the United States.[4] Misdiagnoses occur especially in otherwise healthy younger patients.[5,6] In one study, stroke/transient ischemic attack (TIA) was the final diagnosis in only 3% of patients presenting to the emergency department with dizziness, vertigo, and imbalance.[7] Moreover, CT scan may be normal in the initial stages, complicating recognition.[8,9] Therefore, it is important to keep in mind the possibility of cerebellar stroke, even if the head CT scan is unremarkable, in patients who present with acute headache, vertigo, nausea or vomiting, and ataxia.

Cerebellar strokes can cause serious complications because of their location. The posterior fossa is a small space with virtually no additional room for expansion. Any mass lesion in the cerebellum thus threatens to compress the fourth ventricle and brain stem. According to some studies, approximately 20% of the patients with

Disclosures: None.
Department of Neurology, Mayo Clinic, 200 First Street SW, Rochester, MN 55905, USA
* Corresponding author.
E-mail address: datar.sudhir@mayo.edu

Neurol Clin 32 (2014) 979–991
http://dx.doi.org/10.1016/j.ncl.2014.07.007
neurologic.theclinics.com

cerebellar stroke develop signs of clinical and radiographic deterioration due to mass effect.[9,10]

As in the anterior circulation, ischemia to the cerebellum commonly occurs because of embolism or large vessel atherosclerosis.[1,11,12] Vertebrobasilar dissection is another important cause of cerebellar infarction.[13] There are 3 major vessels supplying the cerebellum: posterior inferior cerebellar artery (PICA), anterior inferior cerebellar artery (AICA), and superior cerebellar artery (SCA). Strokes can occur in any of these vascular territories. Sometimes there is more than one vascular territory involved.[4]

CLINICAL FINDINGS
Patient History

As noted earlier, patients with cerebellar infarction often present with nonspecific symptoms, such as dizziness, nausea, vomiting, and headache. They are summarized in **Table 1**. Many of these symptoms can be seen with benign nonneurologic conditions, such as gastritis or viral enteritis, which are far more common in patients presenting to the emergency department. Careful attention to certain details in the history might point toward cerebellar stroke as the cause. These details in the patient's history include the following:

- Abrupt onset
- Temporal association with head or neck trauma
- Accompanying acute onset neck pain (due to vertebral dissection)
- Presence of stroke risk factors (diabetes mellitus, hypertension, hypercholesterolemia, cigarette smoking, advanced age, atrial fibrillation)
- History of TIAs or strokes
- Gait or limb incoordination out of proportion to nausea and vomiting

Physical Examination

A detailed neurologic examination should be performed with special attention to the level of consciousness, gaze and ocular movements, cranial nerve deficits, speech,

Table 1
Signs and symptoms of cerebellar infarction

Symptoms	Signs
Dizziness	Limb and/or gait ataxia
Nausea	Nystagmus[a]
Vomiting	Intention tremor
Limb and/or gait incoordination	Dysmetria
Headache	Rebound phenomenon[b]
Slurred speech	Dysarthria (scanning speech)
Hearing loss[c]	Hypotonia
Intractable hiccups[d]	Pendular reflexes[e]

[a] Direction changing or vertical, not inhibited by visual fixation and without any associated tinnitus suggests central rather than peripheral cause.
[b] When muscles are contracted against resistance and the resistance is then suddenly removed, the antagonists fail to check the movement and the limb continues to move in the direction of the muscle contraction.
[c] Sometimes seen with AICA territory infarction.
[d] Seen sometimes with PICA territory infarction with simultaneous involvement of the medulla.
[e] Oscillating motion of the extremity after a reflex is elicited.

long tract findings (hemimotor or hemisensory deficits), autonomic changes (heart rate, blood pressure, Horner syndrome), coordination, and, most importantly, gait. Truncal ataxia can be the only manifestation of stroke affecting the vermis of the cerebellum, which can be easily missed if gait is not assessed. Physical signs commonly seen with cerebellar infarctions are summarized in **Table 1**.

Ischemia of the cerebellum may coexist with ischemia of the brain stem due to pathologic abnormality in the vertebrobasilar vasculature. In that case, additional symptoms and signs due to dysfunction of the brain stem may help the clinician with lesion localization and diagnosis:

- Diplopia or skew deviation
- Cranial nerve deficits
- Horner syndrome
- Long tract signs (hemimotor or hemisensory deficits)
- Abnormal pupillary reaction
- Reduced level of consciousness

Alternatively, these clinical features may be present because of obstructive hydrocephalus or brain stem displacement from mass effect. Deterioration due to tissue swelling is often manifested by reduction in the level of consciousness, which is dependent more on the volume of the tissue involved than the vascular territory.[9] Nevertheless, most infarctions necessitating surgical decompression involve the PICA territory and rarely the SCA territory. Isolated, unilateral AICA territory infarctions and infarctions restricted to the lateral cerebellum do not require surgical treatment.[9,14]

DIAGNOSTIC MODALITIES

Noncontrast head CT scan (NCCT) is usually the first-line imaging modality. MR imaging is sometimes needed as NCCT may be normal in as many as 25% of the patients, especially when performed shortly after the onset of symptoms.[9] Advantages and pitfalls of different imaging techniques are outlined in **Table 2**. Occasionally, NCCT may show hyperdensity in the basilar artery, which may indicate an occlusive thrombus.

Cause and Pathogenesis

Common causes of cerebellar stroke are summarized as follows:

- Cardiac embolism
  - Atrial fibrillation
  - Patent foramen ovale (paradoxic embolism)
  - Valvular thrombi or vegetations
  - Severe cardiomyopathy with heart failure
- Atherosclerosis
  - Vertebrobasilar atherosclerosis
  - Aortic arch atherosclerosis with artery-to-artery embolism
- Vertebral or basilar arterial dissection
  - Head or neck trauma
  - Nontraumatic spontaneous dissection
  - Connective tissue disorders (eg, fibromuscular dysplasia)
- Hypercoagulable states
  - Hereditary (such as protein C deficiency, protein S deficiency, or factor V Leiden mutation)
  - Oral contraceptives

Table 2
Diagnostic imaging modalities in patients with cerebellar stroke

Imaging Modality	Pros	Cons
Non-contrast head CT scan (NCCT)	• Quick and widely available study • Helps rule out some of the differential diagnoses, most importantly posterior fossa hemorrhage • Helps exclude complications of cerebellar infarction[a]	• May be normal in the initial stages in as many as 25% or more patients[8,9]
CT Angiogram (CTA) head and neck	• Can help identify mechanism of stroke (eg, embolic occlusion, atherosclerosis, or dissection) • Useful to rule out basilar artery occlusion if clinically suspected	• Uses iodine-based contrast with potential for nephrotoxicity
MRI brain	• Diffusion-weighted imaging can identify infarctions that are missed by NCCT • Can demonstrate additional lesions elsewhere in the brain not visible on NCCT, which may help identify the stroke mechanism (eg, embolic shower vs focal dissection or occlusion) • Helps to rule out differential diagnoses	• Less readily available than NCCT especially after hours • May be contraindicated in certain patients with implanted devices, such as pacemakers or vagal nerve stimulators • More time-consuming study than CT scan and challenging to perform in unstable patients
MR angiogram (MRA) of head and neck	• Provides similar clinical information as CTA but without nephrotoxic iodine contrast • Probably better at defining vascular anatomy in patients with severe calcification of vessel wall compared with CTA[39,40]	• Same as above
Transthoracic echocardiogram (TTE) and transesophageal echocardiogram (TEE)	• Provides detailed assessment of cardiac anatomy and function • Can identify pathologic condition such as thrombi or valvular vegetations which may be a source of embolism	• TTE alone can miss a left atrial appendage thrombus • TEE may be technically difficult in patients with esophageal pathologic condition or previous esophageal surgery • TEE can very rarely lead to esophageal perforation

[a] Such as brain stem displacement from tissue swelling and obstructive hydrocephalus.

- Vasculitis/vasculopathy
  - Infectious (eg, syphilis,[15] Lyme neuroborreliosis[16])
  - Inflammatory (eg, central nervous system vasculitis)
  - Drug induced (eg, cocaine[17] or methamphetamines)
- Migraine[18]
- Cryptogenic

The mechanism of stroke varies depending on the age of the patient. Atherosclerosis is more common in the middle-aged or older population (>45 years for men and >55 years for women) and in the presence of comorbidities, such as hypertension, diabetes mellitus, hyperlipidemia, obesity, and cigarette smoking. Common causes of strokes in younger patients include drug abuse, vascular dissection, infections, and hypercoagulable states. Identification of the correct cause is important for secondary stroke prevention. However, in some cases, the stroke remains cryptogenic even after an exhaustive search.

PROCESS OF ELIMINATION/DIFFERENTIAL DIAGNOSIS

The first step for a clinician is to determine if the presenting symptoms are caused by neurologic disease. Once neurologic origin is suspected, the following differential diagnosis should be considered:

- Central
  - Cerebellar infarction
  - Cerebellar hemorrhage
  - Demyelinating disorders such as multiple sclerosis or acute disseminated encephalomyelitis
  - Cerebellitis (infectious or noninfectious)
  - Medication toxicity (eg, antiseizure medications such as phenytoin or carbamazepine)
  - Illicit drugs and alcohol
  - Cerebellar neoplasm (rarely causes acute symptoms)
- Peripheral
  - Vestibular neuronitis
  - Labyrinthitis
  - Benign paroxysmal positional vertigo
  - Meniere's disease

MANAGEMENT/TREATMENT
Patient Evaluation Overview

Patient evaluation overview is outlined in **Fig. 1**.

Management Principles

Airway management and mechanical ventilation

- Endotracheal intubation may be indicated for the following reasons:
  - Inability to protect the airway and clear the secretions due to depressed level of consciousness (usually with Glasgow coma scale sum score ≤8).
  - Hypoxemic or hypercarbic respiratory failure.
  - Need for posterior fossa decompression.
  - Apneic episodes.
- Normocarbia should be maintained.
- Hyperventilation is used (only for a short period) in cases of impending or progressing brain herniation. There is no role for prophylactic hyperventilation.[19]
- Bronchoscopy may be necessary to remove any foreign bodies if aspiration is suspected.

Blood pressure management

- Acute hypertension is commonly seen after ischemic stroke and cerebellar strokes are no exception.

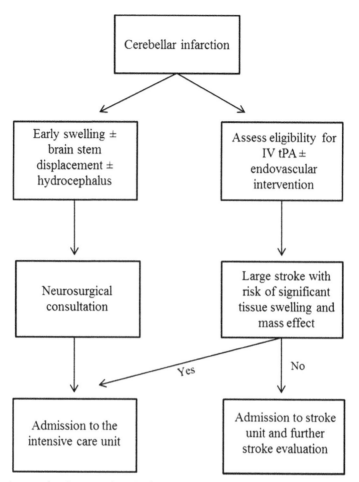

Fig. 1. Patient evaluation overview. IV, intravenous; tPA, tissue plasminogen activator.

- Allow permissive hypertension to optimize perfusion to the penumbra; however, precise blood pressure parameters are unknown.
- Risk of hemorrhagic transformation increases with extreme hypertension (eg, systolic blood pressure >220 mm Hg or diastolic blood pressure >105 mm Hg).[19]
- Blood pressure goals need to be tailored for each individual based on baseline blood pressure. Antihypertensive therapy should be used more cautiously in patients with chronic hypertension who may have the autoregulatory curve shifted to the right and consequently be more susceptible to cerebral hypoperfusion with blood pressure reduction.
- Unless necessary (for reasons such as aortic dissection or myocardial infarction), the usual practice is not to treat systolic blood pressures when less than 180 mm Hg or mean arterial pressures less than 120 mm Hg.

Temperature management

- Fever is detrimental to the injured brain and has been shown to worsen outcome following ischemic stroke.[20,21]

- Maintain normothermia (core temperature ≤37.5 C) and use cooling devices (cooling blankets, ice packs, cooling pads) if pharmacotherapy (acetaminophen) alone is ineffective.
- There is inadequate evidence currently to recommend routine hypothermia for ischemic stroke.
- Fever is not usually caused by cerebellar infarction and instead may be a sign of systemic infection/inflammation (eg, aspiration pneumonitis or pneumonia).[20,21]

Glucose management

- Hyperglycemia has been associated with worse outcomes in patients with ischemic strokes.[22–24]
- The optimal glycemic target is not yet elucidated, but the authors recommend maintaining serum glucose levels between 100 and 180 mg/dL with insulin, which can be given either as a continuous infusion or as a "sliding scale."[19,25]
- Tight sugar control with intensive insulin therapy is not indicated. It can increase the risk of hypoglycemia and in one trial this strategy was associated with greater infarct growth in the first 24 hours.[26]
- Hypoglycemia however should be avoided at all times.

Fluid and electrolyte management

- Avoid hypotonic fluids or fluids containing dextrose.
- Correct dehydration if present and maintain normovolemia using isotonic saline.
- Hyponatremia should always be corrected.
- Consider using mildly hypertonic solutions such as 1.5% saline as maintenance fluids in patients with low normal serum sodium.
- Optimize serum potassium (≥4.0 mmol/L) and magnesium (≥2.0 mg/dL). Cardiac arrhythmias can occur (if the stroke involves the brain stem in addition to the cerebellum), which may be aggravated by hypokalemia and hypomagnesemia.

Anticoagulation and antiplatelet therapy

- Antiplatelet monotherapy (aspirin 81 mg/d or 325 mg/d) can be used, although caution needs to be exercised in patients with hemorrhagic transformation and may be best avoided in some cases during the acute phase.
- There is no role for dual antiplatelet therapy in large cerebellar strokes due to the risk of hemorrhagic transformation.[27]
- Clopidogrel is best avoided in patients with large strokes who may need decompressive surgery or ventriculostomy.
- Subcutaneous heparin should be used for the prevention of deep venous thrombosis.
- With large strokes, full-dose anticoagulation (in patients who are on warfarin or other anticoagulants) may need to be reversed in the acute stage due to the risk of hemorrhagic transformation, after carefully weighing the risks of no anticoagulation.

Treatment of modifiable risk factors

Treatment of risk factors such as hypertension, diabetes mellitus, hyperlipidemia (ideal goal low-density lipoprotein <70 mg/dL), and obesity is important for secondary stroke prevention. Lifestyle modification (increased physical activity and smoking cessation) are vital. The treatment goals do not differ from strokes in the anterior circulation. Detailed overview of secondary stroke prevention is outside the scope of this article, but can be found in recent guidelines.[28]

Complications and Their Management

The following complications can occur with large infarctions:

- Swelling and mass effect resulting in brain stem compression.
- Compression of the fourth ventricle resulting into obstructive hydrocephalus.
- Hemorrhagic conversion of ischemic infarction.

Hyperosmolar agents and decompressive surgery are indicated in patients with symptomatic mass effect.

Hyperosmolar therapy

Osmolar therapy with either mannitol or hypertonic saline is used in the deteriorating patient to reduce the space-occupying effects of the swollen infarcted tissue. These solutions increase osmolality of the serum, which promotes osmotic movement of water into the vasculature, thereby inducing reactive vasoconstriction. The net effect is reduction in ICP and tissue shrinkage. These effects are more prominent on healthy brain tissue than infarcted tissue likely because of preserved blood-brain barrier in healthy tissue.[29]

- Mannitol
  - The usual first dose of mannitol (20% concentration) is variable in the range of 1 to 2 g/kg.[29,30]
  - Additional doses of 0.5 g/kg every 4 to 6 hours can be given while monitoring serum osmolality.
  - As mannitol induces diuresis, it is essential to maintain euvolemia by replacing the lost fluids preferably with isotonic saline.
  - Problems arise with mannitol use in the presence of renal failure because mannitol can lead to volume overload, which may necessitate the use of dialysis to remove three times the given volume 15 to 30 minutes following the infusion.[31]
  - Mannitol has traditionally been used cautiously when the osmolality reaches greater than 320 mOsm for the fear of renal toxicity. This concern comes from a small study in which high doses were used as continuous infusions. Crossing the 320 mOsm threshold is probably safe as long as dehydration is avoided,[32] but caution is advised.
- Hypertonic saline
  - The commonly used concentrations are 3% (250 mL bolus), 10% (75–150 mL bolus), and 23.4% (30 mL bolus). Like mannitol, hypertonic saline boluses can be repeated every 4 to 6 hours while monitoring serum sodium.
  - Potential (but rare) complications with hypertonic saline include transient hypotension, pulmonary edema and heart failure, hypokalemia, hyperchloremic acidemia, coagulopathy, intravascular hemolysis, myelinolysis (only with rapid overcorrection of pre-existing hyponatremia), and encephalopathy.[33,34] Phlebitis can occur if peripheral venous access is used for administration, although this complication is very uncommon with continuous infusion of the 3% concentration.
  - It is generally accepted that hypertonic saline should not be used if the serum sodium level is greater than 160 mmol/L. In a study of 600 patients in the neurointensive care unit, there was an independent increase in mortality in patients with serum sodium greater than 160 mmol/L.[35] In the same study, the incidence of renal failure was also high in patients with this degree of hypernatremia.

Whether to choose mannitol or hypertonic saline depends on the clinical situation. No study has proven superiority of one therapy over the other in patients with large ischemic strokes.

Surgical treatment

- Surgical options are considered when there is clinical deterioration attributed to mass effect from tissue swelling or hemorrhagic conversion.
- Signs of deterioration include a decrease in the level of consciousness, downward displacement of conjugate gaze (sunset eyes), gaze paresis, cranial nerve deficits, and long tract signs.
- Suboccipital decompressive craniectomy (SDC) with dural expansion is the procedure of choice. It creates space for the swollen cerebellum to expand posteriorly instead of compressing the fourth ventricle and brain stem.[19]
- SDC may or may not be combined with resection of the necrotic tissue.[11] When possible, it is preferable to avoid infarctectomy because it can potentially resect recoverable tissue.
- SDC is a relatively safe procedure. However, it should be reserved for patients who fail medical management and those who deteriorate rapidly.
- Ventriculostomy to treat obstructive hydrocephalus may be performed in isolation[11,36] or it may be combined with SDC. The risk of supratentorial cerebellar herniation with ventriculostomy alone is real, but only documented in a few case reports. Nonetheless, it is preferable to pursue SDC, in addition to ventriculostomy, in patients with obstructive hydrocephalus from a swollen cerebellar infarction.

Evaluation of outcome and long-term recommendations

- Outcome can be good if managed appropriately and in the absence of additional brain stem infarction.[12,14,37,38]
- Older patients seem to do worse than younger patients.[36,37] Thus, age and preexisting comorbidities are important considerations when selecting patients for surgical intervention.

Case study

A 59 year-old right-handed woman presented to the emergency room with acute onset of dizziness, intractable nausea, and gait ataxia. Her past medical history was significant only for essential hypertension. NCCT scan demonstrated subtle changes consistent with early cerebellar infarction in the distribution of the left PICA. A CT angiogram of the head and neck showed patent vertebrobasilar vasculature with no evidence of stenosis or dissection. Because her infarction was large, she was admitted to the intensive care unit for close monitoring.

Two days later, her clinical condition worsened with increasing somnolence, up-gaze palsy, and bilateral sixth nerve palsy. Repeat NCCT scan (**Fig. 2**) revealed hydrocephalus and mass effect in the posterior fossa with evidence of displacement of the brain stem. Mannitol was administered without any significant change. She was taken emergently to the operating room for SDC. Following the surgery (**Fig. 3**), her clinical examination improved. Approximately 2 days after the decompression, mild dysmetria and unsteadiness were her only deficits.

Investigations for cause of stroke included transesophageal echocardiogram, which demonstrated a patent foramen ovale. Examination of the deep veins of the legs demonstrated deep venous thrombosis. With the rest of the stroke workup negative, paradoxic embolism was considered a strong possibility. Because of the risk of hemorrhagic transformation, the patient was initially not started on anticoagulation; instead, a filter was placed in the inferior vena cava. Approximately 10 days into her hospital course, she developed hemorrhagic transformation of the ischemic stroke (**Fig. 4**). She was on aspirin 81 mg/d at the time of the hemorrhage.

Her hemorrhage was managed conservatively, and she had excellent recovery. An extensive workup looking for any underlying hypercoagulable state was negative. Because paradoxic embolism was considered the most likely mechanism of the stroke, the patient was anticoagulated with warfarin, which was started approximately 2 months after the stroke onset. In the interim, she was maintained on aspirin.

She is currently living at home and working with physical therapy for gait and balance.

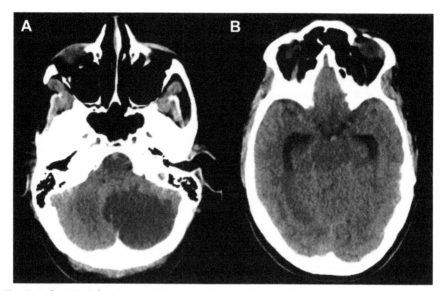

Fig. 2. Left PICA infarction. (*A*) Tissue swelling and mass effect leading to tight posterior fossa and compression of the fourth ventricle. (*B*) Obstructive hydrocephalus with ballooning of the temporal horns, loss of cerebral sulci, and anterior displacement of the brain stem.

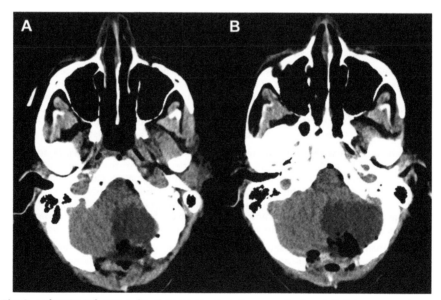

Fig. 3. Left PICA infarction. (*A, B*) Postoperative changes of suboccipital decompressive craniectomy (SDC) and resection of the posterior arch of C1.

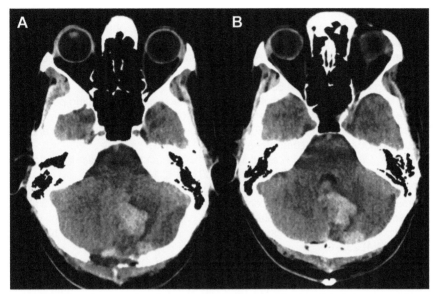

Fig. 4. Left PICA infarction. (*A, B*) Postoperative changes of suboccipital decompressive cra-niectomy (SDC) with hemorrhagic transformation of the infarction.

SUMMARY

Cerebellar infarction is relatively uncommon, but clinicians need to be mindful of this diagnosis in patients presenting with common symptoms such as nausea, vomiting, dizziness, and headache. Careful neurologic examination must be performed in these patients, looking for signs of cerebellar dysfunction.

Mass effect resulting in brain stem displacement and obstructive hydrocephalus are life-threatening complications that must be treated promptly. Patients with large infarctions are at risk of these complications and should be closely monitored in an intensive care unit. Outcome can be good with optimal care, including decompressive surgery in patients with large infarctions producing symptomatic mass effect.

REFERENCES

1. Macdonell RA, Kalnins RM, Donnan GA. Cerebellar infarction: natural history, prognosis, and pathology. Stroke 1987;18(5):849–55.
2. Tohgi H, Takahashi S, Chiba K, et al. Cerebellar infarction. Clinical and neuroimaging analysis in 293 patients. The Tohoku Cerebellar Infarction Study Group. Stroke 1993;24(11):1697–701.
3. Bogousslavsky J, Van Melle G, Regli F. The Lausanne Stroke Registry: analysis of 1,000 consecutive patients with first stroke. Stroke 1988;19(9):1083–92.
4. Edlow JA, Newman-Toker DE, Savitz SI. Diagnosis and initial management of cerebellar infarction. Lancet Neurol 2008;7(10):951–64.
5. Savitz SI, Caplan LR, Edlow JA. Pitfalls in the diagnosis of cerebellar infarction. Acad Emerg Med 2007;14(1):63–8.
6. Masuda Y, Tei H, Shimizu S, et al. Factors associated with the misdiagnosis of cerebellar infarction. J Stroke Cerebrovasc Dis 2013;22(7):1125–30.

7. Kerber KA, Brown DL, Lisabeth LD, et al. Stroke among patients with dizziness, vertigo, and imbalance in the emergency department: a population-based study. Stroke 2006;37(10):2484–7.

8. Hwang DY, Silva GS, Furie KL, et al. Comparative sensitivity of computed tomography vs. magnetic resonance imaging for detecting acute posterior fossa infarct. J Emerg Med 2012;42(5):559–65.

9. Koh MG, Phan TG, Atkinson JL, et al. Neuroimaging in deteriorating patients with cerebellar infarcts and mass effect. Stroke 2000;31(9):2062–7.

10. Kase CS, Norrving B, Levine SR, et al. Cerebellar infarction. Clinical and anatomic observations in 66 cases. Stroke 1993;24(1):76–83.

11. Raco A, Caroli E, Isidori A, et al. Management of acute cerebellar infarction: one institution's experience. Neurosurgery 2003;53(5):1061–5.

12. Pfefferkorn T, Eppinger U, Linn J, et al. Long-term outcome after suboccipital decompressive craniectomy for malignant cerebellar infarction. Stroke 2009;40(9):3045–50.

13. Saeed AB, Shuaib A, Al-Sulaiti G, et al. Vertebral artery dissection: warning symptoms, clinical features and prognosis in 26 patients. Can J Neurol Sci 2000;27(4):292–6.

14. Jauss M, Krieger D, Hornig C, et al. Surgical and medical management of patients with massive cerebellar infarctions: results of the German-Austrian Cerebellar Infarction Study. J Neurol 1999;246(4):257–64.

15. Umashankar G, Gupta V, Harik SI. Acute bilateral inferior cerebellar infarction in a patient with neurosyphilis. Arch Neurol 2004;61(6):953–6.

16. Topakian R, Stieglbauer K, Nussbaumer K, et al. Cerebral vasculitis and stroke in Lyme neuroborreliosis. Two case reports and review of current knowledge. Cerebrovasc Dis 2008;26(5):455–61.

17. Aggarwal S, Byrne BD. Massive ischemic cerebellar infarction due to cocaine use. Neuroradiology 1991;33(5):449–50.

18. Kruit MC, Launer LJ, Ferrari MD, et al. Infarcts in the posterior circulation territory in migraine. The population-based MRI CAMERA study. Brain 2005;128(Pt 9):2068–77.

19. Wijdicks EF, Sheth KN, Carter BS, et al. Recommendations for the management of cerebral and cerebellar infarction with swelling: a statement for healthcare professionals from the American Heart Association/American Stroke Association. Stroke 2014;45(4):1222–38.

20. Castillo J, Davalos A, Marrugat J, et al. Timing for fever-related brain damage in acute ischemic stroke. Stroke 1998;29(12):2455–60.

21. Greer DM, Funk SE, Reaven NL, et al. Impact of fever on outcome in patients with stroke and neurologic injury: a comprehensive meta-analysis. Stroke 2008;39(11): 3029–35.

22. Gilmore RM, Stead LG. The role of hyperglycemia in acute ischemic stroke. Neurocrit Care 2006;5(2):153–8.

23. Kawai N, Keep RF, Betz AL. Effects of hyperglycemia on cerebral blood flow and edema formation after carotid artery occlusion in Fischer 344 rats. Acta Neurochir Suppl 1997;70:34–6.

24. Pulsinelli WA, Waldman S, Rawlinson D, et al. Moderate hyperglycemia augments ischemic brain damage: a neuropathologic study in the rat. Neurology 1982; 32(11):1239–46.

25. Godoy DA, Di Napoli M, Rabinstein AA. Treating hyperglycemia in neurocritical patients: benefits and perils. Neurocrit Care 2010;13(3):425–38.

26. Rosso C, Corvol JC, Pires C, et al. Intensive versus subcutaneous insulin in patients with hyperacute stroke: results from the randomized INSULINFARCT trial. Stroke 2012;43(9):2343–9.

27. Motto C, Ciccone A, Aritzu E, et al. Hemorrhage after an acute ischemic stroke. MAST-I Collaborative Group. Stroke 1999;30(4):761–4.
28. Furie KL, Kasner SE, Adams RJ, et al. Guidelines for the prevention of stroke in patients with stroke or transient ischemic attack: a guideline for healthcare professionals from the American Heart Association/American Stroke Association. Stroke 2011;42(1):227–76.
29. Videen TO, Zazulia AR, Manno EM, et al. Mannitol bolus preferentially shrinks non-infarcted brain in patients with ischemic stroke. Neurology 2001;57(11): 2120–2.
30. Diringer MN, Scalfani MT, Zazulia AR, et al. Cerebral hemodynamic and metabolic effects of equi-osmolar doses mannitol and 23.4% saline in patients with edema following large ischemic stroke. Neurocrit Care 2011;14(1):11–7.
31. Datar S, Wijdicks EF. Neurologic manifestations of acute liver failure. Handb Clin Neurol 2014;120:645–59.
32. Diringer MN, Zazulia AR. Osmotic therapy: fact and fiction. Neurocrit Care 2004; 1(2):219–33.
33. Worthley LI, Cooper DJ, Jones N. Treatment of resistant intracranial hypertension with hypertonic saline. Report of two cases. J Neurosurg 1988;68(3):478–81.
34. Bhardwaj A, Ulatowski JA. Hypertonic saline solutions in brain injury. Curr Opin Crit Care 2004;10(2):126–31.
35. Aiyagari V, Deibert E, Diringer MN. Hypernatremia in the neurologic intensive care unit: how high is too high? J Crit Care 2006;21(2):163–72.
36. Hornig CR, Rust DS, Busse O, et al. Space-occupying cerebellar infarction. Clinical course and prognosis. Stroke 1994;25(2):372–4.
37. Juttler E, Schweickert S, Ringleb PA, et al. Long-term outcome after surgical treatment for space-occupying cerebellar infarction: experience in 56 patients. Stroke 2009;40(9):3060–6.
38. Tsitsopoulos PP, Tobieson L, Enblad P, et al. Clinical outcome following surgical treatment for bilateral cerebellar infarction. Acta Neurol Scand 2011;123(5): 345–51.
39. Hirai T, Korogi Y, Ono K, et al. Prospective evaluation of suspected stenoocclusive disease of the intracranial artery: combined MR angiography and CT angiography compared with digital subtraction angiography. AJNR Am J Neuroradiol 2002;23(1):93–101.
40. Latchaw RE, Alberts MJ, Lev MH, et al. Recommendations for imaging of acute ischemic stroke: a scientific statement from the American Heart Association. Stroke 2009;40(11):3646–78.

Cerebellar Hemorrhage

Sudhir Datar, MD*, Alejandro A. Rabinstein, MD

KEYWORDS

- Cerebellar hemorrhagic stroke • Posterior circulation hemorrhage
- Cerebellar hematoma • Vertigo • Ataxia

KEY POINTS

- The spectrum of clinical presentation of cerebellar hemorrhage depends on the size of the hematoma. Smaller hemorrhages can mimic cerebellar infarction whereas larger ones can present with catastrophic neurologic deterioration.
- The most common cause is hypertension; other causes include coagulopathy, arteriovenous malformation, aneurysm, neoplasm, and hemorrhagic transformation of ischemic infarction.
- Obstructive hydrocephalus, brainstem compression, and cerebellar herniation are life-threatening complications arising from tissue swelling and mass effect.
- Close monitoring is essential in the acute phase for timely recognition and treatment of these complications.
- Prompt surgical evacuation is indicated in patients with neurologic deterioration attributed to mass effect and brainstem compression or hydrocephalus.

INTRODUCTION

Cerebellar hemorrhage accounts for approximately 9% to 10 % of all intracranial hemorrhages (ICH).[1–3] Hypertension and small vessel disease being the most common cause, it is frequently seen in middle-aged to older patients (usually beyond the fifth decade).[3–6] The posterior fossa is a small space with virtually no additional room for expansion. Any mass lesion in the cerebellum thus threatens to compress neighboring structures, most importantly the brainstem and the fourth ventricle. Moreover, the hematoma can extend into the ventricular system via the fourth ventricle, worsening the hydrocephalus. The clinical spectrum of cerebellar hemorrhage is determined by its size and perilesional edema. Preexisting atrophy also plays a role by providing additional space for expansion. Indications for imaging beyond a noncontrast computed tomography (CT) scan, surgical management, and optimal timing of surgery are currently uncertain and controversial.

Disclosures: None.
Department of Neurology, Mayo Clinic, 200 First Street SW, Rochester, MN 55905, USA
* Corresponding author.
E-mail address: datar.sudhir@mayo.edu

Neurol Clin 32 (2014) 993–1007
http://dx.doi.org/10.1016/j.ncl.2014.07.006 neurologic.theclinics.com

Most hemorrhages related to hypertension occur in the area of the dentate nucleus.[1,3] The hemorrhage can further extend into the cerebellar peduncles, to the contralateral side, or to the fourth ventricle. In addition to the cerebellar parenchyma, blood can be present in the subarachnoid space tracking along the cerebellar folia. Rarely, hemorrhage is present predominantly along the superior folia, following neurosurgical manipulation in the supratentorial space; this phenomenon is termed remote cerebellar hemorrhage (see later discussion).

CLINICAL FINDINGS
Patient History

Patients with smaller cerebellar hemorrhage can present with symptoms of cerebellar stroke such as vertigo, ataxia, nausea, vomiting, and headache (**Table 1**). Often the symptoms are sudden in onset, and may happen during strenuous exertion or a stressful situation. If the hemorrhage is large, patients may present with a change in the level of consciousness or may become comatose. Careful attention to the following details in the history is essential.

- History of chronic hypertension
- Presence of coagulopathy or thrombocytopenia
- Use of antiplatelet medications or anticoagulants
- Recent head trauma
- Known arteriovenous malformation (AVM) or posterior circulation aneurysm
- History of systemic or central nervous system (CNS) malignancy
- Use of recreational drugs (eg, cocaine or amphetamines)

Physical Examination

A detailed neurologic examination should be performed with special attention to the level of consciousness, gaze and ocular movements, cranial nerve deficits, autonomic changes (heart rate, blood pressure, Horner syndrome), and long tract findings (hemimotor or hemisensory deficits). Clinical signs are summarized in **Table 1**.

Deterioration following cerebellar hemorrhage can occur at any time between a few hours and 5 days after the onset of symptoms, but is more frequent in the first 2 to

Table 1 Signs and symptoms of cerebellar hemorrhage	
Symptoms	**Signs**
Dizziness	Limb and/or gait ataxia
Nausea	Nystagmus[a]
Vomiting	Intention tremor
Limb and/or gait incoordination	Dysmetria
Headache	Rebound phenomenon[b]
Slurred speech	Dysarthria (scanning speech)
Intractable hiccups[c]	Hypotonia
	Pendular reflexes[d]

[a] Direction changing or vertical, not inhibited by visual fixation, and without any associated tinnitus suggests central rather than peripheral cause.
[b] When muscles are contracted against resistance and the resistance is then suddenly removed, the antagonists fail to check the movement and the limb continues to move in the direction of the muscle contraction.
[c] Seen sometimes with pressure on the brainstem because of involvement of the medulla.
[d] Oscillating motion of the extremity after a reflex is elicited.

3 days.[7] Decrease in the level of consciousness with downward displacement of conjugate gaze ("sunset eyes") signals developing hydrocephalus. Large hemorrhage with surrounding edema may displace the brainstem anteriorly against the clivus. With deterioration, the following focal findings may be present (in addition to decreased level of consciousness) owing to pressure on the brainstem and cranial nerves:

- Dysconjugate gaze or skew deviation
- Cranial nerve deficits, especially facial weakness
- Horner syndrome
- Long tract signs (hemimotor or hemisensory deficits)
- Anisocoria or loss of pupillary reflex

Once a baseline examination is recorded at the time of admission, serial neurologic examinations should be performed to pick up signs of deterioration.

DIAGNOSTIC MODALITIES

Noncontrast head CT (NCCT) is usually the first-line imaging modality. Hemorrhages are easily identified as hyperdense lesions with the following 2 exceptions, which can generate confusion:

1. Occasionally it may be difficult to differentiate parenchymal hemorrhage from contrast extravasation following endovascular procedures, such as mechanical thrombectomy. Dual-energy CT can be helpful in this situation in differentiating the two.[8]
2. Dense calcification of the dentate nucleus can sometimes be confused with hemorrhage, such as in Fahr disease. However, sharply defined margins, absence of mass effect, absence of edema, and involvement of bilateral dentate nuclei and supratentorial structures should point more toward calcification rather than hemorrhage.

NCCT scan alone may suffice in patients with a history of chronic hypertension and typical location of the hemorrhage. However, in certain circumstances patients may need additional imaging with CT angiography (CTA), magnetic resonance (MR) imaging, or catheter angiography to identify the cause of hemorrhage:

- No history of hypertension
- Atypical location of hemorrhage
- Presence of calcification within the lesion with abnormally appearing blood vessels, raising the suspicion for AVM
- Concurrent subarachnoid hemorrhage (can be seen with AVM or cerebral amyloid angiopathy)
- Known history of cancer and perilesional edema out of proportion to the size of the hemorrhage
- Suspected hemorrhagic transformation of ischemic stroke
- Presence of other hemorrhages or lesions of supratentorial location suggesting a cause other than hypertension

Advantages and pitfalls of different imaging techniques are outlined in **Table 2**.

Etiology and Pathogenesis

Common causes of cerebellar hemorrhage are as follows.

- Chronic hypertension
  - Hemorrhage occurs from rupture of microaneurysms in small penetrating vessels
  - Often involves the dentate nucleus

Table 2
Diagnostic imaging modalities in patients with cerebellar hemorrhage

Imaging Modality	Pros	Cons
Noncontrast head CT scan (NCCT)	Quick and widely available Helps exclude complications of cerebellar hemorrhage[a]	Dentate nucleus calcification can sometimes be confused with hemorrhage
CT angiogram (CTA) of head and neck	May help identify arteriovenous malformation (AVM) or aneurysm as a cause of the hemorrhage	Uses iodine-based contrast with potential for nephrotoxicity
MR imaging of brain	Diffusion-weighted imaging can identify ischemic stroke with hemorrhagic transformation Hemosiderin-sensitive sequences help identify microhemorrhages (seen with cerebral amyloid angiopathy but also with hypertension) Contrast studies can help rule out neoplasm	Less readily available than NCCT especially after hours May be contraindicated in certain patients with implanted devices such as pacemakers or vagal nerve stimulators More time-consuming study than CT scan and challenging to perform in unstable patients Presence of the blood and the pressure caused by the mass effect may obscure any underlying vascular malformation or tumor in the acute stage
MR angiogram of head and neck	Provides similar clinical information as CTA but can be done without nephrotoxic iodine contrast Probably better at defining vascular anatomy in patients with severe calcification of vessel wall compared with CTA	Same as above
Catheter cerebral angiogram	Gold-standard test to rule out aneurysms or AVMs Provides an opportunity for endovascular treatment	Carries a risk of stroke, vascular dissection, or rupture Uses iodine contrast with potential for nephrotoxicity

[a] Such as brainstem displacement from tissue swelling, obstructive hydrocephalus, cerebellar herniation, and ventricular extension.

- Coagulopathy
  - Caused by deficiency of coagulation proteins (eg, liver cirrhosis, disseminated intravascular coagulation)
  - Medication-induced (warfarin, heparin, newer oral anticoagulants)
  - Thrombocytopenia or medication-induced platelet dysfunction (eg, aspirin, clopidogrel)
- Hemorrhagic transformation of ischemic infarction[9]
  - Blood-brain barrier disruption and ensuing reperfusion are thought to contribute to the hemorrhagic transformation
  - Can be seen spontaneously or following recombinant tissue plasminogen activator infusion

- In most cases it is asymptomatic and detected only by brain imaging
  - In a few cases, however, it can become symptomatic and lead to neurologic decline
- AVM
  - Subarachnoid hemorrhage may coexist with parenchymal blood
  - Presence of calcification on NCCT can provide a clue
- Dural arteriovenous fistula in the tentorium[10]
- Cerebral amyloid angiopathy (CAA)[11]
  - Usually accompanied by simultaneous hemorrhage in the subarachnoid space
  - Patients may have a history of dementia of Alzheimer type
- Neoplasm
  - Intratumoral hemorrhage should be suspected when the perilesional edema is greater than expected for the size of the hemorrhage
  - Can be due to primary CNS malignancy or metastatic disease[12,13]
- Trauma
- Aneurysm
  - Posterior circulation aneurysms can rupture into the cerebellum
  - Often coexists with subarachnoid hemorrhage in the basal cistern
- Remote hemorrhage[14]
  - Occurs following supratentorial neurosurgical procedures
  - Thought to be venous in origin

Hypertension is the most common cause of cerebellar hemorrhage, and is more common in the middle-aged or older population. Hemorrhage is often located in the dentate nucleus, and may then extend to other areas. Rupture of microaneurysms along the penetrating small vessels, first recognized by Virchow and Gull and later confirmed by Charcot and Bouchard, is thought to be the cause. History of systemic or CNS malignancy may point toward neoplasm as the cause. Metastatic CNS lesions from carcinomas originating in the lung, breast, kidneys, and melanomas are more prone than others to undergo hemorrhagic transformation. Among the primary malignancies, glioblastomas frequently undergo hemorrhagic transformation. Hemorrhages occurring in younger patients may be due to drug abuse, trauma, aneurysms, or AVMs. Remote cerebellar hemorrhages have been described following supratentorial neurosurgical procedures, most commonly craniotomies. Excessive loss of cerebrospinal fluid during these procedures with resultant cerebellar "sag" is thought to be the most likely pathophysiologic mechanism.[14] These hemorrhages track along the superior cerebellar folia and are probably venous in origin. Many cases exhibit a benign course, although remote cerebellar hemorrhages can cause death or major morbidity. Hemorrhages occurring as a result of coagulopathy can sometimes demonstrate a fluid level attributable to inadequate coagulation of extravasated blood.

PROCESS OF ELIMINATION AND DIFFERENTIAL DIAGNOSIS

The differential diagnosis for patients presenting to the emergency room with acute onset of symptoms such as dizziness, nausea, vomiting, headache, or vertigo is outlined here.

- Central
  - Cerebellar infarction
  - Cerebellar hemorrhage
  - Demyelinating disorders such as multiple sclerosis or acute disseminated encephalomyelitis

- ○ Cerebellitis (infectious or noninfectious)
- ○ Medication toxicity (eg, antiseizure medications such as phenytoin or carbamazepine)
- ○ Illicit drugs and alcohol
- ○ Cerebellar neoplasm (rarely causes acute symptoms)
- Peripheral
  - ○ Vestibular neuronitis
  - ○ Labyrinthitis
  - ○ Benign paroxysmal positional vertigo
  - ○ Meniere disease

Any patients with an acute cerebellar syndrome must be examined with NCCT, which typically provides excellent visualization of the hematoma.

MANAGEMENT AND TREATMENT
Overview of Patient Evaluation

The patient evaluation overview is outlined in **Fig. 1.**

Management Principles

Airway management and mechanical ventilation

- Endotracheal intubation may be indicated for the following reasons:
  - ○ Inability to protect the airway and clear the secretions because of the depressed level of consciousness (usually with Glasgow Coma Scale [GCS] sum score ≤8)

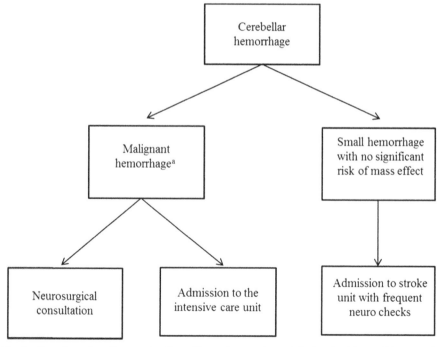

Fig. 1. Overview of patient evaluation. [a] Large hemorrhage (>3–4 cm) with or without early edema, brainstem displacement, intraventricular extension, or hydrocephalus.

○ Hypoxemic or hypercarbic respiratory failure
○ Need for hematoma evacuation
○ Apneic episodes
- Normocarbia should be maintained.
- Hyperventilation is used (only for short period) in cases of impending or progressing brain herniation. There is no role for prophylactic hyperventilation.[15]
- Bronchoscopy may be necessary to remove any foreign bodies if aspiration is suspected.

Anticoagulation and antiplatelet therapy

- All antiplatelet agents and anticoagulants should be discontinued in patients with symptomatic cerebellar hemorrhage. The decision regarding whether to restart antithrombotics and, if so, the timing of reinitiation, should be individualized depending on the balance between the estimated risks of recurrent hemorrhage and thromboembolism.[16]
- With severe bleeding and impending surgical procedure, some prefer using platelet transfusions in patients on antiplatelet therapy at the time of hemorrhage. However, the utility and safety of platelet transfusion in this setting is unknown.
- Platelet transfusion is indicated in patients with thrombocytopenia, but the precise platelet goal is not known (the generally accepted threshold for transfusion is between 50,000 and 100,000/μL).
- For patients who are receiving full-dose intravenous heparin, protamine should be used to reverse the prolongation of activated partial thromboplastin time.[17] Protamine can also be administered to patients receiving low molecular weight heparin, although the efficacy of the drug for this indication is unclear.[18]
- Patients who are on warfarin should receive intravenous vitamin K (10 mg) and replacement of clotting factors. Fresh frozen plasma (FFP) or prothrombin complex concentrate (PCC) can be used for this purpose.[19] There is no evidence that one therapy improves outcome over another, although PCC carries less risk of complications in comparison with FFP.[20,21]
- Factor VIIa does not replace all of the clotting factors and, owing to the increased risk of prothrombotic complications (ischemic stroke, myocardial infarction, deep venous thrombosis [DVT]), it is not recommended.[22,23]
- Specific antidotes for patients receiving newer oral anticoagulants such as direct thrombin inhibitors (dabigatran) or factor Xa inhibitors (rivaroxaban, apixaban) are under development[24] but not yet available. Factor replacement with PCC, 4-factor PCC, or activated PCC should be tried, although the evidence to support their use is limited.[25,26] Hemodialysis has been shown to eliminate a substantial amount of dabigatran (up to 60%), but is not a practical intervention.[27]
- Patients with intracerebral hemorrhage are at increased risk of venous thromboembolism.[28] Subcutaneous low-dose heparin should be used for prevention of DVT, and can be started within 2 to 4 days of hemorrhage onset after confirming cessation of active bleeding.[29,30] Until then, intermittent pneumatic compression devices should be used for the prevention of DVT.

Blood pressure management

- Acute hypertension is common after any intracranial hemorrhage.
- Based on recent data on intracerebral hemorrhage, lowering the blood pressure to less than 140 mm Hg systolic is probably safe.[31–33] Some centers use a goal blood pressure of less than 160/90 mm Hg or mean arterial pressure less than

110 mm Hg as recommended by the 2010 American Heart Association guide-lines on management of intracerebral hemorrhage.[34] Caution is advised in the presence of elevated intracranial pressure, as reduction in blood pressure can compromise cerebral perfusion.

Temperature management

- Fever is detrimental to the injured brain and has been shown to worsen outcome.[35,36]
- Maintain normothermia (core temperature ≤37.5 C) and use cooling devices if pharmacotherapy alone is ineffective.
- There is currently no evidence to recommend routine hypothermia for cerebellar hemorrhage.
- Fever is not usually caused by the hematoma (except in cases of ventricular hem-orrhage),[36] and instead may be a sign of systemic infection/inflammation (eg, aspiration pneumonitis or pneumonia).

Glucose management

- Hyperglycemia has been associated with worse outcomes in patients with intra-cranial hemorrhage.[37–39]
- Insulin is preferred in the intensive care unit over oral hypoglycemic agents. Insu-lin can be used as an infusion or as a "sliding scale."
- Intensive insulin therapy to maintain strict normoglycemia in critically ill patients is associated with an increased risk of hypoglycemia and worse outcomes.[40,41] Therefore, this strategy must not be used when caring for neurocritical patients, including patients with cerebellar hematomas.[42] Hypoglycemia should be avoided at all times.
- Although the optimal serum glucose range has not been established, it is a reasonable practice to maintain serum glucose concentrations between 100 and 180 mg/dL.[42]

Fluid and electrolyte management

- Avoid hypotonic fluids.
- Correct dehydration if present and maintain normovolemia using isotonic saline.
- Hyponatremia should always be corrected.
- Consider using mildly hypertonic solutions such as 1.5% saline as maintenance fluids in patients with low normal serum sodium.
- Optimize serum potassium (≥4.0 mmol/L) and magnesium (≥2.0 mg/dL). Cardiac arrhythmias can occur after cerebellar hemorrhage (owing to pressure on the brainstem), which may be aggravated by hypokalemia and hypomagnesemia.

Complications and Their Treatment

The following complications can occur with large cerebellar hemorrhages:

- Perilesional edema and mass effect causing brainstem compression and cere-bellar herniation
- Compression of the fourth ventricle producing obstructive hydrocephalus
- Extension of the hemorrhage into the ventricular system
- Recurrent hemorrhage (usually within the first 24 hours)

The therapeutic options for symptomatic mass effect include hyperosmolar agents and decompressive surgery.

Hyperosmolar therapy

Osmolar therapy with either mannitol or hypertonic saline is used in the deteriorating patient to reduce the space-occupying effects of the hemorrhage and perilesional edema. These solutions increase osmolality of the serum, which facilitates osmotic movement of water into the vasculature, thereby inducing reactive vasoconstriction. The net effect is reduction in intracranial pressure and shrinkage of tissue. These effects are more prominent on healthy brain tissue than on infarcted tissue, likely because of the preserved blood-brain barrier in healthy tissue.[43]

- Mannitol
  - The usual first dose of mannitol (20% concentration) is variable in the range of 1 to 2 g/kg.[43,44]
  - Additional doses of 0.5 g/kg every 4 to 6 hours can be given while monitoring serum osmolality.
  - As mannitol induces diuresis, it is essential to maintain euvolemia by replacing the lost fluids, preferably with isotonic saline.
  - Problems arise with mannitol use in the presence of renal failure because mannitol can lead to volume overload, which may necessitate the use of dialysis to remove 3 times the given volume 15 to 30 minutes following infusion.[45]
  - Mannitol has traditionally been used cautiously when the osmolality reaches greater than 320 mOsm for the fear of renal toxicity. This concern derives from a small study in which high doses were used as continuous infusions. Crossing the 320-mOsm threshold is probably safe as long as dehydration is avoided,[46] but caution is advised.
- Hypertonic saline
  - The commonly used concentrations are 3% (250 mL bolus), 10% (75–150 mL bolus), and 23.4% (30 mL bolus).
  - It is sometimes used as a continuous infusion of 3% (rather than a bolus) with target sodium 145 to 155 mmol/L and target osmolality of 310 to 320 mOsm/kg.[47]
  - Potential (but rare) complications with hypertonic saline include transient hypotension, pulmonary edema and heart failure, hypokalemia, hyperchloremic acidemia, coagulopathy, intravascular hemolysis, myelinolysis (only with rapid overcorrection of preexisting hyponatremia), and encephalopathy.[48,49] Phlebitis can occur if peripheral venous access is used for infusion, although this is very uncommon with infusion of 3% concentration through a large-bore peripheral line.
  - It is generally accepted that hypertonic saline should not be used if the serum sodium level is greater than 160 mmol/L. In a study of 600 patients in the neurointensive care unit, there was an independent increase in mortality in patients with a serum sodium level greater than 160 mmol/L.[50] In the same study, the incidence of renal failure was also high in patients with this degree of hypernatremia.

Whether to choose mannitol or hypertonic saline depends on the clinical situation. No study has proved superiority of one therapy over the other in the treatment of intracranial hemorrhage.

Surgical treatment

- Surgical options are considered when there is clinical deterioration attributed to mass effect from tissue swelling (**Fig. 2**).
- Deterioration can be due to either obstructive hydrocephalus, brainstem compression, or both. It may be difficult to differentiate the relative contribution

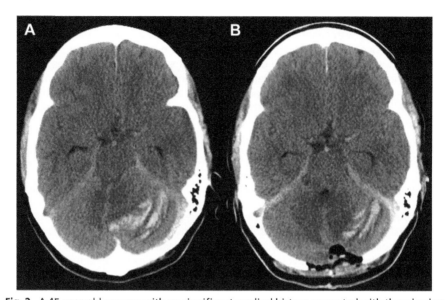

Fig. 2. A 45-year-old-woman with no significant medical history presented with thunderclap headache. Noncontrast head CT (*A*) showed acute intraparenchymal, subarachnoid, and subdural hemorrhage in the left cerebellum with mass effect, midline shift, and effacement of the fourth ventricle and basilar cisterns, and development of obstructive hydrocephalus. She underwent emergent suboccipital decompressive craniectomy and partial evacuation of the hematoma (*B*) with resultant improvement in the mass effect. Arteriovenous malformation was found during surgery, and was fully resected. The patient did well and was discharged home after 5 days.

of these 2 complications to the clinical decline when both are present clinically and radiologically. Surgical evacuation of the hematoma with suboccipital craniectomy is the procedure of choice.[6,51,52]

- External ventricular drain (EVD) is used to treat obstructive hydrocephalus. Although it may be performed in isolation, it is optimally combined with hematoma evacuation. In patients with obliteration of cisterns, it is advisable to evacuate the hematoma as well, because EVD alone may be insufficient to reverse the clinical decline.[53] The risk of supratentorial cerebellar herniation when ventriculostomy is performed in isolation is possible, but the magnitude of this risk remains poorly defined because this complication has been documented in only a few case reports.
- Several different criteria have been proposed to select patients for surgery and/ or EVD placement.[5,52,54,55] These criteria are based on radiographic features (hematoma size, presence of hydrocephalus, ventricular extension, evidence of brainstem compression, and cisternal effacement) and clinical presentation (GCS score and loss of brainstem reflexes).
- If the hemorrhage is less than 3 cm in diameter and there is no brainstem compression or hydrocephalus, reasonable outcomes may be achieved without surgery.
- More recently, stereotactic burr-hole aspiration has been used for selected patients with smaller hemorrhages (mean hematoma volume 21.8 ± 5.8 mL). This procedure is less invasive, and in one study resulted in no surgery-related complications.[56]

EVALUATION OF OUTCOME AND LONG-TERM RECOMMENDATIONS

- Mortality can range anywhere from 25% to 57%.[6,57–59]
- Outcome following surgery is strongly correlated with the preoperative clinical status,[57,60] and can be favorable in more than half of the patients. However, a worse preoperative neurologic examination does not necessarily imply a poor prognosis.[4] Thus, in the absence of multiple comorbidities, surgery should be recommended even in patients with poor preoperative neurologic status.

Case study

A 50-year-old right-handed man presented to the emergency room with a 3-day history of severe headache, dizziness, nausea, and mild gait unsteadiness. His only significant medical history was diabetes mellitus for several years controlled by metformin. He did not have hypertension, coagulopathy, or thrombocytopenia. He took aspirin (81 mg) daily. His level of consciousness was normal at the time of admission. Neurologic examination revealed gait ataxia and left-sided dysmetria. CT scan of the head demonstrated an acute left cerebellar hemorrhage (**Fig. 3**).

He was admitted to the intensive care unit (ICU) for monitoring. MR imaging of the brain with MR angiography did not show any signs of an underlying mass or vascular malformation. Neurosurgery was consulted and the patient underwent a diagnostic cerebral angiogram (**Fig. 4**). This angiogram revealed a small AVM in the left cerebellar hemisphere supplied by a distal left posterior inferior cerebellar artery branch and draining via a vermian vein.

The patient did well throughout his hospital course and did not need any surgical intervention for the hemorrhage. After 2 days of monitoring in the ICU, he was transferred to the floor and was discharged shortly afterward from the hospital. All of his deficits had improved significantly by the time of his discharge. Three weeks later, he underwent suboccipital craniotomy for resection of the AVM.

This case highlights the importance of additional imaging to evaluate the etiology of the hemorrhage in patients without a clear cause.

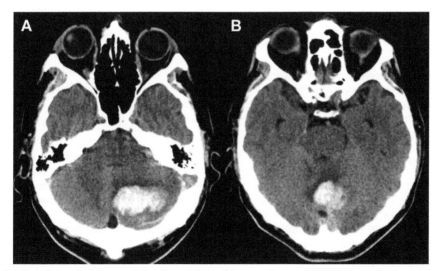

Fig. 3. Left hemisphere cerebellar hemorrhage (*A*) extending to the contralateral side and the vermis. (*B*) There is mild degree of surrounding edema with minimal mass effect on the fourth ventricle and effacement of the quadrigeminal cistern, but no obstructive hydrocephalus.

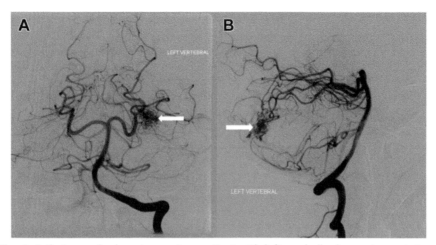

Fig. 4. Catheter cerebral angiogram in a patient with left cerebellar hemorrhage. Antero-posterior view (*A*) and lateral view (*B*), showing small arteriovenous malformation (*white arrows*) in the left cerebellar hemisphere supplied by a distal branch of the left posterior inferior cerebellar artery and draining via a vermian vein.

SUMMARY

Cerebellar hemorrhage (when small) can present with few nonspecific symptoms mimicking ischemic stroke, or (when larger) may present with catastrophic neurologic deterioration. Smaller hemorrhages can further expand or develop perilesional edema extensively enough to cause mass effect with resultant brainstem displacement and obstructive hydrocephalus. These life-threatening complications must be recognized and treated promptly. Any coagulopathy should be corrected immediately to prevent expansion of the hematoma. Most of the hemorrhages are hypertensive in origin, but in select cases vascular imaging or MR imaging may be needed to identify the cause. Patients with large hemorrhages are at risk of complications and are best managed in an ICU. Controversies exist with regard to the choice of surgical procedure (EVD or craniectomy with hematoma evacuation, or both) and the optimal timing. This decision depends on both clinical and radiographic characteristics. Postoperative outcome is influenced by the neurologic preoperative state; however, in the absence of multiple medical comorbidities or advanced age, surgery is recommended for most patients having symptomatic mass effect, including those with severe neurologic deterioration.

REFERENCES

1. Heros RC. Cerebellar hemorrhage and infarction. Stroke 1982;13(1):106–9.
2. Lui TN, Fairholm DJ, Shu TF, et al. Surgical treatment of spontaneous cerebellar hemorrhage. Surg Neurol 1985;23(6):555–8.
3. Dinsdale HB. Spontaneous hemorrhage in the posterior fossa. A Study of primary cerebellar and pontine hemorrhages with observations on their pathogenesis. Arch Neurol 1964;10:200–17.
4. Dahdaleh NS, Dlouhy BJ, Viljoen SV, et al. Clinical and radiographic predictors of neurological outcome following posterior fossa decompression for spontaneous cerebellar hemorrhage. J Clin Neurosci 2012;19(9):1236–41.

5. Kirollos RW, Tyagi AK, Ross SA, et al. Management of spontaneous cerebellar hematomas: a prospective treatment protocol. Neurosurgery 2001;49(6): 1378–86.
6. St Louis EK, Wijdicks EF, Li H, et al. Predictors of poor outcome in patients with a spontaneous cerebellar hematoma. Can J Neurol Sci 2000;27(1):32–6.
7. St Louis EK, Wijdicks EF, Li H. Predicting neurologic deterioration in patients with cerebellar hematomas. Neurology 1998;51(5):1364–9.
8. Gupta R, Phan CM, Leidecker C, et al. Evaluation of dual-energy CT for differentiating intracerebral hemorrhage from iodinated contrast material staining. Radiology 2010;257(1):205–11.
9. Sakamoto Y, Kimura K, Iguchi Y, et al. Hemorrhagic transformation in acute cerebellar infarction. Cerebrovasc Dis 2011;32(4):327–33.
10. Satoh K, Satomi J, Nakajima N, et al. Cerebellar hemorrhage caused by dural arteriovenous fistula: a review of five cases. J Neurosurg 2001;94(3):422–6.
11. Itoh Y, Yamada M, Hayakawa M, et al. Cerebral amyloid angiopathy: a significant cause of cerebellar as well as lobar cerebral hemorrhage in the elderly. J Neurol Sci 1993;116(2):135–41.
12. Kim MS, Kim SW, Chang CH, et al. Cerebellar pilocytic astrocytomas with spontaneous intratumoral hemorrhage in adult. J Korean Neurosurg Soc 2011;49(6): 363–6.
13. Mesiwala AH, Avellino AM, Roberts TS, et al. Spontaneous cerebellar hemorrhage due to a juvenile pilocytic astrocytoma: case report and review of the literature. Pediatr Neurosurg 2001;34(5):235–8.
14. Friedman JA, Piepgras DG, Duke DA, et al. Remote cerebellar hemorrhage after supratentorial surgery. Neurosurgery 2001;49(6):1327–40.
15. Wijdicks EF, Sheth KN, Carter BS, et al. Recommendations for the management of cerebral and cerebellar infarction with swelling: a statement for healthcare professionals from the American Heart Association/American Stroke Association. Stroke 2014;45(4):1222–38.
16. Rabinstein AA, Gupta A. Restarting anticoagulation after intracranial hemorrhage: a risky decision with no recipe. Neurology 2014;82(12):1016–7.
17. Hirsh J, Bauer KA, Donati MB, et al. Parenteral anticoagulants: American College of Chest Physicians Evidence-Based Clinical Practice Guidelines (8th edition). Chest 2008;133(6 Suppl):141S–59S.
18. van Veen JJ, Maclean RM, Hampton KK, et al. Protamine reversal of low molecular weight heparin: clinically effective? Blood Coagul Fibrinolysis 2011;22(7): 565–70.
19. Fredriksson K, Norrving B, Stromblad LG. Emergency reversal of anticoagulation after intracerebral hemorrhage. Stroke 1992;23(7):972–7.
20. Boulis NM, Bobek MP, Schmaier A, et al. Use of factor IX complex in warfarin-related intracranial hemorrhage. Neurosurgery 1999;45(5):1113–8.
21. Sjoblom L, Hardemark HG, Lindgren A, et al. Management and prognostic features of intracerebral hemorrhage during anticoagulant therapy: a Swedish multicenter study. Stroke 2001;32(11):2567–74.
22. Mayer SA, Brun NC, Begtrup K, et al. Efficacy and safety of recombinant activated factor VII for acute intracerebral hemorrhage. N Engl J Med 2008; 358(20):2127–37.
23. Mayer SA, Brun NC, Begtrup K, et al. Recombinant activated factor VII for acute intracerebral hemorrhage. N Engl J Med 2005;352(8):777–85.
24. Ansell J. Blocking bleeding: reversing anticoagulant therapy. Nat Med 2013; 19(4):402–4.

25. Siegal DM, Garcia DA, Crowther MA. How I treat target-specific oral anticoagulant-associated bleeding. Blood 2014;123(8):1152–8.

26. Pernod G, Albaladejo P, Godier A, et al. Management of major bleeding complications and emergency surgery in patients on long-term treatment with direct oral anticoagulants, thrombin or factor-Xa inhibitors. Proposals of the working group on perioperative haemostasis (GIHP) - March 2013. Ann Fr Anesth Reanim 2013;32(10):691–700 [in French].

27. Khadzhynov D, Wagner F, Formella S, et al. Effective elimination of dabigatran by haemodialysis. a phase I single-centre study in patients with end-stage renal disease. Thromb Haemost 2013;109(4):596–605.

28. Masotti L, Godoy DA, Napoli MD, et al. Pharmacological prophylaxis of venous thromboembolism during acute phase of spontaneous intracerebral hemorrhage: what do we know about risks and benefits? Clin Appl Thromb Hemost 2012;18(4):393–402.

29. Wu TC, Kasam M, Harun N, et al. Pharmacological deep vein thrombosis prophylaxis does not lead to hematoma expansion in intracerebral hemorrhage with intraventricular extension. Stroke 2011;42(3):705–9.

30. Boeer A, Voth E, Henze T, et al. Early heparin therapy in patients with spontaneous intracerebral haemorrhage. J Neurol Neurosurg Psychiatry 1991;54(5):466–7.

31. Anderson CS, Huang Y, Wang JG, et al. Intensive blood pressure reduction in acute cerebral haemorrhage trial (INTERACT): a randomised pilot trial. Lancet Neurol 2008;7(5):391–9.

32. Qureshi AI. Antihypertensive treatment of acute cerebral hemorrhage (ATACH): rationale and design. Neurocrit Care 2007;6(1):56–66.

33. Anderson CS, Heeley E, Huang Y, et al. Rapid blood-pressure lowering in patients with acute intracerebral hemorrhage. N Engl J Med 2013;368(25):2355–65.

34. Morgenstern LB, Hemphill JC 3rd, Anderson C, et al. Guidelines for the management of spontaneous intracerebral hemorrhage: a guideline for healthcare professionals from the American Heart Association/American Stroke Association. Stroke 2010;41(9):2108–29.

35. Takagi K. Body temperature in acute stroke. Stroke 2002;33(9):2154–5.

36. Schwarz S, Hafner K, Aschoff A, et al. Incidence and prognostic significance of fever following intracerebral hemorrhage. Neurology 2000;54(2):354–61.

37. Kimura K, Iguchi Y, Inoue T, et al. Hyperglycemia independently increases the risk of early death in acute spontaneous intracerebral hemorrhage. J Neurol Sci 2007;255(1–2):90–4.

38. Passero S, Ciacci G, Ulivelli M. The influence of diabetes and hyperglycemia on clinical course after intracerebral hemorrhage. Neurology 2003;61(10):1351–6.

39. Wu YT, Li TY, Lu SC, et al. Hyperglycemia as a predictor of poor outcome at discharge in patients with acute spontaneous cerebellar hemorrhage. Cerebellum 2012;11(2):543–8.

40. Finfer S, Chittock DR, Su SY, et al. Intensive versus conventional glucose control in critically ill patients. N Engl J Med 2009;360(13):1283–97.

41. van den Berghe G, Wouters P, Weekers F, et al. Intensive insulin therapy in critically ill patients. N Engl J Med 2001;345(19):1359–67.

42. Godoy DA, Di Napoli M, Rabinstein AA. Treating hyperglycemia in neurocritical patients: benefits and perils. Neurocrit Care 2010;13(3):425–38.

43. Videen TO, Zazulia AR, Manno EM, et al. Mannitol bolus preferentially shrinks noninfarcted brain in patients with ischemic stroke. Neurology 2001;57(11):2120–2.

44. Diringer MN, Scalfani MT, Zazulia AR, et al. Cerebral hemodynamic and meta-bolic effects of equi-osmolar doses mannitol and 23.4% saline in patients with edema following large ischemic stroke. Neurocrit Care 2011;14(1):11–7.
45. Datar S, Wijdicks EF. Neurologic manifestations of acute liver failure. Handb Clin Neurol 2014;120:645–59.
46. Diringer MN, Zazulia AR. Osmotic therapy: fact and fiction. Neurocrit Care 2004; 1(2):219–33.
47. Hauer EM, Stark D, Staykov D, et al. Early continuous hypertonic saline infusion in patients with severe cerebrovascular disease. Crit Care Med 2011;39(7): 1766–72.
48. Worthley LI, Cooper DJ, Jones N. Treatment of resistant intracranial hyperten-sion with hypertonic saline. Report of two cases. J Neurosurg 1988;68(3): 478–81.
49. Bhardwaj A, Ulatowski JA. Hypertonic saline solutions in brain injury. Curr Opin Crit Care 2004;10(2):126–31.
50. Aiyagari V, Deibert E, Diringer MN. Hypernatremia in the neurologic intensive care unit: how high is too high? J Crit Care 2006;21(2):163–72.
51. Yanaka K, Meguro K, Fujita K, et al. Immediate surgery reduces mortality in deeply comatose patients with spontaneous cerebellar hemorrhage. Neurol Med Chir (Tokyo) 2000;40(6):295–9 [discussion: 299–300].
52. Kobayashi S, Sato A, Kageyama Y, et al. Treatment of hypertensive cerebellar hemorrhage–surgical or conservative management? Neurosurgery 1994;34(2): 246–50 [discussion: 250–1].
53. van Loon J, Van Calenbergh F, Goffin J, et al. Controversies in the management of spontaneous cerebellar haemorrhage. a consecutive series of 49 cases and review of the literature. Acta Neurochir (Wien) 1993;122(3–4):187–93.
54. Luparello V, Canavero S. Treatment of hypertensive cerebellar hemorrhage–sur-gical or conservative management? Neurosurgery 1995;37(3):552–3.
55. Taneda M, Hayakawa T, Mogami H. Primary cerebellar hemorrhage. Quadrige-minal cistern obliteration on CT scans as a predictor of outcome. J Neurosurg 1987;67(4):545–52.
56. Lee JH, Kim DW, Kang SD. Stereotactic burr hole aspiration surgery for sponta-neous hypertensive cerebellar hemorrhage. J Cerebrovasc Endovasc Neuro-surg 2012;14(3):170–4.
57. Dammann P, Asgari S, Bassiouni H, et al. Spontaneous cerebellar hemorrhage–experience with 57 surgically treated patients and review of the literature. Neu-rosurg Rev 2011;34(1):77–86.
58. Yanaka K, Meguro K, Fujita K, et al. Postoperative brainstem high intensity is correlated with poor outcomes for patients with spontaneous cerebellar hemor-rhage. Neurosurgery 1999;45(6):1323–7 [discussion: 1327–8].
59. Waidhauser E, Hamburger C, Marguth F. Neurosurgical management of cere-bellar hemorrhage. Neurosurg Rev 1990;13(3):211–7.
60. Ott KH, Kase CS, Ojemann RG, et al. Cerebellar hemorrhage: diagnosis and treatment. a review of 56 cases. Arch Neurol 1974;31(3):160–7.

Neuro-ophthalmic Manifestations of Cerebellar Disease

Shin C. Beh, MD[a], Teresa C. Frohman, PA-C[a],
Elliot M. Frohman, MD, PhD[a,b],*

KEYWORDS

- Cerebellum • Neuro-ophthalmology • Eye movements • Nystagmus • Saccades
- Smooth pursuit • Vestibuloocular reflex • Vergence

KEY POINTS

- The cerebellum is intimately involved in all classes of eye movements.
- Ocular motor findings can help localize the cerebellar structure that is dysfunctional.
- The 3 regions of the cerebellum involved in ocular motor control are (1) the oculomotor vermis (lobule VI and VII) and fastigial nuclei, (2) the uvula and nodulus, and (3) the flocculus and paraflocculus. Lesions to each region result in a unique clinical syndrome.
- Certain cerebellar disorders may result in abnormalities of the afferent visual pathway.
- Oscillopsia may arise from nystagmus or saccadic intrusions, and be highly disabling in some patients. Certain therapeutic measures can dampen the nystagmus or saccadic intrusions to improve the visual acuity of these patients.

INTRODUCTION

The cerebellum is responsible for sculpting and refining ocular movements to ensure their precision and accuracy (to bring images to the fovea and keep them stable there), thereby guaranteeing the best possible visual acuity and clarity despite changes in body or head positions or movement of the object of interest. Cerebellar lesions do not abolish eye movements but cause them to become coarse, slow, imprecise, and unreliable, leading to degradation in the quality of vision.

Disclosures: Dr S.C. Beh has no relevant disclosures. T.C. Frohman is a consultant and speaker for Biogen Idec and Novartis. Dr E.M. Frohman has received speaker fees from Biogen Idec, Teva Neuroscience, and Acorda Pharmaceuticals, and consulting fees from Biogen Idec, Teva Neurosciences, Abbott, Acorda Therapeutics, and Novartis.
[a] Department of Neurology, University of Texas Southwestern Medical Center, 5323 Harry Hines Boulevard, Dallas, TX 75390, USA; [b] Department of Ophthalmology, University of Texas Southwestern Medical Center, 5323 Harry Hines Boulevard, Dallas, TX 75390, USA
* Corresponding author. Department of Neurology, University of Texas Southwestern Medical Center, 5323 Harry Hines Boulevard, Dallas, TX 75390.
E-mail address: elliot.frohman@utsouthwestern.edu

Neurol Clin 32 (2014) 1009–1080
http://dx.doi.org/10.1016/j.ncl.2014.07.002　　neurologic.theclinics.com
0733-8619/14/$ – see front matter © 2014 Elsevier Inc. All rights reserved.

CASE VIGNETTE

A 60-year-old man complains of a bouncing of his vision when he walks or drives. As a result, he has to stop in order to read road signs or to look at the facial features of others. He also reports progressively worsening gait imbalance, but denies any cognitive deficits, autonomic symptoms, or parkinsonian features. He has no family history of similar complaints. Examination reveals gaze-evoked nystagmus, rebound nystagmus, and saccadic pursuit. Ophthalmoscopy revealed that his discs were unstable and moved with head oscillations. He lost more than 5 lines of acuity when the examiner oscillated his head in the horizontal and vertical planes. He had some mild dysmetria, dysdiadochokinesia, and heel-shin ataxia. His gait was wide based and he was not able to maintain his stance when his eyes were closed. He had diminution of sensation over his shoulders, posterior torso, and proximal lower extremities. Magnetic resonance imaging (MRI) revealed cerebellar atrophy, most noticeably over the anterior and dorsal vermis. What is his likely diagnosis? What electrophysiologic test can help confirm this diagnosis?

The cerebellum is involved in the control of all classes of eye movements, both in their real-time, immediate modulation, and in their long-term adaptive calibration.[1] When approaching cerebellar neuro-ophthalmic abnormalities, 3 important caveats should be remembered. First, the cerebellum is able to adapt and compensate for lesions, and therefore the ocular motor manifestations of acute cerebellar lesions can change, and usually improve with time. Second, because of the intimate relationship between the brainstem and cerebellar pathways that mediate eye movements, lesions affecting the cerebellar peduncles, or the cerebellar brainstem projections (both efferent and afferent), can also give rise to clinical signs and symptoms suggestive of cerebellar dysfunction. The presence of such phenomenology does not automatically indicate damage to the cerebellum. Furthermore, in disorders that affect both the brainstem and cerebellum, it may be impossible to accurately localize the source of a specific ocular motility disorder. In addition, although eye movement abnormalities are the most prominent neuro-ophthalmic manifestation of cerebellar disease, afferent visual pathway disorders may coexist with some cerebellar disorders; the presence of such findings often provides vital clues regarding the diagnosis.

This article begins with an overview of the role of cerebellar structures in modulating various classes of eye movements, including gaze holding, the vestibular ocular reflex (VOR), saccades, vergence, smooth pursuit, and the optokinetic reflex (OKR). This overview is germane to the later discussion of the different ocular motor abnormalities that can arise from cerebellar disorders. In addition, some treatment options for oscillopsia, a common symptom of cerebellar disease, are discussed.

THE ROLE OF THE CEREBELLUM IN OCULAR MOTOR CONTROL

The goal of all eye movements is to direct and maintain the angle of gaze (ie, the line of sight of the fovea) on an object of interest, to ensure the best visual acuity and clarity. Three distinct mechanisms help the visual system achieve this goal: (1) fixation, which detects (and corrects for) any retinal image drift, and suppresses unwanted saccades; (2) the VOR, by which eye movements compensate for head perturbations at short latency, ensuring visual acuity during locomotion; and (3) the gaze-holding system, which counteracts the elasticity of orbital tissue.[1–3]

The cerebellum continuously uses visual input to calibrate and optimize all categories of eye movements. Neurons in the dorsolateral pontine nuclei and climbing fibers from the inferior olivary nuclei (ION) convey visual signals to the cerebellum.[1,3,4] Another important aspect of the role of the cerebellum in calibrating eye movements involves comparing the afferent visual signals with eye movement commands (efference copies), which are conveyed to the flocculus via the paramedian tract (a pontine structure that receives projections from almost all ocular motor structures).[1,5] The 3 regions of the cerebellum involved in ocular motor control are (1) the oculomotor vermis (lobule VI and VII) and fastigial nuclei, (2) the uvula and nodulus, and (3) the flocculus and paraflocculus. The flocculus-paraflocculus complex and the caudal vermis (nodulus and uvula) together constitute the vestibulocerebellum. Lesions affecting these 3 regions give rise to 3 principal clinical cerebellar syndromes, which are summarized in **Table 1.**[1]

A BRIEF OVERVIEW OF OCULAR MOVEMENTS

Ocular movements are controlled by the 6 extraocular muscles, which are grouped into 3 agonist-antagonist pairs obeying Sherington's law of reciprocal innervations: lateral rectus (LR) and medial rectus (MR), superior rectus (SR) and inferior rectus (IR), and superior oblique (SO) and inferior oblique (IO).[1] The abducens nerve (cranial nerve [CN] VI) innervates the LR, the trochlear nerve (CN IV) innervates the SO, and the oculomotor nerve (CN III) innervates the remaining extraocular muscles. The extraocular muscles are also yoked in pairs that ensure that both eyes move together, and are innervated according to Hering's law of equal innervations. The connections that link the yoked muscles that mediate horizontal eye movements are contained within the medial longitudinal fasciculus (MLF).[1,6]

Table 1	
The 3 principal cerebellar syndromes	
Syndrome	**Features**
Flocculus-Paraflocculus Syndrome	• Saccadic smooth pursuit and VOR suppression • Impaired gaze holding (resulting in gaze-evoked nystagmus, and rebound nystagmus) • Downbeat nystagmus • Impaired VOR adaptation (gain and direction) • Impaired OKRs • Postsaccadic drifts
Nodulus-Ventral Uvula Syndrome	• Impaired velocity storage (leading to prolonged postrotatory nystagmus, failure of tilt suppression of postrotatory nystagmus, perverted head-shaking nystagmus, and/or periodic alternating nystagmus) • Positional nystagmus
Oculomotor Vermis-Caudal Fastigial Nucleus Syndrome	Dorsal vermis damage: bilateral *hypometric* saccades, saccadic smooth pursuit, impaired OKR Caudal fastigial nuclei damage: bilateral *hypermetric* saccades, saccadic smooth pursuit, impaired OKR Unilateral dorsal vermis dysfunction: • Ocular contrapulsion (contraversive ocular deviation) • Saccadic contrapulsion (hypermetric contralateral, and hypometric ipsilateral saccades) • Ipsiversive saccadic pursuit Unilateral caudal fastigial nuclear dysfunction: • Ocular ipsipulsion (ipsiversive ocular deviation) • Saccadic ipsipulsion (hypometric contralateral and hypermetric ipsilateral saccades) • Contraversive saccadic pursuit

All ocular movements that enter this final common pathway consist of 2 main components: the pulse and the step. The pulse, or velocity command, provides the high-frequency phasic discharge, or torque, that overcomes the viscosity of orbital tissue (eg, tendons, muscles), and moves the eyes from one orbital position to another. The step, or position command, provides the steady tonic discharge that helps maintain the stability of the eye in its new position. For horizontal eye movements, the excitatory burst neurons (EBNs) that generate the pulse command are located in the pontine paramedian reticular formation (PPRF); for vertical and torsional eye movements, the EBNs reside in the rostral interstitial nucleus of the MLF (riMLF).[1,6]

The step command is generated by a brainstem network that integrates eye velocity commands, and is referred to as the neural integrator.[7–9] The neural integrator for vertical and torsional gaze is the interstitial nucleus of Cajal (INC) in the midbrain.[10] For horizontal gaze, it is the nucleus prepositus hypoglossi (NPH) and medial vestibular nucleus (MVN), located in the pons.[11,12]

SACCADES

Saccades are rapid eye movements that redirect the fovea from one object of interest to another, and must be fast and accurate to ensure visual clarity. Human saccades follow a target jump within ~200 milliseconds, are fast (~600°/s), brief (~30–100 milliseconds), accurate, and stop abruptly (with little subsequent ocular drift).[1,6]

Saccades are generated by a pulse-step neuronal signal, as discussed earlier. For saccades to be accurate, the pulse command must be of the correct magnitude. To keep the eye still following the saccade, the step command must match that of the pulse, and must be sustained for the duration of the fixation.[1] The superior colliculi and cortical areas responsible for saccade commands (ie, the frontal eye fields, parietal eye field, and supplementary eye field) project to the long-lead burst neurons (LLBNs) in the brainstem. Some LLBNs project to the premotor burst neurons and others (particularly those in the nucleus reticularis tegmenti pontis [NRTP]) convey saccade commands to the cerebellum.[6,13–15] The superior colliculi project to the dorsolateral pontine nucleus (DLPN).[16] Both the NRTP and DLPN project to the oculomotor vermis, as well as the caudal fastigial nuclei.[17,18]

The premotor burst neurons responsible for saccade generation consist of EBNs and inhibitory burst neurons (IBNs). As mentioned previously, the EBNs for horizontal gaze are located in the PPRF, whereas EBNs for vertical and torsional gaze are located in the riMLF.[1,6] In contrast, IBNs are responsible for suppressing the activity in the antagonist pair of extraocular muscles. For example, a rightward saccade command excites the right EBN as well as the right abducens nucleus and right IBNs. These IBNs then inhibit the left abducens nucleus, left EBNs, and left IBNs. For horizontal gaze, the IBNs are located in the medullary reticular formation; for vertical and torsional gaze, they reside in the region of the INC and riMLF.[1,6] Omnipause neurons (OPNs), located close to the midline in the raphe interpositus nucleus, project to all 4 groups of burst neurons and tonically inhibit them, but pause firing just before a saccade is generated.[1,6,19] They maintain the stability of saccade-related neurons, and prevent high-frequency conjugate eye oscillations.[1,6,20]

Disorders of Saccadic Accuracy

The oculomotor vermis is responsible for saccadic control and adaptation. Purkinje cells from the oculomotor vermis project to the ipsilateral caudal fastigial nucleus (CFN),[17,18,21] which in turn conveys saccade commands to the premotor burst neurons in the contralateral brainstem.[6] Conjugate saccade pulse dysmetria is a classic sign of cerebellar disease.[1,22–25] Oculomotor vermal lesions that spare the CFN result in hypometric saccades.[26–33] In contrast, unilateral CFN lesions result in hypometric contralesional, and hypermetric ipsilesional saccades,[34,35] and severe saccadic hypermetria arises from total cerebellectomy and bilateral CFN inactivation.[24,34,36] The function of the CFN, therefore, must be to overcome the inherent hypermetria of the brainstem saccade pulse generator,[27] presumably by balancing the activity between EBNs and IBNs located in the left and right pontine and medullary formation.[37–40]

Saccade-related neurons within the CFN fire before the onset of contraversive saccades, and following the onset of ipsiversive saccades[41]; this pattern of firing suggests that the CFN provides the push for contraversive saccades to move the eyes toward a target, and apply the brakes for ipsiversive saccades to stop the eye when it reaches the desired position. Therefore, in unilateral fastigial lesions, contralesional saccades are hypometric because of insufficient push, and ipsilesional saccades are hypermetric as a result of impaired slowing. In contrast, bilateral oculomotor vermal lesions remove their inhibitory effect on the CFN (thereby *disinhibiting the inhibitors*) and result in bilateral hypometric saccades.

CFN damage also affects vertical saccades and gaze position, because both CFN are active during vertical saccades.[40,42,43] In unilateral CFN lesions, the push from the unaffected CFN is unopposed, causing an ipsilesional horizontal deviation of vertical saccades. During fixation, the eyes are often deviated slightly toward the side of the lesion.[34,40] This asymmetry in CFN activity provides the pathobiological mechanism for ocular and saccadic lateropulsion (discussed later).

The ventral posterior interposed nuclei (VPIN) fire for every saccade.[44] The VPIN receive projections from saccade-related pontine nuclei via the paraflocculus.[45,46] Each VPIN in turn conveys efferent projections to the contralateral superior colliculi and contralateral INC.[47] In primates, VPIN inactivation results in hypermetric upward saccades, and hypometric downward saccades, as well as upward deviation of horizontally directed saccades,[48] akin to the horizontal saccadic lateropulsion.

It is important to distinguish saccadic dysmetria from postsaccadic drifts. Unlike the corrective quick phase that follows saccade pulse dysmetria, the postsaccadic drift usually occurs in the same direction as the pulse command (even if the pulse was hypermetric) and is attributed to a pulse-step mismatch in which the step command is larger than the pulse.[25]

Slow Saccades

Slow saccades may arise from disorders of the extraocular muscles, their CNs, MLF, or brainstem. Slow saccades do not occur in isolated cerebellar lesions but may be present in conditions in which cerebellar ataxia is prominent. Quick phases are typically slow or absent, but smooth pursuit and VOR are normal; in such situations, a moving target is needed to generate volitional pursuit movements.[1] Slow saccades are a prominent feature of spinocerebellar ataxia (SCA) type 2 (SCA2) and SCA7 (discussed later), and often distinguish them from the other SCAs. Selective slowing of horizontal or vertical saccades may occur in certain disorders and as a result, when patients attempt diagonal saccades, the trajectories of these movements are strongly curved. Horizontal saccades may be selectively affected early in SCA2.[1] Vertical saccades may be slowed early in the course of Whipple disease,[49] progressive supranuclear palsy (PSP),[50] and neuroacanthocytosis.[51] As a paraneoplastic manifestation, slow horizontal saccades have been associated with prostate carcinoma,[52] and slow vertical saccades have been observed in conjunction with anti-Ma2 antibodies.[53]

Decelerating (Stuttering) Saccades

Healthy subjects are normally able to make a single saccade to a target of interest; these saccades have smooth velocity profiles that are bell-shaped for small movements, but get progressively positively skewed for larger ones.[6] Stuttering saccades refers to the abrupt, premature, partial deceleration of the eyes, followed by successful resumption of the original movement.[1,6] During large-amplitude saccades, transient decelerations may be seen in normal individuals,[54] but these decelerations are more prominent in certain diseases.

In late-onset Tay-Sachs disease (LOTS), saccadic waveforms often show transient decelerations, which are difficult to appreciate at the bedside.[6,55] Because LOTS affects both the brainstem and cerebellum, it is not possible to pinpoint the precise neural pathway that results in this phenomenon. One hypothesis is that vermal Purkinje cell dysfunction disinhibits the FOR, resulting in the saccade being choked off prematurely.[6] Stuttering saccades have also been observed in a case of stiff person syndrome (SPS) associated with cerebellar ataxia in the presence of anti–glutamic acid decarboxylase (anti-GAD) antibodies.[56] The selective loss of cerebellar Purkinje cells in anti-GAD ataxia,[57] affirms the role of Purkinje cell dysfunction in stuttering saccades. Other disorders with decelerating saccades are Wernicke encephalopathy and Wilson disease.[1]

Saccadic Intrusions and Oscillations

Although saccadic intrusions are a normal finding, in certain neurologic disorders they may manifest at a higher frequency and/or amplitude, reflecting dysfunction of the brainstem, cerebellum, superior colliculus, basal ganglia, and/or cerebral hemispheres.[58] Saccadic intrusions may be distinguished from oscillations by the presence of an intersaccadic interval in the former.[1,58] Saccadic intrusions include square wave jerks (SWJ), square wave pulses, macrosaccadic oscillations, and saccadic pulses. Saccadic oscillations (ie, without any intersaccadic interval) include ocular flutter and opsoclonus.[58]

SWJ and square wave pulses

The most common of saccadic intrusions, SWJs are small, conjugate couplets of horizontal saccades (about 0.5° in size) that take the eyes away from a fixation point, before a refixation saccade moves them back, after a normal intersaccadic interval of 200 to 400 milliseconds.[1,58]

They can be seen in healthy adults (especially in the elderly), but are a prominent finding in PSP and Huntington chorea, as well as certain ataxic disorders, including SCAs (particularly SCA3), Friedreich ataxia (FRDA), multiple system atrophy (MSA), and ataxia with ocular motor apraxia type 2 (AOA2).[1,58–67] SWJs may also be increased following opioid use[68] and cigarette smoking.[69]

Although the precise neural mechanisms that generate SWJs is unclear, some clinicians have hypothesized that a dysfunctional inhibitory system, which includes the cerebellum, fails to suppress unwanted saccades.[1,58] The coexistence of downbeat nystagmus (DBN) and SWJs (resulting in conspicuous eye movement abnormality termed bow-tie nystagmus) supports the role of cerebellar networks in the genesis of SWJs.[58,70]

Macro-SWJs (also called square wave pulses) consist of large-amplitude saccadic intrusions followed by a large-amplitude return saccade at a short intersaccadic interval of 80 milliseconds.[1,58,71,72] Macro-SWJs may result from impaired input from the CFN or superior colliculi to the OPN.[73,74]

Macrosaccadic oscillations

Macrosaccadic oscillations (MSO) refer to runs of horizontal saccades, with a crescendo buildup followed by a decrescendo in amplitude, and an intersaccadic interval of 200 milliseconds.[1,6,75] They are usually precipitated by gaze shifts and reattempted fixation.[6] MSO reflect saccadic dysmetria in which both the primary and corrective saccades are so hypermetric that they overshoot the target continuously in both directions, therefore oscillating around the fixation point.[1] They differ from SWJs, which take the eye less than 2° away from the target, and return it within a normal intersaccadic interval.[76] MSO can be distinguished from opsoclonus and ocular flutter by the presence of the intersaccadic period of 200 milliseconds.[6]

Studies in nonhuman primates have suggested that excessive activity in the caudal superior colliculi, or inactivation of the rostral superior colliculi, may be responsible for MSO.[77–79] In humans, MSO have been observed in hereditary cerebellar ataxia,[80] and are also attributed to CFN and occasionally pontine lesions.[1,3,6,75,81]

Saccadic pulses

Saccadic pulses are brief saccadic intrusions that move the eyes off target, immediately followed by a slower drift that returns them to position.[1] Saccadic pulses may occur in runs or as doublets.[58] They have been reported in multiple sclerosis (MS) and traumatic brain injuries,[81–83] or as a side effect of opioids.[68]

Opsoclonus and ocular flutter

Opsoclonus refers to bursts of high-frequency, arrhythmic, chaotic, saccadic oscillations with horizontal, vertical, and torsional components. Ocular flutter consists of high-frequency bursts of oscillations limited to the horizontal plane. Both are thought to be saccadic in origin; hence, each burst of oscillations consists of back-to-back saccades without any intersaccadic interval. These oscillations persist during fixation, smooth pursuit, convergence, sleep, and eyelid closure. Opsoclonus is usually continuous and is associated with ataxia, encephalopathy, behavioral disturbances, as well as myoclonus.[1,6,58,84]

The pathophysiologic mechanisms of ocular flutter and opsoclonus are unknown. Some clinicians have proposed a cerebellar origin, specifically failure of the Purkinje cells to inhibit the CFN, with subsequent failure of the OPN to prevent saccadic burst neurons from oscillating.[58,85–87] Causes for ocular flutter and opsoclonus include parainfectious (presumably autoimmune) brainstem encephalitis; toxic metabolic states; demyelinating disorders; and, most importantly, as a paraneoplastic manifestation (usually neuroblastomas in children, and lung, breast, or ovarian malignancies in adults).[1,58,84,88–91] Conditions associated with opsoclonus and ocular flutter are listed in **Table 2**.

Small, brief, horizontal saccadic oscillations may be seen in normal subjects, particularly during blinking, when combining saccades with vergence, and with large vertical saccades.[6] Some individuals are even able to generate volitional conjugate oscillations, usually with convergence effort (voluntary nystagmus).[87]

Ocular and Saccadic Lateropulsion

Ocular lateropulsion refers to horizontal conjugate gaze deviation during eye closure, either toward (ipsipulsion) or away from (contrapulsion) the side of the lesion, that is corrected by a saccade toward the midline when the eyes are opened. Ocular lateropulsion is usually accompanied by saccadic lateropulsion and horizontal misdirection of vertical saccades. The role of the CFN in saccades, as discussed earlier, is important in understanding the pathophysiology of ocular and saccadic lateropulsion.

Table 2
Causes of opsoclonus/ocular flutter

	Causes	References
Neoplasms	Children: neuroblastoma and neural crest tumors	1,58,88
	Adults: small cell lung cancer, breast cancer, ovarian cancer, ovarian teratoma, pancreatic carcinoma, renal cell carcinoma, renal adenocarcinoma, non-Hodgkin lymphoma, melanoma, parietal glioma	1,92–99
Paraneoplastic manifestation	Antibodies: anti-Ri (ANNA-2); anti-Yo (PCA-1); anti-Hu (ANNA-1); anti-Ma1; anti-Ma2; antiamphiphysin; anti-CRMP-5; anti-Zic2; antineurofilaments; anti-VGCC; antirostral interstitial	85,89,100–112
Parainfectious encephalitis	Viral: Coxsackie B3; Epstein-Barr; Enterovirus; influenza A; West Nile; HIV/AIDS; Varicella-Zoster; hepatitis A; hepatitis C; Cytomegalovirus; St Louis encephalitis; mumps	92,113–138
	Bacterial: *Mycoplasma pneumoniae*; *Salmonella*; *Rickettsia*; *Chlamydophila psittaci*; *Borrelia burgdorferi*; *Streptococcus*; *Haemophilus influenzae*	
Postvaccination complication	Antirubella vaccine; human papilloma virus vaccine	139,140
Autoimmune disorders	MS; neuromyelitis optica; sarcoidosis; celiac disease; anti-NMDA receptor antibody encephalitis; antiganglioside Q1b antibodies; anti-GAD antibodies	124,141–148
Strokes	Thalamic hemorrhage; pontine hemorrhage; locked-in syndrome	149,150
Toxin exposure	Thallium; chlordecone; strychnine; toluene; organophosphates; cocaine	151–157
Drug toxicity	Opioids; lithium; amitriptyline; phenytoin and diazepam; phenelzine and imipramine	68,158–161
Inherited disorders	Krabbe disease; KCTD7 gene mutation	162,163
Miscellaneous causes	Nonketotic hyperosmolar coma	164,165
	Amyotrophic lateral sclerosis	166
	Hydrocephalus	167
	Allogeneic hematopoietic stem cell transplantation	168
	Head trauma	92
	Pregnancy	169

Abbreviations: AIDS, acquired immunodeficiency syndrome; HIV, human immunodeficiency virus; NMDA, *N*-methyl-D-aspartate; VGCC, voltage-gated calcium channel.

Ocular/saccadic ipsipulsion most commonly occurs in the setting of a Wallenberg (lateral medullary) syndrome.[170–172] It is hypothesized that damage to the inhibitory climbing fibers from the contralateral ION (traveling via the inferior cerebellar peduncle) to the vermal Purkinje cells leads to increased inhibition of the ipsilateral CFN (ie, mimicking the effects of an ipsilateral CFN lesion).[172,173] This reduced drive for contraversive saccades, and failure to slow ipsiversive saccades, results in hypometric contraversive saccades and hypermetric ipsiversive saccades, respectively.

In contrast, ocular/saccadic contrapulsion results from damage to fibers traveling in the uncinate fasciculus (within the superior cerebellar peduncle) from the contralateral CFN to the ipsilateral PPRF,[174,175] which leads to decreased drive for ipsilesional saccades, and failure to slow contralesional saccades results in hypometric ipsilesional saccades and hypermetric contralesional saccades, respectively. Note that ocular contrapulsion may arise from medullary lesions if the climbing fibers from the ION are compromised before crossing the midline.[176,177]

Cross-coupling of horizontal eye movements into vertical saccades resulting in a curved trajectory also occurs in saccadic lateropulsion. In saccadic contrapulsion, the horizontal bias is directed contralesionally, whereas an ipsilesional horizontal misdirection characterizes saccadic ipsipulsion.[1,175,178] The amplitude of horizontal deviation may be greater in upward compared with downward saccades.[177] The cross-coupling of inappropriate vertical components into horizontal saccades has been observed with pontine lesions,[179] perhaps reflecting damage to the pathways of the VPIN.

An unusual phenomenon termed saccadic torsipulsion, in which inappropriate torsional components (with the superior poles of the eyes beating contralesionally) emerge during attempted horizontal saccades, has also been reported in Wallenberg syndrome. This pattern of cross-coupling may be a result of a central imbalance of the anterior and posterior semicircular canals (SCC) pathways.[180]

SMOOTH PURSUIT

Smooth pursuit helps reduce image slip on the fovea to ensure clear vision. The neural network for smooth pursuit partially overlaps with that of the saccadic system. The neural substrate for smooth pursuit includes the lateral geniculate nuclei, the striate cortex, a neocortical network (including the middle temporal [MT] area, medial superior temporal [MST] area, parietal eye field [PEF; also called the lateral intraparietal area], supplementary eye field, and frontal eye field [FEF]), brainstem nuclei (the nucleus of the optic tract [NOT], DLPN, NRTP, ION, NPH, MVN), and cerebellar structures.[1]

The cerebellum plays a crucial role in the gain (gain equals eye velocity divided by target velocity) and adaptation of smooth eye tracking of a moving target, either when the head is still (ie, smooth pursuit) or when the head is passively moving (ie, VOR suppression). Complete cerebellectomy abolishes smooth pursuit in humans and monkeys.[181–183] The main cerebellar structures involved in control of smooth pursuit eye movements are the flocculus-paraflocculus, oculomotor vermis, and CFN. Other cerebellar structures involved in pursuit tracking include the nodulus, uvula, and more lateral cerebellar hemispheres.[26,184–192]

A common finding in cerebellar disease is diminished smooth pursuit gain (ie, eye velocity less than target velocity). The patient compensates for this with catch-up saccades, leading to saccadic (choppy or cogwheel) pursuit. In general, saccadic pursuit tracking is non-localizing, and may be caused by dysfunction of a variety of neural structures, and has to be interpreted in the context of other neuro-ophthalmic deficits. In patients with cerebellar disorders, downward pursuit may be more severely impaired than upward pursuit.[193] This finding may be explained by the fact that most floccular Purkinje cells are activated during downward, as opposed to upward, pursuit.[186,194]

Cross-coupling of eye movements refers to inappropriately produced eye movements that rotate the globe around an axis orthogonal to the correct one.[178] A conspicuous manifestation of cavernous angiomas of the middle cerebellar peduncle (MCP) is cross-coupling of torsional into vertical eye movements during vertical smooth pursuit, resulting in a direction-changing torsional nystagmus during vertical pursuit tracking, with the upper poles of the eyes beating contralesionally during upward pursuit (and ipsilesionally during downward pursuit), and with the slow phase velocity of the torsional eye movements proportional to that of the vertical component.[178] One possible explanation for this finding is that smooth pursuit uses a neural network based on a vestibular labyrinthine coordinate system. When stimulated, the anterior canals produce upward slow phases with a torsional component that rotates the upper poles contralaterally, whereas the posterior canals produce downward slow phases (but the torsional component also rotates upper poles of the eyes contralaterally).[1,178] Pure vertical slow phases occur when the SCC on both sides are activated simultaneously, thereby canceling the torsional components within the vestibular nuclei.[178] Signals from the pontine vestibular nuclei (which control the vertical VOR and vertical pursuit signals) are encoded in anterior SCC coordinates and conveyed to the vestibulocerebellum via the MCP.[195–197] Therefore, a unilateral MCP lesion causes an imbalance in the torsional components during vertical pursuit, resulting in contralesional-beating torsional nystagmus during upward tracking (from the activity of the unopposed contralateral anterior canal), and ipsilesional-beating torsional component during downward tracking (caused by the lack of inhibitory signals from the ipsilateral anterior SCC).[178]

GAZE HOLDING

The neural integrator is inherently imperfect (leaky) and the eye position signal is a decaying exponential that results in the eye slowly drifting centripetally until a corrective saccadic quick phase moves the eye back to target. This condition is the basis for gaze-evoked nystagmus (GEN).[1] The cerebellum, in particular the flocculus-paraflocculus, is responsible for improving the performance of this inherently leaky neural integrator.[184,198] Positive feedback loops between the cerebellum and the brainstem, most likely via connections from the NPH-MVN region to the vestibulocerebellum and paramedian tract (PMT) input into the flocculus, optimize the performance of the neural integrator, and therefore maintain eccentric gaze positions.[1,9] Floccular-parafloccular lesions therefore result in GEN because of increased neural integrator leakiness.[1] The most common cause of GEN is medication/drug effects, including alcohol, antiepileptics, and sedatives. Other causes include myasthenia gravis (fatigue nystagmus) and brainstem lesions that damage the neural integrator, as in Wernicke encephalopathy.[1]

After persistent effort at maintaining eccentric gaze, returning to central position may result in nystagmus that beats in the opposite direction; this is referred to as rebound nystagmus.[1,199] Rebound nystagmus is characteristic of flocculus-paraflocculus lesions. Another form of nystagmus in some patients with cerebellar disorders is a centripetal nystagmus in eccentric gaze that consists of centrifugally directed slow phases and centripetally directed quick phases.[200]

GEN should be distinguished from vestibular nystagmus. Nystagmus arising from peripheral vestibular imbalance is characterized by a unilateral jerk nystagmus that obeys Alexander's law (ie, its amplitude is greatest when the patient is looking in the direction of the fast phase). In contrast, the amplitude of horizontal GEN changes direction with gaze direction and its amplitude is almost always nearly the same in both directions of gaze. In some situations, GEN and vestibular nystagmus coexist. A cerebellopontine angle tumor may cause low-frequency, high-amplitude GEN (from flocculus-paraflocculus compression) when looking ipsilesionally, and a high-frequency, low-amplitude vestibular nystagmus (from vestibular nerve impingement) when looking contralesionally. In primary position, there may be horizontal contralesional-beating nystagmus caused by the vestibular imbalance. This finding is referred to as Brun's nystagmus.[1,201] Although it is most commonly seen in patients with vestibular schwannomas exceeding 3.5 cm in diameter,[201] it may rarely be seen in paramedian basis pontis infarction.[202]

It is also important to differentiate GEN from physiologic (end-gaze) nystagmus, which is a common finding in healthy individuals. In comparison, end-gaze nystagmus is typically unsustained, conjugate, brought out in extreme lateral gaze, has a smaller amplitude and frequency, and is unaccompanied by other ocular motor abnormalities. In contrast, GEN may be elicited with as little as 15° eccentricity, and may be disconjugate.[1,25]

DBN

DBN is characterized by slow upward drifts and corrective downward quick phases. It is typically increased with convergence, and with eccentric gaze, particularly by having the patient look downward and laterally (ie, side-pocket nystagmus). Although it mostly obeys Alexander's law (ie, intensifies with downgaze), the reverse is occasionally observed. In general, DBN is accompanied by other ocular motor abnormalities, such as horizontal GEN, rebound nystagmus, saccadic pursuit, impaired OKR, dysmetric saccades, and/or perverted (cross-coupled head-shaking nystagmus [HSN]), as well as a tendency to fall backwards (retropulsion).[1,203–208]

In theory, the upward drift consists of 2 components: an upward bias drift, and a gaze-evoked drift.[203] The gaze-evoked drift is caused by a leaky neural integrator,[203,206] but the cause of the bias drift remains unclear.[203–205] This bias drift hypothetically consists of gravity-dependent and gravity-independent components.[204,205] The gravity-dependent component may be caused by otolith-ocular reflex hyperactivity,[205] and may explain why DBN is amplified in the prone, straight head hanging, and head pitched forward positions but is diminished in the supine position.[209] The pathophysiologic basis of the gravity-independent component is less clear. The most favored hypothesis[210] is that the geometric configuration of the SCCs predisposes to an upward ocular drift (because of the relative predominance of the anterior SCC pathways compared with the posterior SCC projections), which is normally suppressed by the flocculus-paraflocculus. Cerebellar disease unmasks this upward bias, resulting in DBN.[210–214] Other clinicians have proposed that neural integrator dysfunction results in a shift of the Listing plane for static eye positions (ie, an upward shift in the eyes' null position for vertical gaze holding).[203,206] However, based on the observation that patients with cerebellar disorders have fairly intact upward, but impaired downward, pursuit tracking, some clinicians propose that floccular damage results in an asymmetry of vertical smooth-pursuit signals, in which a preponderance of upward velocity results in spontaneous upward drifts.[1,193,194,204,215]

Most clinicians agree that DBN is a prominent manifestation of floccular-parafloccular dysfunction.[184,204,205,215–217] However, lesions of the oculomotor vermis[218] or PMT[219] may also result in DBN. The PMT receive input from the anterior SCCs (via vestibular secondary neurons from the superior vestibular nuclei [SVN]) and convey vertical eye position signals to the flocculus. Damage to the PMT may result in DBN.[219] Because of their proximity to the MLF, pathologic processes that affect the PMT may cause both DBN and internuclear ophthalmoparesis (INO).[220] Otherwise, it seems that focal brainstem lesions by themselves do not cause DBN.[221] The causes of DBN are summarized in **Box 1**.[1,68,100,141,207,213,218,222–240]

We propose categorizing DBN patients clinically as (1) isolated DBN (for those with only ocular motor signs attributable to floccular-parafloccular dysfunction), (2) DBN with central signs (for patients with brainstem and cerebellar signs, but not those with cranial neuropathies), and (3) DBN with central and peripheral signs (for those with evidence of peripheral involvement; eg, vestibulopathy, peripheral neuropathy). This system is based on the suggested classification scheme by Wagner and colleagues.[207] This method may be helpful in directing a clinician's diagnostic work-up, and because

---

Box 1
Causes of DBN

Most common causes:

- Idiopathic
- Cerebellar degeneration (usually from SCA or MSA)
- Chiari I malformation

Important considerations:

- Gluten ataxia
- Episodic ataxia type 2
- Paraneoplastic cerebellar degeneration
- Anti-GAD antibodies
- Drug toxicity (lithium, amiodarone, antiepileptics, opioids, and metronidazole)
- Vertebrobasilar arterial dolichoectasia
- Multiple sclerosis
- Stroke
- Hypomagnesemia

Rare causes reported in the literature:

- Neuromyelitis optica
- Herpes simplex encephalitis
- Ciguatera poisoning
- Cephalic tetanus
- Heat stroke
- Vitamin B_{12} deficiency
- Miller-Fisher syndrome
- Human T-lymphotropic virus infection
- West Nile encephalomyelitis
- Legionnaires' disease

---

patients with idiopathic DBN usually have a better prognosis and a very slow disease progression.[241]

UPBEAT NYSTAGMUS

In upbeat nystagmus (UBN), downward slow phases in primary position are followed by corrective upward quick phases. UBN typically increases with upgaze, diminishes with downgaze, and is unaffected by horizontal gaze. UBN has been described in lesions of the caudal medulla, ventral pontine tegmentum, anterior cerebellar vermis, and thalamus.[1,221]

The nucleus of Roller in the medulla receives projections from the posterior SCCs (via the SVN) and conveys inhibitory signals to the flocculus. The nucleus intercalatus of Staderini, located in the dorsal caudal medulla, is connected to the MVN and vestibulocerebellum. Paramedian tegmental caudal medullary lesions that damage these structures result in disinhibition of the flocculus (causing hyperinhibition of the downstream pathway), and therefore predisposes to downward ocular drifts.[221,242–248] In contrast, UBN may result from damage to the pontine ventral tegmentum and/or posterior basis pontis that disrupts the vestibulooculomotor pathways that mediate upward eye movements; namely the MLF (conveying signals from the MVN) crossing the ventral tegmental tract (originating from the SVN), and to a lesser degree the superior cerebellar peduncle (also carrying afferent fibers from the SVN).[221,246,249,250] UBN has been observed infrequently in lesions of the anterior vermis or thalamus.[1,246,251] The presence of concurrent ocular motor abnormalities may help localize the lesion responsible for UBN. For instance, ocular/saccadic contrapulsion and skew deviation suggest a medullary lesion, an INO indicates pontine damage, and vertical gaze palsy suggests mesencephalic dysfunction.

Like DBN, UBN has a gravity-dependent component (likely mediated by otolithic projections to the nodulus and uvula traveling in the crossing ventral tegmental tract), accounting for its variation with changes in head position and vergence.[221,249,252,253] UBN may be attenuated by convergence, and with head-hanging, Dix-Hallpike, supine, or prone positions; it may even convert to DBN when the patient is prone.[244,246,247,249,251,254–256] In unusual cases (especially caudal medullary lesions), the amplitude of UBN increases with downgaze.[244,257]

Two important causes of UBN should be emphasized. First, nicotine exposure (from smoking or from nicotine-replacement products) can cause transient UBN.[258–261] Second, Wernicke encephalopathy is a potentially severe, easily treated cause of UBN (discussed later); UBN that converts to DBN with convergence is particularly concerning for thiamine deficiency.[262] Other causes of UBN are summarized in **Table 3**.[141,246,247,250,263–271]

POSITIONAL NYSTAGMUS

In certain disorders, specific head movements evoke a nystagmus that outlasts the head movement. Positioning refers to nystagmus caused by the head movements,

Table 3 Causes of UBN	
Cause	**Comments**
Toxin exposure	Nicotine Organoarsenic Organophosphates
Drugs	Amitriptyline withdrawal Barbiturates
Immune mediated	MS Neuromyelitis optica Paraneoplastic syndrome Anti-GAD antibodies
Chiari malformation	UBN may occur with neck flexion and extension An unusual case of UBN triggered by optic flow stimulation was reported in a patient with a Chiari malformation[263]
Other causes	Pseudotumor cerebri Epileptic phenomenon Creutzfeldt-Jakob disease Neurocysticercosis

whereas positional indicates that the new head position causes the nystagmus.[272] Three positions are typically tested: right Dix-Hallpike, left Dix-Hallpike, and straight head hanging.

Positional/positioning nystagmus can be divided into 2 general types, although a rigid distinction between central and peripheral causes cannot always be made: (1) central positional nystagmus, in which the nystagmus persists as long as the head remains in the inciting position, and may not be associated with vertigo; (2) peripheral positional nystagmus, or benign paroxysmal positional vertigo (BPPV), which is usually transient but is associated with a significant vertigo component. However, exceptions are common, and a peripheral pattern may be seen with central causes.[272,273] Peripheral causes (especially BPPV) are far more common than central causes but central lesions carry more sinister ramifications.[273,274] Other peripheral causes of positional vertigo include disorders that cause a specific gravity gradient between the cupula and endolymph (eg, macroglobulinemia, certain toxins [alcohol, glycerol, heavy water]), perilymphatic fistulae, Meniere disease, vestibular atelectasis, vestibular migraine, and physiologic (head extension or bending over) vertigo.[275]

Nystagmus and vertigo (with nausea and vomiting) are highly correlated in BPPV. Sustained nystagmus without vertigo is more characteristic of a central lesion. Positional vomiting without intense nystagmus is similarly atypical for peripheral causes. Diagnostic difficulty arises in the case of central paroxysmal positional vertigo (CPPV), in which the clinical picture mimics BPPV. The presence of neurologic deficits, especially ataxia and ocular motor manifestations, as well as abnormal imaging, can help identify central causes.[272,274,276]

Central positional nystagmus (particularly positional DBN) is a valuable clinical sign indicating vestibulocerebellar or pontomedullary dysfunction; it is not accompanied by primary gaze DBN in some patients. In contrast with DBN that occurs in the head-upright position (ie, caused by floccular-parafloccular dysfunction), positional DBN occurs in lesions involving uvulonodular dysfunction, as well as dorsolateral to the fourth ventricle.[272–274] Uvulonodular damage typically results in transient positional DBN in cats[277] and in humans.[205,212,278–280] By contrast, when there is a persistent and dramatic increase in DBN with head-hanging, compression of neural structures in the posterior fossa (eg, Chiari malformation) during neck hyperextension must be excluded.[205]

Chiari I malformation is an important consideration in every patient with central positional nystagmus.[281,282] Other disorders associated with central positioning nystagmus are summarized in **Table 4**.[273,274,276,278,283–294]

A rare but important differential diagnosis in patients with positional vertigo and nystagmus induced by neck rotation or hyperextension is Bowhunter syndrome, in which neck movement causes dynamic obstruction of the dominant vertebral artery at the atlantoaxial level, resulting in nystagmus, vertigo, and incoordination that stop when the head is returned to neutral position.[295–300] Classic findings include vertigo with horizontal nystagmus with the slow phase away from the compressed vertebral artery,[299] but DBN may occur.[300,301] It is most commonly associated with cervical spondylosis, but may be a complication of surgical positioning, chiropractic manipulation, and atlantoaxial subluxation. Close follow-up and neurosurgical evaluation (including dynamic angiographic studies) are needed because nearly half of patients go on to have strokes.[296]

In the absence of vascular insufficiency, structural lesions, or other neurologic deficits, positional DBN may be a manifestation of anterior canal BPPV (the rarest form of BPPV),[276] or an apogeotropic variant of posterior canal BPPV (caused by an otoconial mass within the distal nonampullary arm of the canal).[302] In these cases, the positional nystagmus typically consists of a downbeating nystagmus (toward

Table 4
Conditions associated with central positional nystagmus

Cause	Comments
Cerebellar lesions	Uvulonodular damage: vermian arachnoid cysts, infarction, metastases, hematomas, hemangioblastomas, and astrocytomas Cerebellar degeneration: spinocerebellar type 6, MSA Superior cerebellar peduncle demyelination: possibly caused by disrupted otolithic pathways
Fourth ventricle tumors	Central positional nystagmus likely results from the tumor causing obstructive hydrocephalus in certain head positions
Brainstem lesions	Demyelination Infarctions
Toxic metabolic disorders	Severe hypomagnesemia Drug toxicity: carbamazepine, amiodarone, lamotrigine, pregabalin
Autoimmune disorders	MS Celiac disease
Paraneoplastic syndrome	Anti-VGCC antibodies
Vestibular migraine	Possibly caused by uvulonodular dysfunction

the patient's feet) and a variable torsional component that can be difficult to appreciate. It also has a brief latency, adapts, and habituates.[276,302] In both anterior canal and the apogeotropic posterior canal BPPV, vertigo and nystagmus may be triggered by the straight head-hanging position, or by a bilateral, ipsilesional, or contralesional Dix-Hallpike maneuver.[276,302,303] It is also important to remember that the straight head-hanging position may provoke DBN in normal, healthy subjects.[259]

ACQUIRED PENDULAR NYSTAGMUS

Acquired pendular nystagmus (APN) consists of involuntary, pseudosinusoidal ocular oscillations typically ranging from 2 to 6 Hz that may be horizontal, vertical, or a combination thereof (ie, circular, elliptical, or windmill). The oscillations may be symmetric, dissociated (different amplitude in each eye), or monocular.[113] APN may arise from lesions affecting the dentate-rubro-olivary pathways (Guillain-Mollaret triangle), pontine tegmentum, ION, cerebellum, and MVN.[1,113,304]

There are 3 principal APN syndromes: (1) APN associated with brainstem/cerebellar demyelinating disease (eg, MS, adrenoleukodystrophy, toluene toxicity, Pelizaeus-Merzbacher disease, Cockayne syndrome, peroxisomal assembly disorders), (2) APN as part of the oculopalatal tremor (OPT) syndrome, and (3) APN in Whipple disease (discussed later).[1,113,305–308]

In demyelinating diseases, APN usually oscillates at a low amplitude and high frequency (at least 4 Hz), and mainly consists of horizontal and torsional oscillations; it is usually symmetric and can be transiently suppressed by saccades and/or convergence.[304,308–311] It is commonly associated with INO, ataxia, and vergence defects.[304,309,310] Demyelinating plaques are frequently seen in the paramedian tegmental region of the brainstem.[304] In these cases, APN may arise from an unstable neural integrator, presumably caused by PMT damage (which conveys ocular motor efference copies to the flocculus).[311,312] Optic neuropathy in demyelinating disease may alternatively impair visual feedback to the cerebellar brainstem networks that calibrate eye position[313]; however, this cannot explain why APN persists in darkness.[1]

In contradistinction, OPT-related APN is more irregular and oscillates at a higher amplitude and lower frequency (1–3 Hz). The oscillations usually occur in the vertical and torsional planes, and may be disconjugate.[1,81,308] OPT is a delayed manifestation of brainstem/cerebellar damage (eg, pontine hemorrhage, Alexander disease, central pontine myelinolysis),[1] or may be a feature of the progressive ataxia and palatal tremor syndrome.[314] Hypertrophic degeneration of the ION occurs several weeks to months after an insult to the central tegmental tract (connecting the ION and deep cerebellar nuclei via the superior cerebellar peduncle); this disrupts gamma-aminobutyric acid (GABA)–mediated cerebellar inhibition of the ION, and as a consequence soma-somatic gap junctions proliferate between adjacent neurons, increasing the strength of their electrotonic coupling.[1,305,315,316] When this electrotonic coupling is sufficiently strong, the normal physiologic oscillations of ION neurons become abnormally synchronized, generating oscillating pulses that are then amplified by the cerebellum to produce the conspicuous clinical manifestations of OPT.[312,315] OPT may be associated with a synchronous contraction of the branchiomeric muscles (ie, muscles derived ontologically from the branchial arch), the diaphragm, and/or distal appendicular muscles.[1,317] OPT onset is associated with the emergence of abnormal hyperintense signal and enlargement of the ION on MRI.[318]

VOR

The integration of visual and vestibular information is critical to maintaining visual stability when in motion. The confluence of visual and vestibular signals occurs in the parietal cortex (at the dorsal medial superior temporal area, the ventral intraparietal area, and the visual posterior sylvian area), as well as in the cerebellum; specifically the nodulus and uvula.[319–324]

The nodulus and uvula receive visual and vestibular information via mossy and climbing fibers. Primary afferent signals to the nodulus and uvula come from the labyrinths, secondary projections arise from the vestibular nuclei, and tertiary input projects from the ION via climbing fibers.[324–345] Efferent fibers from the nodulus and ventral uvula project in a topographic fashion back to the vestibular nuclei.[19] These reciprocal connections attest to the critical role of the vestibulocerebellum in mediating VOR responses.

By detecting head motion and position and generating compensatory eye movements, the VOR ensures that the line of sight for each fovea continues to be directed at a target even when the head is moved.[1,346] The labyrinth contains 2 types of motion detectors: the SCCs and the otolith organs, which consist of the saccule and macula.

The Angular VOR

The angular VOR (AVOR) is tasked with stabilizing the eyes in space during angular head acceleration.[1,347] The human SCCs are almost orthogonal in both their anatomic array and physiologic responses.[348–350] Each head rotation activates a unique combination of SCCs (which are commonly grouped in 3 coplanar pairs) that is contingent on the orientation of each individual canal relative to the axis of head velocity.[347] For example, a leftward yaw rotation with the head upright excites the left horizontal SCC, as well as the right anterior and posterior SCC, and inhibits the remaining 3 SCCs. Because the precise orientation of the SCCs and extraocular muscles varies between individuals, the connections between them must be calibrated accurately to ensure a fully compensatory AVOR.[351]

The VOR is a highly modifiable reflex.[352] With image motion across the retina during head movements, the VOR undergoes gain changes and/or phase shifts to ensure its accuracy. The vestibulocerebellum plays a vital role in this calibration; damage to this structure results in abnormal VOR gain and direction.[189,346,347,352–359] A VOR gain greater than 1 (ie, eye velocity exceeding head velocity) with low-frequency stimulation usually occurs in cerebellar lesions, and results from disinhibition of brainstem circuits that control the VOR.[184,346,347,352] By contrast, peripheral vestibulopathy typically results in low gain in VOR (ie, <1), and results in oscillopsia during locomotion because the AVOR gain is too low to ensure gaze stabilization.[209] However, certain cerebellar disorders may cause low VOR gain, notably CANVAS (cerebellar ataxia, neuropathy, and vestibular areflexia syndrome), SCA3, FRDA, and Wernicke encephalopathy (discussed later). At high frequencies of stimulation (ie, with the head-impulse test), the VOR gain is decreased with flocculus-paraflocculus lesions.[184,352] In humans, the head-impulse test is a highly sensitive and specific bedside method of differentiating peripheral from central vestibulopathies,[101,360–362] and is usually normal in cerebellar disease.[113,363–365] However, a positive head-impulse test (ie, with a corrective catch-up saccade) occurs rarely in pontine and cerebellar infarctions.[362,366]

Vestibulocerebellar lesions may also cause directional errors (cross-coupling) in vestibular and optokinetic responses (OKRs).[346,347] Horizontal VOR responses may be cross-coupled with inappropriate disconjugate upward slow phases (most prominent in the abducting eye), akin to a dynamic skew that resembles a static alternating skew deviation (discussed later).[346,347] This cross-coupling results in an oblique ocular trajectory that requires a corrective quick phase to return the eye to target. During yaw rotations with the head upright, the contralateral vertical SCCs are excited, whereas the ipsilateral vertical canals are inhibited.[347] In healthy individuals, the inhibitory signals from the flocculus and paraflocculus (to the anterior and horizontal SCC pathways) prevent vertical eye velocity in the absence of pitch head motion.[195,346,347,367] The loss of floccular-parafloccular inhibition of activated contralateral anterior SCC signals during yaw rotations is thought to be the cause of these inappropriate vertical eye movements.[346,347]

The Translational VOR

The otolith organs play an essential role in spatial orientation by detecting the direction of the head vertical with respect to a gravitational reference. The sensory epithelium of the utricle (macula utriculi) lies in the horizontal plane, and detects earth-horizontal linear acceleration in any direction, as well as changes in head position with respect to gravity (eg, static head tilt). The sensory epithelium of the saccule is oriented vertically and as such detects vertical head motion that occurs during locomotion.[19,368]

The translational VOR (TVOR), or linear VOR, which relies on the otolithic system to transform linear head acceleration into angular eye rotation, stabilizes eye position to compensate for translational head movements. The normal TVOR varies with the target proximity; its sensitivity is inversely proportional to fixation distance.[369–371]

Vestibular neurons with otolithic input project to the anterior cerebellar lobe, nodulus, and uvula.[341] Dynamic utricular responses are diminished in cerebellar disease.[197,371,372] Patients with CACNA1A mutations have reduced otolithic sensitivity, and almost absent modulation of the TVOR by vergence angle,[371] which is likely to be a consequence of degenerative loss of uvulonodular Purkinje cells.[373]

The Velocity Storage Mechanism

After an initial deflection, when the head moves at a constant angular velocity, the SCC cupula passively returns to its resting position, resulting in a decay of the firing rate of the vestibular nerve; the SCC cupula time constant has been estimated to be between 3 and 7 seconds.[1,374] However, the compensatory vestibular nystagmus that emerges following a constant-velocity rotation in darkness outlasts the duration of the SCC input (ie, the SCC cupula time constant).[1,374–376] A central brainstem and cerebellar neural network, known as the velocity storage mechanism, prolongs the SCC afferent signal and extends the duration of the reflexive eye responses, thus improving the compensatory response to low-frequency head rotations.[1,368,374]

Velocity storage maintains the spatial orientation of the AVOR by realigning the eye velocity vector toward the gravitoinertial acceleration vector (ie, the vector sum of gravitational and linear acceleration). Movement in a terrestrial environment activates SCCs and otoliths, producing signals that are processed in a head-based canal-coordinate frame that is rotated relative to the cardinal axes of the head. In contrast, velocity storage processes information in a spatially linked coordinate frame, whose yaw axis is related to a combination of the head vertical and the gravitoinertial acceleration vector. The velocity storage mechanism transforms sensory signals from a head-fixed reference frame into a spatially linked reference frame.[1,363,368,374,377–382]

The nodulus and ventral uvula are critical components of the vestibulocerebellum that modulate the velocity storage mechanism.[368,383–385] GABAergic Purkinje fibers from the nodulus and ventral uvula project to the ipsilateral vestibular nuclear complex.[384–387] The ability of baclofen, a GABA-B receptor agonist, to reduce the time constant of postrotatory nystagmus provides further proof of Purkinje cell involvement in the velocity storage mechanism.[388] The vestibulocerebellum is also able to discharge the velocity storage mechanism by means of otolithic input[383,389]; head tilts are therefore able to decrease the postrotatory VOR time constant (and nystagmus).[390–392] This tilt suppression nystagmus is lost in vestibulocerebellar disease.

Cerebellar diseases that perturb the velocity storage mechanism cause 2 conspicuous forms of nystagmus: HSN and periodic alternating nystagmus (PAN).

HSN

Head shaking at 2 to 3 Hz for about 20 seconds may provoke nystagmus in peripheral and central vestibular dysfunction.[1,393–395] HSN is attributed to the asymmetrical accumulation of activity from the peripheral vestibular organs within the velocity storage system.[1,346,396]

HSN is most commonly seen following unilateral peripheral vestibulopathy, in which horizontal head shaking induces a horizontal nystagmus with ipsiversive quick phases that decays over 20 seconds, and then undergoes a weak reversal.[346,396] In contradistinction, central vestibular lesions give rise to various patterns of HSN, often in planes other than that being stimulated during head shaking (the so-called perverted HSN). Other central HSN patterns include a disproportionally strong HSN in response to weak head shaking, ipsilesional HSN, strongly biphasic HSN, and HSN in the absence of caloric paresis.[1,178,359,395,397,398]

Uvulonodular damage is most frequently associated with central vestibular HSN. The most common form of perverted HSN is DBN following horizontal head shaking,[346,395] which may be the consequence of inappropriate accumulation of upward bias from asymmetrical anterior canal signals within the velocity storage system during horizontal head shaking.[346] Impaired AVOR adaptation may alternatively lead to inappropriately directed VOR slow phases following horizontal head shaking.[178,346,395] Lateral medullary infarction may cause unilateral uvulonodular dysfunction, resulting in asymmetric inhibition of velocity storage (favoring contralesional velocity storage) during head shaking, leading to an ipsiversive horizontal jerk HSN.[359,395,399]

Dentate lesions occasionally cause HSN.[395,400] Unilateral dentate lesions often cause contraversive ocular deviation, possibly by disinhibiting the ipsilesional vestibular nuclear complex. Head shaking may increase this contraversive bias (as well as contraversive slow phases), resulting in ipsiversive corrective quick phases, which are observed as an ipsiversive horizontal jerk HSN.[395,401]

PAN

PAN is a spontaneous, conjugate horizontal jerk nystagmus that changes direction periodically. Congenital PAN has a null region that is constantly shifting from side to side, resulting in head turns in the direction away from the shifting null zone in order to maintain the null in straight-ahead position and ensure the best visual acuity.[402] Congenital PAN is frequently associated with albinism.[402]

In contradistinction, acquired PAN is characterized by a spontaneous, primary position, horizontal jerk nystagmus with a changes direction regularly (typically ~90–120 seconds). The nystagmus beats in one direction with an increasing and then decreasing intensity, followed by a brief transitional period (which may be punctuated by UBN, DBN, or saccadic intrusions), and then beats in the opposite direction. Acquired PAN is usually caused by nodular dysfunction that causes disinhibition of the GABA-mediated velocity storage mechanism.[1,383,402,403] Acquired PAN is typically associated with impaired smooth pursuit and OKR.[404,405] It may be suppressed by vestibular stimuli (eg, with head turns), and with convergence.[1] In rare cases, PAN may be associated with bilateral visual loss[406,407] and peripheral vestibulopathies like Meniere disease.[408] PAN arising from peripheral vestibular dysfunction is suppressed by visual fixation, has a more irregular periodicity, and is associated with hearing loss but not central neurologic signs.[408] Conditions associated with acquired PAN are summarized in **Table 5**.[1,70,199,271,403–407,409–418]

In rare cases, PAN is associated with periodic alternating skew deviation. This unusual combination has been reported in MS,[419] vertebral artery dolichoectasia,[301] brainstem abscess,[420] mesencephalic stroke,[421] iatrogenic uvula injury,[422] hereditary

Table 5 Conditions associated with acquired PAN	
Cerebellar lesions	• Degeneration: SCA type 6; FRDA; ataxia-telangiectasia • Mass lesions: arachnoid cyst, tumors, abscesses • Chiari malformation
Brainstem lesions	• Strokes • Syringobulbia • Brainstem encephalitis
Drugs	• Lithium • Antiepileptic medications (eg, primidone, phenytoin)
Infections	• Neurosyphilis • Neurocysticercosis • Creutzfeldt-Jakob disease
Autoimmune disorders	• MS • Anti-GAD antibodies • Antiganglioside antibodies
Bilateral severe visual loss	• Cataracts • Vitreous hemorrhage
Peripheral vestibulopathy	• Meniere disease
Miscellaneous	• Trauma • Hepatic encephalopathy

ataxia (without a specific genetic diagnosis),[423] and SCA6.[424] The etiopathophysiologic underpinnings of periodic alternating skew deviation remain unclear, but may be related to otolithic imbalance and maladaptive attempts by the cerebellum to recalibrate this asymmetry.

Periodic alternating gaze deviation (with a periodicity of about 90–120 seconds) results if concomitant brainstem disease abolishes quick phases.[412,425] It is important to distinguish this finding from ping-pong gaze, which occurs in comatose patients with bihemispheric lesions, and has a periodicity of a few seconds.[1,402]

Vestibular Migraine

Migraineurs often report symptoms that suggest vestibular dysfunction, including instability, dizziness, and motion sickness. In addition, they frequently show signs of vestibular dysfunction, including HSN, positional nystagmus, GEN, impaired smooth pursuit, postural instability, and evidence of peripheral vestibulopathy.[426–437] The relationship between dysfunctional velocity storage and motion sickness,[438–440] as well as hypersensitivity to integration of visual and vestibular signals,[441] suggests a role for uvulonodular dysfunction in vestibular migraine. Some clinicians have argued that vestibulocerebellar adaptive mechanisms are augmented to suppress the inherent vestibular hypersensitivity of migraneurs, as shown by enhanced VOR tilt suppression.[437] The role of the cerebellum in the etiopathobiological underpinnings of vestibular migraine is unclear, but is intriguing.

OPTOKINETIC NYSTAGMUS

The VOR and OKR ensure image stabilization on the fovea during self-movement and environmental movement. Under most conditions, both reflexes cooperate but the working range of each differs; the retinal direction-selective cells mediating the OKR respond to low-frequency motion, and it therefore complements the VOR, which is effective at high-frequency movements. Moreover, the OKR system can react to constant velocities, whereas the VOR does not. The OKR may have evolved phylogenetically to improve the VOR's ability to stabilize images on the fovea during spontaneous head movements in the light.[1,442]

Optokinetic nystagmus (OKN) is induced clinically by moving high-contrast patterns (eg, alternating black and white stripes) across the patient's central and peripheral visual fields. The OKN consists of smooth pursuit tracking (slow phases) in the direction of the moving stimulus, and automatic resetting saccades (quick phases) in the opposite direction. OKR relies on both the smooth pursuit and saccadic systems. Look OKN is elicited by instructing patients to follow the individual stripes of the moving stimulus; stare OKN is tested by instructing patients to stare at the center of the moving optokinetic display and not to follow the individual elements.[443] Look OKN, a voluntary response that involves cortical activation, is characterized by large-amplitude, low-frequency, alternating voluntary pursuit and saccadic eye movements. In contrast, stare OKN is an involuntary, more subcortical response that consists of low-amplitude, high-frequency alternating eye movements.[443–446]

Various cortical, subcortical, and cerebellar structures are involved in the OKR, including those related to saccadic and smooth pursuit pathways.[216,442,447] Many cerebellar structures participate in the OKR, including the oculomotor vermis, flocculus, deep nuclei (including the dentate and caudal fastigial nuclei), MCP, and various hemispheric regions.[216,443,448,449] As such, an impaired OKR is not location specific and has to be interpreted in the context of associated neuro-ophthalmic deficits.

Cross-coupled OKN is a more conspicuous manifestation of cerebellar disease. Inappropriate torsional responses with horizontal optokinetic stimulation may be observed.[346] This finding may be caused by horizontal visual stimuli being transformed into a horizontal canal frame of reference, and subsequently evoking a mixed horizontal-torsional nystagmus as though the horizontal SCC were being activated.[346] MCP cavernous angiomas that cause inappropriate torsional components during vertical pursuit also can cause a cross-coupled OKN characterized by inappropriate torsional components during vertical quick phases.[178]

OCULAR ALIGNMENT AND VERGENCE
Vergence and Horizontal Ocular Misalignment

The cerebellum plays an important role in vergence eye movements.[191,450,451] The neurons controlling vergence in the MST, SEF, and FEF project to the NRTP, which also receives input from the superior colliculi and mesencephalic pretectum. The neurons of the NRTP in turn project to the oculomotor vermis and deep cerebellar nuclei.[191,452–454] The cerebellar pathways for convergence and divergence are anatomically distinct.[191,451,453–456] There is evidence that the ventral paraflocculus, vermis, and VPIN mediate divergence,[1,456,457] whereas the oculomotor vermis and CFN control convergence.[451] In addition, divergence-related vermal neurons may be more vulnerable to injury and convergence is better compensated for.[191] As such, cerebellar disease frequently results in divergence insufficiency and excessive convergence tone,[25,450,458,459] and may explain why incomitant esodeviation is common in cerebellar disease, especially with oculomotor vermal lesions.[25,191] Acute-onset esotropia may be the first sign of cerebellar disorder, especially in children.[460–464]

Vertical Ocular Misalignment

Skew deviation has long been recognized as a feature of cerebellar disease.[25,465] It often changes with horizontal position, with the abducting eye being higher; this is referred to as the alternating skew deviation.[22,25,466–470] In addition, downgaze increases the degree of vertical misalignment, although to a lesser degree than lateral gaze.[25] The pathobiological basis of this phenomenon is unclear but may be related to impaired cerebellar calibration of eye position. Depriving the cerebellum of visual disparity errors by patching 1 eye for a few days in healthy patients leads to alternating skew deviations.[25,471,472] Cerebellar lesions similarly may impair the mechanisms needed to accurately calibrate ocular alignment using visual feedback. Cerebellar disorders alternatively may affect the vestibular response to different lateral eye positions in the orbit and result in misalignment.[25,470]

The cerebellum is an integral part of the neural network involved in the integration of graviceptive signals to ensure the accuracy of the internal representation of the earth vertical.[400] More specifically, the nodulus, biventer lobe, and dentate are involved in graviceptive processing.[400,473] Ocular tilt reaction (OTR; a combination of skew deviation, ocular torsion, as well as head and perceptual tilts) may result from cerebellar disease, presumably causing otolithic imbalance.[400,474] In general, lesions affecting the biventer, inferior semilunar lobule, or vestibular nerve root entry zone cause an ipsiversive OTR. In contrast, uvulonodular and dentate lesions disinhibit the ipsilateral vestibular nuclei and cause a contraversive OTR.[400] Degenerative ION hypertrophy alternatively leads to overexcitation of the contralateral dentate, resulting in an OTR away from the hypertrophic ION.[475]

CEREBELLAR DISORDERS WITH AFFERENT VISUAL PATHWAY MANIFESTATIONS
Autosomal Dominant Disorders

SCA7 is an autosomal dominant ataxic disorder associated with retinitis pigmentosa and blindness.[476–478] Central visual field deficits and diminished visual acuity are usually the initial visual complaint. However, blue-yellow dyschromatopsia arising from cone dystrophy precedes these symptoms.[479,480] On fundoscopy, an initially near-normal appearance progresses to macular pigmentary degeneration (resulting in a bull's-eye appearance on fluorescein angiography); the degenerative changes spread outwards, and eventually only an atrophic macula with optic pallor and attenuated retinal vasculature remain.[480–482] Peripheral vision is spared until late in the disease course.[479] Electroretinographic studies are almost always abnormal, indicating outer retinal damage initially and inner retinal dysfunction later.[479,482,483] Optical coherence tomography (OCT) may reveal thinning of the macula and peripapillary retinal nerve fiber layer (RNFL).[484] The temporal quadrant of the peripapillary RNFL is often spared even in the presence of severe disease,[484] in contrast with MS, which predominantly affects the temporal quadrant.

There are rare reports of SCA1 associated with optic atrophy,[485] rod-cone dystrophy,[486] and maculopathies.[487] Very infrequently, patients with SCA2 and SCA6 develop retinitis pigmentosa with visual loss.[488–492] In the first OCT study comparing SCA1, SCA2, SCA3, SCA6, and MSA, peripapillary RNFL thinning was more pronounced in SCA2 and SCA3, but macular thinning was more prominent in SCA1, SCA3, SCA6, and MSA.[493] These findings suggest that changes in retinal architecture detected by OCT metrics may mirror the neurodegenerative changes that occur in the rest of the nervous system, and may be a promising biomarker of disease activity and the effectiveness of neuroprotective therapies.

Autosomal Recessive Disorders

Adult Refsum disease is an autosomal recessive peroxisomal disease caused by phytanic acid accumulation. It is progressive disease beginning in early adulthood with nyctalopia. Marked disability arises from cerebellar ataxia, peripheral neuropathy, and retinitis pigmentosa.[494] An autosomal recessive disorder similar to Refsum disease (but without phytanic acid increase), called polyneuropathy, hearing loss, ataxia, retinitis pigmentosa, and cataract, was recently described.[495]

Cerebrotendinous xanthomatosis (CTX) is an autosomal recessive disorder that results in cholestanol accumulation in tendons and nervous tissue, causing cerebellar ataxia, pyramidal signs, extrapyramidal findings, seizures, cognitive impairment, and peripheral neuropathy.[496,497] Neuro-ophthalmic manifestations of CTX include presenile cataracts, myelinated retinal nerve fibers, premature retinal senescence with retinal vessel sclerosis, cholesterol deposits in retinal vessels, palpebral xanthelasma, blepharospasm, proptosis, and optic atrophy.[497–501] Another rare ataxic disorder that is often associated with myelinated retinal nerve fibers is autosomal recessive spastic ataxia of Charlevoix-Saguenay.[502]

Mitochondrial Disorders

Many mitochondrial disorders are characterized by ataxia and ophthalmic manifestations. A few salient disorders are shown in **Table 6**.[1,504–519]

Miscellaneous Disorders

Neurologic dysfunction in the setting of vitamin E deficiency is most commonly caused by malabsorption syndromes, but may also be inherited (eg, ataxia with vitamin E

Table 6
Neuro-ophthalmic features of mitochondrial disorders with ataxia

Disorder	Neuro-ophthalmic Findings	Associated Features/Comments
MERRF	Optic atrophy (rare)	Cerebellar ataxia (common); myopathy; dementia; deafness; lipomas; foot deformities; parkinsonism
LHON	Optic atrophy (characteristic feature)	Cerebellar ataxia is rare
NARP	Retinitis pigmentosa	Motor neuropathy, cerebellar ataxia, and retinitis pigmentosa are cardinal features. Other findings include deafness, dementia, seizures, and sensory neuropathy
KSS	CPEO Retinitis pigmentosa Others: glaucoma, ptosis	Cardiac arrhythmia; diabetes mellitus; amenorrhea; myopathy; deafness; pyramidal dysfunction; increased CSF protein
MSL	CPEO	Deafness; myopathy; neuropathy
Leigh syndrome	Nystagmus Ophthalmoparesis (similar to Wernicke encephalopathy) Optic atrophy OTR See-saw nystagmus	Mental retardation; seizures; dystonia; respiratory failure; myopathy; neuropathy A variant of the MTATP6 mutation (which causes Leigh syndrome) was recently reported to cause adult-onset spinocerebellar syndrome[503]
Autosomal dominant CPEO	CPEO	Deafness; myopathy
SANDO	Ophthalmoparesis	Cerebellar or sensory ataxia, dysarthria, and ophthalmoparesis form the triad of SANDO. Other features include myopathy, neuropathy, and dysphagia
MNGIE	Ophthalmoparesis	Cardinal features: nausea, vomiting, diarrhea, ascites, dysmotility, neuropathy, myopathy Other features: cerebellar ataxia, deafness, facial palsy, hepatosplenomegaly, orthostatic hypotension, dysarthria, dysphonia, urinary dysfunction
Autosomal dominant optic atrophy and deafness	Optic atrophy CPEO	Deafness; cerebellar ataxia; sensorimotor axonal neuropathy; myopathy
Wolfram syndrome	Optic atrophy	DIDMOAD. Other findings include cerebellar ataxia, joint contractures, autonomic neuropathy, hypogonadism, psychiatric disorders

Abbreviations: CPEO, chronic progressive external ophthalmoplegia; CSF, cerebrospinal fluid; DIDMOAD, diabetes insipidus, diabetes mellitus, optic atrophy, and deafness; KSS, Kearns-Sayre syndrome; LHON, Leber hereditary optic neuropathy; MERRF, myoclonic epilepsy and ragged red fibers; MNGIE, mitochondrial neuro-gastrointestinal encephalomyopathy; MSL, multiple symmetric lipomatosis; NARP, neurogenic muscle weakness, ataxia, and retinitis pigmentosa; SANDO, sensory ataxia with neuropathy, dysarthria, and ophthalmoparesis.

deficiency).[520] Cerebellar ocular motor abnormalities are frequent, but retinitis pigmentosa may also occur.[520]

Cerebellar ataxia and atrophy is a rare manifestation of Sjögren syndrome.[521–525] Sjögren syndrome causes many neuro-ophthalmic manifestations, including keratoconjunctivitis sicca, Adie tonic pupil, optic neuropathy, ischemic choroidopathy, and cranial neuropathies.[526–529] Hydroxychloroquine, a common treatment of Sjögren syndrome, also may cause ophthalmic toxic side effects, including pigmentary retinopathy, keratopathy, ciliary body dysfunction, and lens opacities.[530]

Creutzfeldt-Jakob disease (CJD) often mimics the clinical course of paraneoplastic cerebellar degeneration (PCD; discussed later). Various visual manifestations, including visual hallucinations and cortical visual dysfunction (eg, Anton syndrome, simultanagnosia, prosopagnosia, optic apraxia, optic ataxia, cerebral achromatopsia) may occur, especially in the Heidenhain variant of CJD.[531–534] Eye movement disturbances in CJD include progressive supranuclear gaze palsy,[535] PAN (and periodic alternating gaze deviation),[411] slowed saccades,[411] and centripetal nystagmus.[536] Another prion disease that often shows cerebellar eye signs is Gerstmann-Straussler-Scheinker disease.[1] Lithium or bismuth toxicity may also mimic the clinical presentation of CJD.[1]

NEURO-OPHTHALMIC ABNORMALITIES IN SELECTED CEREBELLAR DISORDERS
Chiari Malformations

Chiari I malformations are among the most common cause of spontaneous DBN, most likely as the consequence of floccular compression.[212,213,537] The neuro-ophthalmic manifestations of Chiari I malformation are summarized in **Box 2**.[538–544] In

---

Box 2
Neuro-ophthalmic manifestations of Chiari I malformation

DBN (most common)

Positional nystagmus

UBN

GEN

PAN

Convergence nystagmus

See-saw nystagmus

Nystagmus of skew

Comitant esotropia

Saccadic pursuit

Dysmetric saccades

Impaired OKRs

Internuclear ophthalmoparesis

Tunnel vision and subjective visual field defects

Optic disc pallor

Anisocoria

Ptosis

contradistinction with Chiari I, Chiari II malformations rarely cause DBN, but frequently cause saccadic smooth pursuit, impaired OKN, and horizontal nystagmus.[543–547] Saccades and VOR gain are infrequently affected.[546,548,549] Brainstem kinking in Chiari II malformations may cause INO.[550–562]

FRDA

The most common autosomal recessive ataxic disorder, FRDA typically presents in childhood to adolescence with hyporeflexia, upgoing plantar reflexes, dorsal column findings, and cerebellar ataxia.[553,554] A prominent finding in FRDA is saccadic intrusions, which are usually SWJs but sometimes ocular flutter may be observed.[61,555,556,559] Other neuro-ophthalmic and nonneurologic manifestations of FRDA are summarized in **Table 7**.[61,554–562]

Ataxia-Telangiectasia

Ataxia-telangiectasia (AT) is an autosomal recessive ataxic disorder that presents in childhood with cerebellar ataxia, oculomotor apraxia, telangiectasias, recurrent infections, and increased serum alpha fetoprotein (AFP) levels.[563–567] AT results in diffuse cerebellar cortical degeneration, with relative sparing of the deep cerebellar nuclei.[568–573]

The neuro-ophthalmic hallmark in AT, telangiectatic vessels confined to the light-exposed, interpalpebral portions of the bulbar conjunctiva, often precedes the development of neurologic deficits by a few years.[563,567,574] These telangiectatic vessels are often asymptomatic and not associated with increased intraocular pressure, unlike Sturge-Weber syndrome, Osler-Weber-Rendu syndrome, and caroticocavernous fistula.[574] Another highly conspicuous finding, oculomotor apraxia, is characterized

Table 7 Neuro-ophthalmic and nonneurologic manifestations of FRDA	
Efferent visual system	• Saccadic intrusions (most commonly horizontal SWJ, but sometimes vertical/oblique SWJ or ocular flutter) • Decreased VOR gain • Reduced smooth pursuit gain • Dysmetric saccades • Impaired OKRs • Gaze-evoked and rebound nystagmus • Ptosis
Afferent visual system	• Diminished visual acuity • Bilateral visual loss mimicking Leber hereditary optic neuropathy • Visual field defects (central, paracentral, and arcuate scotomas) • Optic pallor • RNFL thinning on OCT
Neurologic	• Hyporeflexia with upgoing plantar reflexes • Dorsal column signs • Cerebellar ataxia • Dysphagia • Hearing loss • Sphincteric dysfunction
Nonneurologic	• Scoliosis • Cardiomyopathy • Diabetes mellitus • Foot deformities

by delayed saccadic initiation followed by slow target-directed gaze shifts.[575–577] To make horizontal refixations (by taking advantage of their normal or increased VOR gain), patients use head thrusts to tonically move the eyes in the opposite direction; the eyes continue to fixate on the desired target as the head slowly turns back to primary position.[1,575,576] During optokinetic and vestibular stimulation, tonic ocular deviation occurs in the direction of the slow phase, with no corrective quick phase in the opposite direction to reset the eyes.[1,575] This distinct clinical finding (in which head turns produce involuntary tonic contraversive eye movements without corrective quick phases) is sometimes called the Roth-Bielschowsky phenomenon.[575]

Other eye movement abnormalities in AT are related to cerebellar dysfunction, and include convergence insufficiency, positional nystagmus, PAN, impaired pursuit, hypometric saccades, and cross-coupled VOR.[312,574,575,578–580] Rare neuro-ophthalmic findings associated with AT include eyelid vitiligo and optic disc drusen.[581]

SCA

The most common SCAs are SCA1, SCA2, SCA3, SCA6, and SCA7, and as such this article focuses on these disorders. They usually present in adulthood and pursue a progressive clinical course with an average disease duration of 15 to 30 years.[582]

Although there is considerable overlap in their eye movement findings, certain patterns may help guide the diagnostic work-up:

- Slowed saccades are a prominent hallmark of SCA2 and SCA7, but are uncommon in SCAs 1, 3, and 6.[479,481,483,583–587]
- GEN and saccadic dysmetria are common in SCA1, SCA3, and SCA6 but are unusual in SCA2 and SCA7.[479,481,483,584,586,587]
- Saccadic intrusions and lid retraction (bulging eyes) suggest SCA3.[586–589]
- Decreased VOR gain, perverted HSN, positional vertigo, and DBN suggest SCA6.[587,590,591]
- Saccadic pursuit is more common in SCA3 and SCA6 than in SCA2 and SCA1.[586,587]

The neurologic and neuro-ophthalmic features of SCA1, SCA2, SCA3, SCA6, and SCA7[70,479,481,483,582,584,586–595] are summarized in **Table 8**.

CANVAS

Cerebellar ataxia with bilateral vestibulopathy characterized by impaired visually enhanced VOR (VVOR) was first proposed as a distinct disorder in 2004.[596] Later, the presence of neuropathy in this syndrome was recognized as part of this syndrome, which was called CANVAS.[597]

The neuro-ophthalmic hallmark of CANVAS is reduced VVOR gain. Other findings include DBN, GEN, diminished high-frequency VOR gain, and saccadic pursuit.[596,597] A non–length-dependent multimodal sensory neuropathy with absent sensory nerve action potentials (SNAPs), suggesting a ganglionopathy, is characteristic of CANVAS.[597] MRI reveals cerebellar atrophy, involving the anterior and dorsal vermis, as well as hemispheric crus.[597] CANVAS seems to follow a late-onset autosomal recessive pattern of inheritance,[597] but the etiopathogenetic underpinnings have yet to be elucidated.

Important differential diagnoses of CANVAS are SCA3, FRDA, and MSA.[597] The salient and distinguishing features of each disorder are summarized in **Table 9**.

Episodic Ataxia Type 2

Episodic ataxia type 2 (EA2) is an autosomal dominant disorder (caused by CACNA1A gene mutation) is characterized by recurrent attacks of ataxia lasting for hours to days

Table 8
Features of SCA types 1, 2, 3, 6, and 7

	Neuro-ophthalmic Abnormalities	Other Features
SCA1	Saccadic pursuit GEN Rebound nystagmus Decreased VOR gain Impaired OKN Optic atrophy (rare)	Dysphagia, pyramidal dysfunction, extrapyramidal symptoms, peripheral neuropathy, cognitive decline
SCA2	Slowed saccades Impaired OKN Retinitis pigmentosa (rare)	Areflexia, myoclonus, kinetic and postural tremor, peripheral neuropathy, dysphagia, sleep disturbances, cognitive decline, hypogonadism, hearing loss, autonomic dysfunction
SCA3	Saccadic intrusions Lid retraction (bulging eyes) GEN Reduced VOR gain Positional horizontal nystagmus Impaired OKN External ophthalmoparesis	Faciolingual myokymia, peripheral neuropathy, spasticity, pyramidal dysfunction, impaired temperature sensation, dystonia, amyotrophy, sleep disturbances, mood and cognitive disorders. Carriers of the mutation may have GEN
SCA6	Saccadic pursuit Dysmetric saccades DBN GEN Rebound nystagmus Perverted HSN Positional DBN Positional vertigo Impaired OKN	Considered a pure cerebellar syndrome but may be accompanied by extrapyramidal, pyramidal, sensory, and swallowing deficits. Some patients with SCA6 may experience episodes of ataxia and dizziness precipitated by stress and fatigue, similar to that of episodic ataxia type 2
SCA7	Retinitis pigmentosa Ptosis Slowed saccades Saccadic pursuit Restricted upgaze and convergence progresses to horizontal and downgaze limitation Impaired VOR (late in disease) Impaired OKN	SCA7 usually presents with ataxia followed by progressive visual loss. Other manifestations include dysphagia, cognitive deficits, sensory signs, and pyramidal dysfunction

that are provoked by physical exertion, stress, heat, caffeine, or alcohol; the disease typically begins before the age of 20 years, but sometimes presents in patients more than 50 years of age.[598,599] More than half of patients also have migraines.[600]

Patients interictally show central ocular motor abnormalities including DBN, positional nystagmus, GEN, rebound nystagmus, saccadic pursuit, and even bilateral INO.[600–602] Other findings may include strabismus, SO palsy, abducens palsy, and limited upgaze.[26,603–605] During attacks, patients experience vertigo, nausea, vomiting, spontaneous nystagmus, incoordination, and/or headaches,[606] similar to vestibular migraine. CACNA1A gene mutations also cause familial hemiplegic migraine and SCA6, explaining the clinical overlap between these syndromes.[598]

Imaging may reveal cerebellar atrophy, particularly of the anterior vermis.[598] The drug of choice for EA2 is acetazolamide.[607] Side effects of acetazolamide include

Table 9
Salient features of CANVAS, SCA3, FRDA, and MSA

	Inheritance	Age of Onset	Vestibular Loss	Neuropathy	Other Features
CANVAS	Possibly late-onset autosomal recessive	Mean age 60 y	Present	Painless, non–length-dependent, multimodal sensory loss (absent SNAPs). Motor action potentials preserved	—
SCA3	Autosomal dominant	Fourth to seventh decade	Possible	Length-dependent, predominantly sensory axonal neuropathy with motor involvement	SWJ
FRDA	Autosomal recessive	Before age 20 y. Rarely, more than 50 y	Possible	Large-fiber sensory neuropathy with diminished SNAPs	Scoliosis, cardiomyopathy, diabetes mellitus
MSA	Sporadic	Sixth decade of life	Very rare	Absent	Autonomic dysfunction, extrapyramidal findings, RBD

Abbreviation: RBD, rapid eye movement sleep behavior disorder.

nephrolithiasis, paresthesias, dysgeusia, and gastrointestinal upset. Sulthiame, a central carbonic anhydrase inhibitor, has fewer side effects than acetazolamide.[599] Topiramate, a weak carbonic anhydrase inhibitor with the additional benefit of migraine prophylaxis, is another useful alternative.[608] Attacks of EA2 were recently shown to be mitigated by 4-aminopyridine (4-AP; discussed later).

Ataxia with Oculomotor Ataxia Type 2

Ataxia with oculomotor ataxia type 2 (AOA2) is an autosomal recessive disorder caused by mutation of the senataxin gene that typically presents in the second decade of life. It is characterized by progressive cerebellar ataxia, peripheral neuropathy (usually axonal sensorimotor neuropathy), and increased serum AFP levels.[609–612] Despite its name, only about half of patients with AOA2 show oculomotor apraxia.[612] Other neuro-ophthalmic manifestations include strabismus, saccadic pursuit, GEN, increased saccade latencies, and dysmetric saccades.[611,612]

MSA

MSA is a sporadic, adult-onset, neurodegenerative disorder resulting from alpha-synuclein accumulation in glial cytoplasmic inclusions within the central nervous system. It consists of 2 phenotypes: one with predominant parkinsonism (MSA-P), and the other with predominant cerebellar ataxia (MSA-C). A history of autonomic dysfunction and rapid eye movement–sleep behavior disorder is typically present in both groups, as well as some elements of parkinsonism or ataxia.[613] The ocular motor abnormalities in MSA reflect the underlying striatonigral and olivopontocerebellar degeneration. These findings are summarized in **Box 3**.[50,67,276,493,556,591,614–624]

Wernicke Encephalopathy

Wernicke encephalopathy, caused by thiamine deficiency, is classically characterized by the triad of confusion, ophthalmoparesis, and ataxia. However, only 16% to 38% of cases show the classic triad; it is far more common to show 1 or 2 of these cardinal features.[625,626] The neuropathologic changes that characterize Wernicke encephalopathy affect the periaqueductal gray matter, mamillary bodies, medial thalamus, superior vermis, pontine tegmentum, mesencephalic reticular formation, posterior corpora quadrigemina, ocular motor nuclei, vestibular nuclei, and cerebral cortex.[627,628] The neuro-ophthalmic manifestations of Wernicke encephalopathy are summarized in **Table 10**.[1,246,254,262,628–644]

When treating Wernicke encephalopathy, it is vital to remember that magnesium is an important cofactor of transketolase and thiamine pyrophosphokinase and is therefore crucial to thiamine metabolism.[645] Severe hypomagnesemia may prevent any response to thiamine replacement therapy until magnesium is repleted.[646] Severe hypomagnesemia may alternatively precipitate Wernicke encephalopathy by impeding thiamine metabolism.[647]

Wilson Disease

Wilson disease is an autosomal recessive disorder caused by mutations in the ATP7B gene on chromosome 13 that results in abnormal accumulation of copper, causing neurologic, hepatic, renal, and corneal manifestations.[648,649] The neuro-ophthalmic manifestations of Wilson disease involves both the afferent and efferent visual pathways and are summarized in **Table 11**.[1,648,650–671]

Box 3
Neuro-ophthalmic manifestations of MSA

DBN

Gaze-evoked and rebound nystagmus

Positional nystagmus

Saccadic intrusions (usually SWJ)

Saccadic pursuit tracking

Dysmetric saccades

Saccade velocities are often spared

Impaired OKRs

Vergence paresis

Horner syndrome

Mild supranuclear vertical gaze palsy

Impaired VOR gain

OCT: macular and nasal peripapillary RNFL thinning

Pupillary autonomic dysfunction (with 0.02% dipivefrine hydrochloride)

Table 10
Neuro-ophthalmic manifestations of Wernicke encephalopathy

Ophthalmoparesis	• Most commonly abducens palsy • May be asymmetric • Affects horizontal eye movements before vertical eye movements • Complete ophthalmoplegia may occur late • Other findings include internuclear ophthalmoparesis, convergence insufficiency, and convergence spasm
Nystagmus	• Most commonly GEN • UBN (especially if it converts to DBN with convergence) • UBN may transition to DBN with recovery • DBN
Vestibular hypofunction	• Decreased visually enhanced VOR gain • Decreased high-frequency VOR gain • Diminished caloric responses • Signs of vestibular hypofunction usually improve partially with thiamine replacement
Saccades	• Decelerating (stuttering) saccades • Dysmetric saccades
Smooth pursuit	• Decreased gain
Pupillary dysfunction	• Anisocoria • Sluggish pupils • Light-near dissociation • Pupillary areflexia
Visual loss	• Infrequent finding • Usually associated with papilledema, as well as peripapillary RNFL thickening, telangiectasias, and retinal hemorrhages • Rarely, cortical visual loss may occur

Table 11	
Neuro-ophthalmic abnormalities in Wilson disease	
Kayser-Fleischer ring	• Greenish brown discoloration of the peripheral cornea caused by copper deposition in Descemet membrane • Considered a pathognomonic sign of neurologic involvement • Begins as a crescent on the superior corneal arc, then involves the inferior arc, before involving the lateral aspects to eventually form the ring • Best visualized with slit lamp examination
Other afferent visual pathway manifestations	• Sunflower cataracts • Abnormal visual evoked potential latencies • Abnormal electroretinographic responses • Reduced macular and peripapillary RNFL thicknesses (especially in the ganglion cell, inner plexiform, and inner nuclear layers)
Distractability of gaze	• Unusual but striking clinical finding in which patients are unable to voluntarily fixate on a target unless competing visual stimuli are removed
Saccadic abnormalities	• Vertical saccades are affected earlier and more severely than horizontal saccades • Slowed saccades • Dysmetric saccades • Saccadic intrusions
Smooth pursuit abnormalities	• Vertical pursuit is impaired earlier and more severely than horizontal pursuit • Decreased vertical pursuit gain is an early finding in Wilson disease
Other findings	• Accommodation defects • Eyelid-opening apraxia • Oculogyric crisis

Whipple Disease

Whipple disease, caused by infection by *Tropheryma whipplei*, typically results in constitutional symptoms, gastrointestinal manifestations, lymphadenopathy, and migratory polyarthralgias.[672–674] A wide range of neurologic manifestations (ataxia is common) may occur, sometimes in the absence of other features.[674,675] Whipple disease may affect both the afferent and efferent visual pathways; these findings are summarized in **Table 12**.[49,674,676–683]

Celiac Disease (Gluten Ataxia)

Celiac disease is characterized by intolerance to dietary gluten. The term gluten sensitivity refers to patients with circulating antigliadin antibodies without any gastrointestinal histologic abnormalities.[684] Neurologic manifestations (the most common being ataxia) may occur in about 10% of patients, and may exist without gastrointestinal features.[289,685–687] Neuro-ophthalmic abnormalities in celiac disease include saccadic pursuit, dysmetric saccades, UBN, DBN, impaired VOR, GEN, slowed saccades, palatal tremor, opsoclonus, and diplopia.[142,289,684,688,689] The response to elimination of dietary gluten depends on the duration of the cerebellar manifestations; prolonged gluten exposure leads to irreversible Purkinje cell damage, and as such prompt recognition of gluten ataxia is imperative.[687] It is important to screen for any concomitant

Table 12
Neuro-ophthalmic manifestations of Whipple disease

Oculomasticatory myorhythmia	• 1-Hz pendular vergence oscillations with synchronous masticatory muscle contractions that persist during sleep and coma • Considered the pathognomonic feature of Whipple disease but is only seen in 20% of cases
Ocular findings	• Uveitis (frequent) • Vitritis • Retinitis • Retinal hemorrhage • Retinal periphlebitis • Retinal vasculitis • Macular edema • Choroiditis • Papillitis • Optic atrophy • Keratitis • Orbital pseudotumor
Vertical supranuclear gaze palsy	• Most common ocular motor abnormality in Whipple disease • Begins with slowed upward saccades, followed by downward saccade slowing • Mimics PSP • Lack of smooth pursuit impairment and saccadic intrusions can help differentiate Whipple disease (a treatable disorder) from PSP (an incurable neurodegenerative disease)
Other neuro-ophthalmic findings	• Internuclear ophthalmoparesis • Nonreactive pupils • Ptosis • Parinaud syndrome • Convergence insufficiency • Vertical nystagmus • Pendular nystagmus • Cranial neuropathies

malabsorption-related nutritional deficiencies because these may cause neurologic deficits as well.

Anti-GAD Ataxia

Anti-GAD antibodies are classically associated with diabetes mellitus type 1, SPS, and progressive encephalomyelitis with rigidity and myoclonus.[690–693] Other neurologic syndromes associated with anti-GAD antibodies include seizures, limbic encephalitis, palatal tremor, subacute cerebellar ataxia, and peripheral neuropathy.[694–699] Neuro-ophthalmic manifestations reported in anti-GAD ataxia (or in rare cases with coexisting SPS) include alternating esotropia, vertical ocular misalignment, limited abduction, DBN, PAN, GEN, saccadic pursuit, macular degeneration, and slowed vertical saccades.[418,698,700] Isolated DBN has also been reported.[701] Anti-GAD autoimmunity is sometimes associated with myasthenia gravis, especially in the presence of a thymoma; as such, the clinician should take note of any ocular signs of myasthenia.[702–704]

Paraneoplastic Ataxic Syndromes

Paraneoplastic cerebellar ataxia may arise in setting of PCD or paraneoplastic brainstem encephalitis. When paraneoplastic onconeural antibodies target cerebellar

Purkinje cells, a syndrome characterized by progressive ataxia and/or vertigo, termed PCD, results.[705] **Table 13** summarizes the details of PCD.[100,102,103,706–718]

Onconeural antibodies involved in paraneoplastic brainstem encephalitis include anti-Hu, anti-Ri, anti-CRMP-5, anti-Ma2, and anti-N-methyl-D-aspartate receptor. Ataxia and opsoclonus-myoclonus has been reported in a newly discovered paraneoplastic antibody, the anti-GABA$_B$ receptor antibody.[719] **Table 14** summarizes the features of anit-Ma2, anti-Hu, and anti-Ri paraneoplastic brainstem encephalitis.[53,252,706,707,720–733]

TREATMENT OF OCULAR MOTOR ABNORMALITIES IN CEREBELLAR DISEASE

Although most patients with cerebellar disorders do not complain of symptoms arising from their ocular motor abnormalities, some manifestations cause oscillopsia and/or may be cosmetically displeasing, impairing the patients' social interactions. As such, symptomatic management may be required in these cases. We do not

Table 13 Features of PCD	
Malignancy	• Lung (especially small cell lung cancer) • Breast • Ovary • Hodgkin lymphoma
Findings	• Progressive subacute cerebellar ataxia • DBN • UBN • GEN • Rebound nystagmus • Saccadic intrusions, Impaired pursuit • Dysmetric saccades
Onconeural antibodies	Anti-Yo: • Most common antibody in PCD (40% of cases) • Usually causes a pure cerebellar syndrome • Typically in postmenopausal women with breast or ovarian cancer • Other neuro-ophthalmic findings: opsoclonus, visual loss, anterior uveitis, abducens palsy, skew deviation, and lid retraction Anti-Hu: • Second most common onconeural antibody in PCD (18%–23% of cases) • Usually associated with extracerebellar neurologic manifestations • Infrequently associated with optic neuropathy Anti–CRMP-5: • Infrequent • May be associated with optic neuropathy, uveitis, and/or retinitis Anti-Tr: • Associated with Hodgkin lymphoma • May be associated with optic neuropathy • Case report of positional periodic alternating vertical nystagmus Anti-VGCC: • PCD may coexist with Lambert-Eaton myasthenic syndrome Other paraneoplastic antibodies: • Anti-Ri • Anti–metabotropic glutamate receptor-1 • Anti-Zic 1 to 4 • Anti-Ma1/Ma2 • Anti-ANNA3 • Anti-GABA

Table 14
Neuro-ophthalmic manifestations of anti-Ma2, anti-Hu, and anti-Ri paraneoplastic brainstem encephalitis

Onconeural Antibody	Features
Anti-Ma2 antibodies	• Typically affect upper brainstem, resulting in progressive supranuclear vertical gaze paresis that later involves horizontal gaze • As the disease advances, vestibuloocular reflexes and Bell phenomenon are impaired • Other neuro-ophthalmic findings: ptosis; skew deviation; opsoclonus; ocular flutter; saccadic pursuit; DBN; UBN in downgaze; horizontal nystagmus; monocular pendular nystagmus; Horner syndrome; oculogyric crisis • A case of anti-Ma1/Ma2 encephalitis causing ocular motor apraxia, eyelid-opening apraxia, impaired vergence, saccadic pursuit, and blepharospasm has been reported • Neurologic manifestations: limbic encephalitis; diencephalic encephalitis; hypokinetic extrapyramidal features; cranial neuropathies; and pyramidal signs
Anti-Hu antibodies	• Typically affects the medulla • Findings include blepharospasm, eyelid-opening apraxia, ptosis, supranuclear gaze palsy, GEN, UBN, DBN, saccadic intrusions, impaired pursuit, Adie tonic pupils, lid nystagmus, and ocular motor cranial neuropathies
Anti-Ri antibodies	• Neurologic findings: extrapyramidal features, cerebellar ataxia, jaw dystonia, and laryngospasm • Neuro-ophthalmic findings: opsoclonus, slowed saccades, ophthalmoparesis, blepharospasm, and saccadic pursuit

Box 4
4AP in cerebellar disorders

4AP is a nonselective voltage-activated potassium channel antagonist that hypothetically enhances Purkinje cell excitability and synaptic transmission.

Benefits:

• Useful in the symptomatic management of oscillopsia resulting from downbeat and UBN

• Also improves smooth pursuit gain, vertical VOR gain, time constants of the neural integrators, visual acuity, and locomotion

• 4AP also diminishes, or even abolishes, attacks of episodic ataxia type 2, and central positional nystagmus

• Dalfampridine, a sustained-release form of 4AP, has shown similar efficacy to 4AP in treating DBN

• In patients with MS and demyelinating disorders, 4AP has the added benefits of improving ambulation and energy levels

Contraindications: 4AP should not be given to patients with abnormal renal function or a prior history of seizures.

Adverse effects: dizziness, nervousness, paresthesias, and most importantly seizures (which occur at toxic serum levels).

Data from Refs.[280,286,734–743]

recommend treating ocular movement abnormalities unless they cause disabling or highly bothersome symptoms, because the potential side effects of some therapeutic choices are worse than the symptoms. There have been no large randomized controlled trials to evaluate the efficacy of the drugs discussed here; most are based on observations in small groups of patients, and from anecdotal reports. Of particular interest is 4AP, which has been found to be effective in treating several ocular motor abnormalities and ataxic disorders (summarized in **Box 4**). **Table 15** lists some treatment options for cerebellar ocular motor abnormalities.

Table 15
Treatment of ocular motility abnormalities in cerebellar disorders

	Treatment Options	References
SWJ and macrosaccadic oscillations	• Benzodiazepines • Gabapentin • Memantine • Phenobarbital • Sodium valproate	1,58,73,150,744,745
Ocular flutter and opsoclonus	• Propranolol • Gabapentin • Levetiracetam • Ethosuximide • Topiramate • All patients with ocular flutter and opsoclonus should be worked up and followed for any evidence of occult malignancies • Children: ACTH, corticosteroids, IVIg, B cell–depleting monoclonal antibodies (eg, rituximab, ofatumumab) • Adults: corticosteroids, IVIg, and plasmapheresis	6,104,147,150,746–753
DBN	• Clonazepam • Baclofen • Gabapentin • 4AP • Chlorzoxazone • Anticholinergic drugs (eg, scopolamine) • Base-down prisms • Laying supine may help reduce oscillopsia while reading • Resting or sleeping in the upright position may help diminish the amplitude of DBN	209,754–759
UBN	• Baclofen • 4AP	755,760
PAN	• Baclofen (most effective) • Memantine • Extraocular muscle resection	410,761–765
Acquired pendular nystagmus	• Gabapentin • Memantine • Anticholinergic drugs (eg, scopolamine, trihexyphenidyl) • Cannabis • A recent report details how mastoid vibration dampens APN in a patient with MS[766]	312,412,757,767–774

Abbreviations: ACTH, adrenocorticotropic hormone; IVIg, intravenous immunoglobulin.

SUMMARY

Cerebellar diseases result in many neuro-ophthalmic abnormalities that most prominently affect ocular movements, but may also cause concurrent afferent visual pathway manifestations. Familiarity with the 3 principal cerebellar syndromes (the floccular-parafloccular syndrome, the ventral uvula-nodular syndrome, and the oculomotor vermis-caudal fastigial nuclei syndromes) as well as the ataxic disorders that involve the anterior visual system helps to refine the diagnostic focus. More cerebellar disorders are being discovered, so clinicians should be familiar with these manifestations as well as the medications that may be used to ameliorate the oscillopsia that results from these disorders.

ACKNOWLEDGMENTS

The authors thank Dr David S. Zee for his guidance and help in preparing this article.

REFERENCES

1. Leigh RJ, Zee DS. The neurology of eye movements. 4th edition. New York: Oxford University Press; 2006.
2. Stahl JS, Leigh RJ. Nystagmus. Curr Neurol Neurosci Rep 2001;1:471–7.
3. Averbuch-Heller L, Leigh RJ. Nystagmus. Curr Opin Ophthalmol 1996;7:42–7.
4. Sato Y, Kawasaki T. Identification of the Purkinje cell/climbing fiber zone and its target neurons responsible for eye-movement control by the cerebellar flocculus. Brain Res Dev Brain Res 1991;16:39–64.
5. Buttner-Ennever JA, Horn AK, Schmidtke K. Cell groups of the medial longitudinal fasciculus and paramedian tracts. Rev Neurol (Paris) 1989;145:533–9.
6. Ramat S, Leigh RJ, Zee DS, et al. What clinical disorders tell us about the neural control of saccadic eye movements. Brain 2007;130:10–35.
7. Robinson DA. Eye movement control in primates. The oculomotor system contains specialized subsystems for acquiring and tracking visual targets. Science 1968;161:1219–24.
8. Robinson DA. Oculomotor control signals. In: Lennerstrand G, Bach-y-Rita P, editors. Basic mechanisms of ocular motility and their clinical implications. Oxford (United Kingdom): Pergamon; 1975. p. 337–74.
9. Arnold DB, Robinson DA. The oculomotor integrator: testing of a neural network model. Exp Brain Res 1997;113:57–74.
10. Helmchen C, Rambold H, Fuhry L, et al. Deficits in vertical and torsional eye movements after uni- and bilateral muscimol inactivation of the interstitial nucleus of Cajal of the alert monkey. Exp Brain Res 1998;119:436–52.
11. Cannon SC, Robinson DA. Loss of the neural integrator of the oculomotor system from brain stem lesions in monkey. J Neurophysiol 1987;57:1383–409.
12. Mettens P, Godaux E, Cheron G, et al. Effects of muscimol microinjections into the prepositus hypoglossi and the medial vestibular nuclei on eye movements. J Neurophysiol 1994;72:785–802.
13. Scudder CA. A new local feedback model of the saccadic burst generator. J Neurophysiol 1988;59:1455–75.
14. Scudder CA, Moschovakis AK, Karabelas AB, et al. Anatomy and physiology of saccadic long-lead burst neurons recorded in the alert squirrel monkey I. Descending projections from the mesencephalon. J Neurophysiol 1996;76:332–52.

15. Scudder CA, Moschovakis AK, Karabelas AB, et al. Anatomy and physiology of saccadic long-lead burst neurons recorded in the alert squirrel monkey II. Pontine neurons. J Neurophysiol 1996;76:353–70.

16. Harting JK. Descending pathways from the superior colliculus: an autoradiographic analysis in rhesus monkeys (*Macaca mulatta*). J Comp Neurol 1997; 173:583–612.

17. Noda H, Sugita S, Ikeda Y. Afferent and efferent connections of the oculomotor region of the fastigial nucleus in the macaque monkey. J Comp Neurol 1990; 302:330–48.

18. Yamada J, Noda H. Afferent and efferent connections of the oculomotor cerebellar vermis in the macaque monkey. J Comp Neurol 1987;265:224–41.

19. Buttner-Ennever JA, Horn AK, Cohen B. Projections from the superior colliculus motor map to omnipause neurons in monkey. J Comp Neurol 1999;413:55–67.

20. Miura K, Optican LM. Membrane channel properties of premotor excitatory burst neurons may underlie saccade slowing after lesions of omnipause neurons. J Comput Neurosci 2006;20:25–41.

21. Noda H, Fujikado T. Topography of the oculomotor area of the cerebellar vermis in macaques as determined by microstimulation. J Neurophysiol 1987;58: 359–78.

22. Goldstein JE, Cogan DG. Lateralizing value of ocular motor dysmetria and skew deviation. Arch Ophthalmol 1961;66:517–8.

23. Zee DS, Yee RD, Cogan DG, et al. Ocular motor abnormalities in hereditary cerebellar ataxia. Brain 1976;99:207–34.

24. Buttner U, Fuhry L. Eye movements. Curr Opin Neurol 1995;8:77–82.

25. Versino M, Hurko O, Zee DS. Disorders of binocular control of eye movements in patients with cerebellar dysfunction. Brain 1996;119:1933–50.

26. Vahedi K, Joutel A, Von Bogaert P, et al. A gene for hereditary paroxysmal cerebellar ataxia maps to chromosome 19p. Ann Neurol 1995;37:289–93.

27. Takagi M, Zee DS, Tamargo RJ. Effects of lesions of the oculomotor vermis on eye movements in primate: saccades. J Neurophysiol 1998;80:1911–31.

28. Aschoff J, Cohen B. Changes in saccadic eye movements produced by cerebellar cortical lesions. Exp Neurol 1971;32:123–33.

29. Sato H, Noda H. Saccadic dysmetria induced by transient functional decortications of the cerebellar vermis. Neurosci Res 1992;12:583–95.

30. Waespe W, Muller-Meisser E. Directional reversal of saccadic dysmetria and gain adaptivity in a patient with a superior cerebellar artery infarction. Neuroophthalmology 1996;16:65–74.

31. Barash S, Melikyan A, Sivakov A, et al. Saccadic dysmetria and adaptation after lesions of the cerebellar cortex. J Neurosci 1999;19:10931–9.

32. Golla H, Tziridis K, Haarmeier T, et al. Reduced saccadic resilience and impaired saccadic adaptation due to cerebellar disease. Eur J Neurosci 2008;27:132–44.

33. Ignashchenko A, Dash S, Dicke PW, et al. Normal spatial attention but impaired saccades and visual motion perception after lesions of the monkey cerebellum. J Neurophysiol 2009;102:3156–68.

34. Robinson FR, Straube A, Fuchs AF. Role of the caudal fastigial nucleus in saccade generation. II. Effects of muscimol inactivation. J Neurophysiol 1993; 70:1741–58.

35. Ohtsuka K, Sato H, Noda H. Saccadic burst neurons in the fastigial nucleus are not involved in compensating for orbital nonlinearities. J Neurophysiol 1994;71: 1976–80.

36. Optican LM, Robinson DA. Cerebellar-dependent adaptive control of primate saccadic system. J Neurophysiol 1980;44:1058–76.

37. van Gisbergen JA, Robinson DA, Gielen S. A quantitative analysis of generation of saccadic eye movements by burst neurons. J Neurophysiol 1981;45:417–42.

38. Sparks DL, Barton EJ. Neural control of saccadic eye movements. Curr Opin Neurobiol 1993;3:966–72.

39. Sparks DL. The brainstem control of saccadic eye movements. Nat Rev Neurosci 2002;3:952–64.

40. Goffart L, Chen LL, Sparks DL. Deficits in saccades and fixation during muscimol inactivation of the caudal fastigial nucleus in the rhesus monkey. J Neurophysiol 2004;92:3351–67.

41. Kleine JF, Guan Y, Büttner U. Saccade-related neurons in the primate fastigial nucleus: what do they encode? J Neurophysiol 2003;90:3137–54.

42. Ohtsuka K, Noda H. Saccadic burst neurons in the oculomotor region of the fastigial nucleus of macaque monkeys. J Neurophysiol 1991;65:1422–34.

43. Fuchs AF, Robinson FR, Straube A. Role of the caudal fastigial nucleus in saccade generation. I. Neuronal discharge patterns. J Neurophysiol 1993;70: 1723–40.

44. Robinson FR, Fuchs AF, Straube A, et al. The role of the interpositus nucleus in saccades is different from the role of the fastigial nucleus. Soc Neurosci Abstr 1996;22:1200.

45. Glickstein M, Gerrits N, Kralj-Hans I, et al. Visual pontocerebellar projections in the macaque. J Comp Neurol 1994;349:51–72.

46. Swales C, Glickstein M, Gibson A. Floccular complex projections to the cerebellar nuclei of macaques. Soc Neurosci Abstr 1997;23:1828.

47. May PJ, Hartwich-Young R, Nelson J, et al. Cerebellotectal pathways in the macaque: implications for collicular generation of saccades. Neuroscience 1990;36:305–24.

48. Robinson FR. Role of the cerebellar posterior interpositus nucleus in saccades I. Effect of temporary lesions. J Neurophysiol 2000;84:1289–302.

49. Averbuch-Heller L, Paulson GW, Daroff RB, et al. Whipple's disease mimicking progressive supranuclear palsy: the diagnostic value of eye movement recording. J Neurol Neurosurg Psychiatry 1999;66:532–5.

50. Rottach KG, Riley DE, DiScenna AO, et al. Dynamic properties of horizontal and vertical eye movements in parkinsonian syndromes. Ann Neurol 1996;39: 368–77.

51. Gradstein LD, Grafman J, Fitzgibbon EJ. Eye movements in chorea-acanthocytosis. Invest Ophthalmol Vis Sci 2005;46:1979–87.

52. Baloh RW, Derossett SE, Cloughesy TF, et al. Novel brainstem syndrome associated with prostate carcinoma. Neurology 1993;43:2591–6.

53. Dalmau J, Graus F, Villarejo A, et al. Clinical analysis of anti-Ma2-associated encephalitis. Brain 2004;127:1831–44.

54. Abel LA, Traccis BT, Troost BT, et al. Saccadic trajectories change with amplitude, not time. Neuroophthalmology 1987;7:309–14.

55. Rucker JC, Shapiro BE, Han YH, et al. Neuro-ophthalmology of late-onset Tay-Sachs disease (LOTS). Neurology 2004;63:1918–26.

56. Zivotofsky AZ, Siman-Tov T, Gadoth N, et al. A rare saccade velocity profile in stiff-person syndrome with cerebellar degeneration. Brain Res 2006;1093:135–40.

57. Ishida K, Mitoma H, Wada Y, et al. Selective loss of Purkinje cells in a patient with anti-glutamic acid decarboxylase antibody-associated cerebellar ataxia. J Neurol Neurosurg Psychiatry 2007;78:190–2.

58. Lemos J, Eggenberger E. Saccadic intrusions: review and update. Curr Opin Neurol 2013;26:59–66.
59. Otero-Millan J, Serra A, Leigh RJ, et al. Distinctive features of saccadic intrusions and microsaccades in progressive supranuclear palsy. J Neurosci 2011; 31:4379–87.
60. Altiparmak UE, Eggenberger E, Coleman A, et al. The ratio of square wave jerk rates to blink rates distinguishes progressive supranuclear palsy from Parkinson disease. J Neuroophthalmol 2006;26:257–9.
61. Fahey MC, Cremer PD, Aw ST, et al. Vestibular, saccadic and fixation abnormalities in genetically confirmed Friedreich ataxia. Brain 2008;131:1035–45.
62. Ribai P, Pousset F, Tanguy ML, et al. Neurological, cardiological, and oculomotor progression in 104 patients with Friedreich ataxia during long-term follow-up. Arch Neurol 2007;64:558–64.
63. Spieker S, Schulz JB, Petersen D, et al. Fixation instability and oculomotor abnormalities in Friedreich's ataxia. J Neurol 1995;242:517–21.
64. Sharpe JA, Herishanu YO, White OB. Cerebral square wave jerks. Neurology 1982;32:57–62.
65. Donaghy C, Pinnock R, Abrahams S, et al. Ocular fixation instabilities in motor neurone disease. A marker of frontal lobe dysfunction? J Neurol 2009;256: 420–6.
66. Clausi S, De Luca M, Chiricozzi FR, et al. Oculomotor deficits affect neuropsychological performance in oculomotor apraxia type 2. Cortex 2013;49: 691–701.
67. Anderson T, Luxon L, Quinn N, et al. Oculomotor function in multiple system atrophy: clinical and laboratory features in 30 patients. Mov Disord 2008;23: 977–84.
68. Rottach KG, Wohlgemuth WA, Dzaja AE, et al. Effects of intravenous opioids on eye movements in humans: possible mechanisms. J Neurol 2002;249:1200–5.
69. Sibony OA, Evinger C, Manning KA. The effects of tobacco smoking on smooth pursuit eye movements. Ann Neurol 1988;23:238–41.
70. Bour LJ, van Rootselaar AF, Koelman JH, et al. Oculomotor abnormalities in myoclonic tremor: a comparison with spinocerebellar ataxia type 6. Brain 2008;131:2295–303.
71. Sharpe JA, Fletcher WA. Saccadic intrusions and oscillations. Can J Neurol Sci 1984;11:426–33.
72. Dell'Osso LF, Troost BT, Daroff RB. Macro square wave jerks. Neurology 1975; 25:975–9.
73. Fuzakawa T, Tashiro K, Hamada T, et al. Multisystem degeneration: drugs and square wave jerks. Neurology 1986;36:1230–3.
74. Klotz L, Klockgether T. Multiple system atrophy with macrosquare-wave jerks. Mov Disord 2005;20:253–4.
75. Selhorst JB, Stark L, Ochs AI, et al. Disorders in cerebellar ocular control II. Macrosaccadic oscillations, an oculographic, control system and clinicoanatomic analysis. Brain 1976;99:509–22.
76. Abadi RV, Gowen E. Characteristics of saccadic intrusions. Vision Res 2004;44: 2675–90.
77. Hikosaka O, Wurtz RH. Modification of saccadic movements by GABA-related substances I. Effect of muscimol and bicuculline in monkey superior colliculus. J Neurophysiol 1985;53:266–91.
78. Munoz DP, Wurtz RH. Fixation cells in monkey superior colliculus II. Reversible activation and deactivation. J Neurophysiol 1993;70:576–89.

79. Carasig D, Paul K, Fucito M, et al. Irrepressible saccades from a tectal lesion in a Rhesus monkey. Vision Res 2006;46:1161–9.

80. Swartz BE, Li S, Bespalova I, et al. Pathogenesis of clinical signs in recessive ataxia with saccadic intrusions. Ann Neurol 2003;54:824–8.

81. Kim JS, Choi KD, Oh SY, et al. Double saccadic pulses and macrosaccadic oscillations from a focal brainstem lesion. J Neurol Sci 2007;263:118–23.

82. Herishanu YO, Sharpe JA. Saccadic intrusions in internuclear ophthalmoplegia. Ann Neurol 1983;14:67–72.

83. Doslak MJ, Dell'Osso LF, Daroff RB. Multiple double saccadic pulses occurring with other saccadic intrusions and oscillations. Neuroophthalmology 1983;3: 109–16.

84. Wong A. An update on opsoclonus. Curr Opin Neurol 2007;20:25–31.

85. Wong AM, Musallam S, Tomlinson RD, et al. Opsoclonus in three dimensions: oculographic, neuropathologic and modeling correlates. J Neurol Sci 2001; 189:71–81.

86. Helmchen C, Rambold H, Sprenger A, et al. Cerebellar activation in opsoclonus: an fMRI study. Neurology 2003;61:412–5.

87. Ramat S, Leigh RJ, Zee DS, et al. Ocular oscillations generated by coupling of brainstem excitatory and inhibitory saccadic burst neurons. Exp Brain Res 2005;160:89–106.

88. Tate ED, Allison TJ, Pranzatelli MR, et al. Neuroepidemiologic trends in 105 US cases of pediatric opsoclonus-myoclonus syndrome. J Pediatr Oncol Nurs 2005;22:8–19.

89. Bataller L, Rosenfeld MR, Graus F, et al. Autoantigen diversity in the opsoclonus-myoclonus syndrome. Ann Neurol 2003;53:347–53.

90. Gorman MP. Update on diagnosis, treatment, and prognosis in opsoclonus-myoclonus-ataxia syndrome. Curr Opin Pediatr 2010;22:745–50.

91. Pranzatelli MR, Slev PR, Tate ED, et al. Cerebrospinal fluid oligoclonal bands in childhood opsoclonus-myoclonus. Pediatr Neurol 2011;45:27–33.

92. Digre KB. Opsoclonus in adults. Report of three cases and review of the literature. Arch Neurol 1986;43:1165–75.

93. Kawachi I, Saji E, Toyoshima Y, et al. Treatment responsive opsoclonus-ataxia associated with ovarian teratoma. J Neurol Neurosurg Psychiatry 2010;81:581–2.

94. Aggarwal A, Williams D. Opsoclonus as a paraneoplastic manifestation of pancreatic carcinoma. J Neurol Neurosurg Psychiatry 1997;63:687–8.

95. Koukoulis A, Cimas I, Gomara S. Paraneoplastic opsoclonus associated with papillary renal cell carcinoma. J Neurol Neurosurg Psychiatry 1998;64:137–8.

96. Kumar A, Lajara-Nanson WA, Neilson RW. Paraneoplastic opsoclonus-myoclonus syndrome: initial presentation of non-Hodgkins lymphoma. J Neurooncol 2005;73: 43–5.

97. Berger JR, Mehari E. Paraneoplastic opsoclonus-myoclonus secondary to malignant melanoma. J Neurooncol 1999;41:43–5.

98. Jung KY, Youn J, Chung CS. Opsoclonus-myoclonus syndrome in an adult with malignant melanoma. J Neurol 2006;253:942–3.

99. Gimeno Campos MJ, Sanchis Minguez C, Diez de Diego P, et al. Opsoclonus-myoclonus: paraneoplastic syndrome associated with renal adenocarcinoma. Rev Esp Anestesiol Reanim 2006;53:54–5.

100. Ko MW, Dalmau J, Galetta SL. Neuro-ophthalmologic manifestations of paraneoplastic syndromes. J Neuroophthalmol 2008;28:58–68.

101. Weber KP, Aw ST, Todd MJ, et al. Head impulse test in unilateral vestibular loss: vestibulo-ocular reflex and catch-up saccades. Neurology 2008;70:454–63.

102. Peterson K, Rosenblum MK, Kotanides H, et al. Paraneoplastic cerebellar degeneration. I. A clinical analysis of 55 anti-Yo antibody-positive patients. Neurology 1992;42:1931–7.
103. Yu Z, Kryzer TJ, Greismann GE, et al. CRMP-5 neuronal autoantibody: marker of lung cancer and thymoma-related autoimmunity. Ann Neurol 2001;49:146–54.
104. Bataller L, Graus F, Saiz A, et al. Clinical outcome in adult onset idiopathic or paraneoplastic opsoclonus-myoclonus. Brain 2001;124:437–43.
105. Pranzatelli MR, Travelstead AL, Tate ED, et al. B- and T-cell markers in opsoclonus-myoclonus syndrome: immunophenotyping of CSF lymphocytes. Neurology 2004;62:1526–32.
106. Zaro-Weber O, Galldiks N, Dohmen C, et al. Ocular flutter, generalized myoclonus, and trunk ataxia associated with anti-GQ1b antibodies. Arch Neurol 2008;65:659–61.
107. Anderson NE, Budde-Steffen C, Rosenblum MK, et al. Opsoclonus, myoclonus, ataxia, and encephalopathy in adults with cancer: a distinct paraneoplastic syndrome. Medicine (Baltimore) 1988;67:100–9.
108. Antunes NL, Khakoo Y, Matthay KK, et al. Antineuronal antibodies in patients with neuroblastoma and paraneoplastic opsoclonus-myoclonus. J Pediatr Hematol Oncol 2000;22:315–20.
109. Rosenfeld MR, Eichen JG, Wade DF, et al. Molecular and clinical diversity in paraneoplastic immunity to Ma proteins. Ann Neurol 2001;50:339–48.
110. Saiz A, Dalmau J, Butler MH, et al. Antiamphiphysin I antibodies in patients with paraneoplastic neurological disorders associated with small cell lung carcinoma. J Neurol Neurosurg Psychiatry 1999;66:214–7.
111. Noetzel MJ, Cawley LP, James VL, et al. Antineurofilaments protein antibodies in opsoclonus-myoclonus. J Neuroimmunol 1987;15:137–45.
112. Simister RJ, Ng K, Lang B, et al. Sequential fluctuating paraneoplastic ocular flutter-opsoclonus-myoclonus syndrome and Lambert-Eaton myasthenic syndrome in small-cell lung cancer. J Neurol Neurosurg Psychiatry 2011;82:344–6.
113. Lee AG, Brazis PW. Localizing forms of nystagmus: symptoms, diagnosis, and treatment. Curr Neurol Neurosci Rep 2006;6:414–20.
114. Kuban KC, Ephros MA, Freeman RL, et al. Syndrome of opsoclonus-myoclonus caused by Coxsackie B3 infection. Ann Neurol 1983;13:69–71.
115. Delreux V, Kevers L, Sindic CJ, et al. Opsoclonus secondary to Epstein-Barr virus infection. Neuroophthalmology 1988;8:179–89.
116. Wiest G, Safoschnik G, Schnaberth G, et al. Ocular flutter and truncal ataxia may be associated with enterovirus infection. J Neurol 1997;244:288–92.
117. Morita A, Ishihara M, Kamei S, et al. Opsoclonus-myoclonus syndrome following influenza A infection. Intern Med 2012;51:2429–31.
118. Alshekhlee A, Sultan B, Chandar K. Opsoclonus persisting during sleep in West Nile encephalitis. Arch Neurol 2006;63:1324–6.
119. Jabs DA, Green WR, Fox R, et al. Ocular manifestations of acquired immune deficiency syndrome. Ophthalmology 1989;96:1092–9.
120. Kaminski HJ, Zee DS, Leigh RJ, et al. Ocular flutter and ataxia associated with AIDS-related complex. Neuroophthalmology 1991;11:163–7.
121. van Toorn R, Rabie H, Warwick JM. Opsoclonus-myoclonus in an HIV-infected child on antiretroviral therapy–possible immune reconstitution inflammatory syndrome. Eur J Paediatr Neurol 2005;9:423–6.
122. Kanjanasut N, Phanthumchinda K, Bhidayasiri R. HIV-related opsoclonus-myoclonus-ataxia syndrome: report on two cases. Clin Neurol Neurosurg 2010;112:572–4.

123. Medrano V, Royo-Villanova C, Flores-Ruiz JJ, et al. Parainfectious opsoclonus-myoclonus syndrome secondary to varicella-zoster virus infection. Rev Neurol 2005;41:507–8.

124. Salonen R, Nikoskelainen E, Aantaa E, et al. Ocular flutter associated with sarcoidosis. Neuroophthalmology 1988;8:77–9.

125. Ertekin V, Tan H. Opsoclonus-myoclonus syndrome attributable to hepatitis C infection. Pediatr Neurol 2010;42:441–2.

126. Zaganas I, Prinianakis G, Xirouchaki N, et al. Opsoclonus-myoclonus syndrome associated with cytomegalovirus encephalitis. Neurology 2007;68:1636.

127. Evans RW, Welch K. Opsoclonus in a confirmed case of St. Louis encephalitis. J Neurol Neurosurg Psychiatry 1982;45:660–1.

128. Mesraoua B, Abbas M, D'Souza A, et al. Adult opsoclonus-myoclonus syndrome following *Mycoplasma pneumoniae* infection with dramatic response to plasmapheresis. Acta Neurol Belg 2011;111:136–8.

129. Nunes JC, Bruscato AM, Walz R, et al. Opsoclonus-myoclonus syndrome associated with *Mycoplasma pneumoniae* infection in an elderly patient. J Neurol Sci 2011;305:147–8.

130. Vejjajiva A, Lerdverasirikul P. Opsoclonus in salmonella infection. Br Med J 1977; 2:1260.

131. Flabeau O, Meissner W, Foubert-Samier A, et al. Opsoclonus myoclonus syndrome in the context of Salmonellosis. Mov Disord 2009;24:2306–8.

132. Kobayashi K, Mizukoshi C, Aoki T, et al. Borrelia burgdorferi-seropositive chronic encephalomyelopathy: Lyme neuroborreliosis? An autopsied report. Dement Geriatr Cogn Disord 1997;8:384–90.

133. Vukelic D, Bozinovic D, Morovic M, et al. Opsoclonus-myoclonus syndrome in a child with neuroborreliosis. J Infect 2000;40:189–91.

134. Peter L, Jung J, Tilikete C, et al. Opsoclonus-myoclonus as a manifestation of Lyme disease. J Neurol Neurosurg Psychiatry 2006;77:1090–1.

135. Skeie GO, Eldoen G, Skeie BS, et al. Opsoclonus myoclonus syndrome in two cases with neuroborreliosis. Eur J Neurol 2007;14:e1–2.

136. Candler PM, Dale RC, Griffin S, et al. Poststreptococcal opsoclonus-myoclonus syndrome associated with antineuroleukin antibodies. J Neurol Neurosurg Psychiatry 2006;77:507–12.

137. Jones CE, Smyth DP, Faust SN. Opsoclonus-myoclonus syndrome associated with group A streptococcal infection. Pediatr Infect Dis 2007;26:358–9.

138. Rivner MH, Jay WM, Green JB, et al. Opsoclonus in *Haemophilus influenzae* meningitis. Neurology 1982;32:661–3.

139. Lapenna F, Lochi L, De Mari M, et al. Post-vaccinic opsoclonus–myoclonus syndrome: a case report. Parkinsonism Relat Disord 2000;6:241–2.

140. McCarthy JE, Filiano J. Opsoclonus myoclonus after human papilloma virus vaccine in a pediatric patient. Parkinsonism Relat Disord 2009;15:792–4.

141. Hage R Jr, Merle H, Jeannin S, et al. Ocular oscillations in the neuromyelitis optica spectrum. J Neuroophthalmol 2011;31:255–9.

142. Deconinck N, Scaillon M, Segers V, et al. Opsoclonus-myoclonus associated with celiac disease. Pediatr Neurol 2006;34:312–4.

143. Francis DA, Heron JR. Ocular flutter in suspected multiple sclerosis: a presenting paroxysmal manifestation. Postgrad Med J 1985;61:333–4.

144. Schon F, Hodgson TL, Mort D, et al. Ocular flutter associated with a localized lesion in the paramedian pontine reticular formation. Ann Neurol 2001;50:413–6.

145. de Seze J, Vukusic S, Viallet-Marcel M, et al. Unusual ocular motor findings in multiple sclerosis. J Neurol Sci 2006;243:91–5.

146. Kurian M, Lalive PH, Dalmau JO, et al. Opsoclonus-myoclonus syndrome in anti-N-methyl-D-aspartate receptor encephalitis. Arch Neurol 2010;67:118–21.

147. Smith JH, Dhamija R, Moseley BD, et al. N-methyl-D-aspartate receptor autoimmune encephalitis presenting with opsoclonus-myoclonus: treatment response to plasmapheresis. Arch Neurol 2011;68:1069–72.

148. Markakis I, Alexiou E, Xifaras M, et al. Opsoclonus-myoclonus-ataxia syndrome with autoantibodies to glutamic acid decarboxylase. Clin Neurol Neurosurg 2008;110:619–21.

149. Keane JR. Transient opsoclonus with thalamic hemorrhage. Arch Neurol 1980; 37:423–4.

150. Pistoia F, Conson M, Sara M. Opsoclonus-myoclonus syndrome in patients with locked-in syndrome: a therapeutic porthole with gabapentin. Mayo Clin Proc 2010;85:527–31.

151. Maccario M, Seelinger D, Snyder R. Thallotoxicosis with coma and abnormal eye movements. Electroencephalogr Clin Neurophysiol 1975;38:98–9.

152. Taylor JR, Selhorst JB, Houff SA, et al. Chlordecone intoxication in man. I Clinical observations. Neurology 1978;28:626–30.

153. Blain PG, Nightingale S, Stoddart JC. Strychnine poisoning: abnormal eye movements. J Toxicol Clin Toxicol 1982;19:215–7.

154. Lazar RB, Ho SU, Melen O, et al. Multifocal central nervous system damage caused by toluene abuse. Neurology 1983;33:1337–40.

155. Pullicino P, Aquilina J. Opsoclonus in organophosphate poisoning. Arch Neurol 1989;46:704–5.

156. Scharf D. Opsoclonus-myoclonus following the intranasal usage of cocaine. J Neurol Neurosurg Psychiatry 1989;52:1447–8.

157. Elkardoudi-Pijnenburg Y, Van Vliet AG. Opsoclonus, a rare complication of cocaine misuse. J Neurol Neurosurg Psychiatry 1996;60:592.

158. Cohen WJ, Cohen NH. Lithium carbonate, haloperidol, and irreversible brain damage. JAMA 1974;230:1283–7.

159. Au WJ, Keltner JL. Opsoclonus with amitriptyline overdose. Ann Neurol 1979;6:87.

160. Dehaene I, Van Vleymen B. Opsoclonus induced by phenytoin and diazepam. Ann Neurol 1987;21:216.

161. Fisher CM. Ocular flutter. J Clin Neuroophthalmol 1990;10:155–6.

162. Brodsky MC, Hunter JS. Positional ocular flutter and thickened optic nerves as sentinel signs of Krabbe disease. J AAPOS 2011;15:595–7.

163. Blumkin L, Kivity S, Lev D, et al. A compound heterozygous missense mutation and a large deletion in the KCTD7 gene presenting as an opsoclonus-myoclonus ataxia-like syndrome. J Neurol 2012;259:2590–8.

164. Matsumura K, Sonoh M, Tamaoka A, et al. Syndrome of opsoclonus-myoclonus in hyperosmolar nonketotic coma. Ann Neurol 1985;18:623–4.

165. Weissman B, Devereaux MW, Chandar K. Opsoclonus and hyperosmolar stupor. Neurology 1989;39:1401–2.

166. Balaratnam MS, Leschziner GD, Seemungal BM, et al. Amyotrophic lateral sclerosis and ocular flutter. Amyotroph Lateral Scler 2010;11:331–4.

167. Shetty T, Rosman NP. Opsoclonus in hydrocephalus. Arch Ophthalmol 1972;88: 585–9.

168. Bishton MJ, Das Gupta E, Byrne JL, et al. Opsoclonus myoclonus following allogeneic haematopoietic stem cell transplantation. Bone Marrow Transplant 2005;36:923.

169. Koide R, Sakamoto M, Tanaka K, et al. Opsoclonus-myoclonus syndrome during pregnancy. J Neuroophthalmol 2004;24:273.

170. Baloh RW, Yee RD, Honrubia V. Eye movements in patients with Wallenberg's syndrome. Ann N Y Acad Sci 1981;374:600–13.
171. Crevits L, vander Eecken H. Ocular lateropulsion in Wallenberg's syndrome: a prospective clinical study. Acta Neurol Scand 1982;65:219–22.
172. Waespe W, Wichmann W. Oculomotor disturbances during visual-vestibular interaction in Wallenberg's lateral medullary syndrome. Brian 1990;113: 821–46.
173. Straube A, Helmchen C, Robinson F, et al. Saccadic dysmetria is similar in patients with a lateral medullary lesion and in monkeys with a lesion of the deep cerebellar nucleus. J Vestib Res 1994;4:327–33.
174. Ranalli PJ, Sharpe JA. Contrapulsion of saccades and ipsilateral ataxia: a unilateral disorder of the rostral cerebellum. Ann Neurol 1986;20:311–6.
175. Frohman EM, Frohman TC, Fleckenstein J, et al. Ocular contrapulsion in multiple sclerosis: clinical features and pathophysiological mechanisms. J Neurol Neurosurg Psychiatry 2001;70:688–92.
176. Tilikete C, Hermier M, Pelisson D, et al. Saccadic lateropulsion and upbeat nystagmus: disorders of caudal medulla. Ann Neurol 2002;52:658–62.
177. Kaski D, Bentley P, Lane R, et al. Up-down asymmetry of saccadic contrapulsion in lateral medullary syndrome. J Neuroophthalmol 2012;32:224–6.
178. Fitzgibbon EJ, Calvert PC, Dieterich M, et al. Torsional nystagmus during vertical pursuit. J Neuroophthalmol 1996;16:79–90.
179. Johnston JL, Sharpe JA, Rannalli PJ, et al. Oblique misdirection and slowing of vertical saccades after unilateral lesions of the pontine tegmentum. Neurology 1993;43:2238–44.
180. Morrow MA, Sharpe JA. Torsional nystagmus in the lateral medullary syndrome. Ann Neurol 1988;24:390–8.
181. Estanol B, Romero R, Corvera J. Effects of cerebellectomy on eye movements in man. Arch Neurol 1979;36:281–4.
182. Burde RM, Stroud MH, Roper-Hall G, et al. Oculomotor dysfunction in total and hemicerebellectomized monkeys. Br J Ophthalmol 1975;59:560–5.
183. Westheimer G, Blair S. Oculomotor defects in cerebellectomized monkeys. Invest Ophthalmol 1973;12:618–21.
184. Zee DS, Yamazaki A, Butler PH, et al. Effects of ablation of flocculus and paraflocculus of eye movements in primate. J Neurophysiol 1981;46:878–99.
185. Suzuki DA, Keller EL. The role of the posterior vermis of monkey cerebellum in smooth-pursuit eye movement control. II. Target velocity-related Purkinje cell activity. J Neurophysiol 1988;59:19–40.
186. Stone LS, Lisberger SG. Visual responses of Purkinje cells in the cerebellar flocculus during smooth-pursuit eye movements in monkeys. II. Complex spikes. J Neurophysiol 1990;63:1262–75.
187. Heinen SJ, Keller EL. The function of the cerebellar uvula in monkey during optokinetic and pursuit eye movements: single-unit responses and lesion effects. Exp Brain Res 1996;110:1–14.
188. Belton T, Suh M, Simpson JI. The nonvisual complex spike signal in the flocculus responds to challenges to the vestibule-ocular reflex gain. Ann N Y Acad Sci 2002;978:503–4.
189. Rambold H, Churchland A, Selig Y, et al. Partial ablations of the flocculus and ventral paraflocculus in monkeys cause linked deficits in smooth pursuit eye movements and adaptive modification of the VOR. J Neurophysiol 2002;87: 912–24.

190. Ohki M, Kitazawa H, Hiramatsu T, et al. Role of primate cerebellar hemisphere in voluntary eye movement control revealed by lesion effects. J Neurophysiol 2009;101:934–47.
191. Sander T, Sprenger A, Neumann G, et al. Vergence deficits in patients with cerebellar lesions. Brain 2009;132:103–15.
192. Xiong G, Nagao S, Kitazawa H. Mossy and climbing fiber collateral inputs in monkey cerebellar paraflocculus lobules petrosus and hemispheric lobule VII and their relevance to oculomotor functions. Neurosci Lett 2010;468:282–6.
193. Zee DS, Friendlich AR, Robinson DA. The mechanism of downbeat nystagmus. Arch Ophthalmol 1974;30:227–37.
194. Glasauer S, Stephan T, Kalla R, et al. Up-down asymmetry of cerebellar activation during vertical pursuit eye movements. Cerebellum 2009;8:385–8.
195. Zhang Y, Partsalis AM, Highstein SM. Properties of superior vestibular nucleus flocculus target neurons in the squirrel monkey. I. General properties in comparison with flocculus projecting neurons. J Neurophysiol 1995;73:2261–78.
196. Zhang Y, Partsalis AM, Highstein SM. Properties of superior vestibular nucleus flocculus target neurons in the squirrel monkey. II. Signal components revealed by reversible flocculus inactivation. J Neurophysiol 1995;73:2279–92.
197. Zee DS, Yee RD, Ramat S. The cerebellar contribution to eye movements based upon lesions: binocular three-axis control and the translational vestibulo-ocular reflex. Ann N Y Acad Sci 2002;956:178–89.
198. Robinson DA. The effect of cerebellectomy on the cat's vestibule-ocular integrator. Brain Res 1974;71:195–207.
199. Hashimoto T, Sasaki O, Yoshida K, et al. Periodic alternating nystagmus and rebound nystagmus in spinocerebellar ataxia type 6. Mov Disord 2003;18:1201–4.
200. Leech J, Gresty M, Hess K, et al. Gaze failure, drifting eye movements, and centripetal nystagmus in cerebellar disease. Br J Ophthalmol 1977;61:774–81.
201. Lloyd SK, Baguley DM, Butler K, et al. Bruns' nystagmus in patients with vestibular schwannoma. Otol Neurotol 2009;30:625–8.
202. Chen JJ, Li WH, Hsieh KY, et al. Bruns-Cushing nystagmus due to hypertensive unilateral paramedian pontine base infarction. Am J Emerg Med 2012;30: 1326.e5–7.
203. Straumann D, Zee DS, Solomon D. Three-dimensional kinematics of ocular drift in humans with cerebellar atrophy. J Neurophysiol 2000;83:1125–40.
204. Marti S, Bockish CJ, Straumann D. Prolonged asymmetric smooth-pursuit leads to downbeat nystagmus in healthy human subjects. Invest Ophthalmol Vis Sci 2005;46:143–9.
205. Marti S, Palla A, Straumann D. Gravity dependence of ocular drift in patients with cerebellar downbeat nystagmus. Ann Neurol 2002;52:712–21.
206. Glasauer S, Hoshi M, Kempermann U, et al. Three-dimensional eye position and slow phase velocity in humans with downbeat nystagmus. J Neurophysiol 2003; 89:338–54.
207. Wagner JN, Glaser M, Brandt T, et al. Downbeat nystagmus: aetiology and comorbidity in 117 patients. J Neurol Neurosurg Psychiatry 2008;79:672–7.
208. Buchele W, Brandt T, Degner D. Ataxia and oscillopsia in downbeat-nystagmus vertigo syndrome. Adv Otorhinolaryngol 1983;30:291–7.
209. Straube A, Bronstein A, Straumann D, European Federation of Neurologic Societies. Nystagmus and oscillopsia. Eur J Neurol 2012;19:6–14.
210. Bohmer A, Straumann D. Pathomechanism of mammalian downbeat nystagmus due to cerebellar lesion: a simple hypothesis. Neurosci Lett 1998;250:127–30.

211. Ito M, Nisimaru N, Yamamoto M. Specific patterns of neuronal connexions involved in the control of the rabbit's vestibulo-ocular reflexes by the cerebellar flocculus. J Physiol (Lond) 1977;265:833–54.

212. Baloh RW, Spooner JW. Downbeat nystagmus: a type of central vestibular nystagmus. Neurology 1981;31:304–10.

213. Halmagyi GM, Rudge P, Gresty MA, et al. Downbeating nystagmus: a review of 62 cases. Arch Neurol 1983;40:777–84.

214. Gresty M, Barratt H, Rudge P, et al. Analysis of downbeat nystagmus: otolithic vs semicircular canal influences. Arch Neurol 1986;43:52–5.

215. Marti S, Straumann D, Buttner U, et al. A model-based theory on the origin of downbeat nystagmus. Exp Brain Res 2008;188:613–31.

216. Bense S, Best C, Buchholz HG, et al. 18F-fluorodeoxyglucose hypometabolism in cerebellar tonsil and flocculus in downbeat nystagmus. Neuroreport 2006;17: 599–603.

217. Kalla R, Deutschlander A, Hufner K, et al. Detection of floccular hypometabolism in downbeat nystagmus by fMRI. Neurology 2006;66:281–3.

218. Hufner K, Stephan T, Kalla R, et al. Structural and functional MRIs disclose cerebellar pathologies in idiopathic downbeat nystagmus. Neurology 2007;69:1128–35.

219. Nakamagoe K, Shimizu K, Koganezawa T, et al. Downbeat nystagmus due to a paramedian medullary lesion. J Clin Neurosci 2012;19:1597–9.

220. Nakamagoe K, Fujizuka N, Koganezawa T, et al. Downbeat nystagmus associated with damage to the medial longitudinal fasciculus of the pons: a vestibular balance control mechanism via the lower brainstem paramedian tract neurons. J Neurol Sci 2013;328:98–101.

221. Pierrot-Deseilligny C, Milea D. Vertical nystagmus: clinical facts and hypotheses. Brain 2005;128:1237–46.

222. Jacobson DM, Corbett JJ. Downbeat nystagmus associated with dolichoectasia of the vertebrobasilar artery. Arch Neurol 1989;46:1005–8.

223. Graus F, Saiz A, Dalmau J. Antibodies and neuronal autoimmune disorders of the CNS. J Neurol 2010;257:509–17.

224. Henderson RD, Widjicks EF. Downbeat nystagmus associated with intravenous patient-controlled administration of morphine. Anesth Analg 2000;91:691–2.

225. Etxeberria A, Lonneville S, Rutgers MP, et al. Metronidazole-cerebellopathy associated with peripheral neuropathy, downbeat nystagmus, and bilateral ocular abduction deficit. Rev Neurol (Paris) 2012;168:193–5.

226. Saul RF, Selhorst JB. Downbeat nystagmus with magnesium depletion. Arch Neurol 1981;38:650–2.

227. Du Pasquier R, Vingerhoets F, Safran AB, et al. Periodic downbeat nystagmus. Neurology 1998;51:1478–80.

228. Oh SY, Kim DH, Seo MW, et al. Reversible cerebellar dysfunction associated with ciguatera fish poisoning. J Emerg Med 2012;43:674–6.

229. Deleu D, El Siddiq A, Kamran S, et al. Downbeat nystagmus following classical heat stroke. Clin Neurol Neurosurg 2005;108:102–4.

230. Van Stavern GP, Biousse V, Newman NJ, et al. Downbeat nystagmus from heat stroke. J Neurol Neurosurg Psychiatry 2000;69:403–4.

231. Orwitz JI, Galetta SL, Teener JW. Bilateral trochlear palsy and downbeat nystagmus in a patient with cephalic tetanus. Neurology 1997;49:894–5.

232. Shaikh AG, Termsarasab P, Riley DE, et al. The floccular syndrome in herpes simplex type 1 encephalitis. J Neurol Sci 2013;325:154–5.

233. Mayfrank L, Thoden U. Downbeat nystagmus indicates cerebellar or brain-stem lesions in vitamin B12 deficiency. J Neurol 1986;233:145–8.

234. Akdal G, Yener GG, Ada E, et al. Eye movement disorders in vitamin B12 deficiency: two new cases and a review of the literature. Eur J Neurol 2007;14: 1170–2.

235. Prasad S, Brown MJ, Galetta SL. Transient downbeat nystagmus from West Nile virus encephalomyelitis. Neurology 2006;66:1599–600.

236. Castillo LC, Garcia F, Roman GC, et al. Spinocerebellar syndrome in patients infected with human T-lymphotropic virus types I and II (HTLV-I/HTLV-II): report of 3 cases from Panama. Acta Neurol Scand 2000;101:405–12.

237. Minoda R, Uno K, Toriya T, et al. Neurologic and otologic finding in Fisher's syndrome. Auris Nasus Larynx 1999;26:153–8.

238. Gans MS, Melmed CA. Downbeat nystagmus associated with doichoectasia of the vertebrobasilar artery. Arch Neurol 1990;47:843.

239. Himi T, Kataura A, Tokuda S, et al. Downbeat nystagmus with compression of the medulla oblongata by the dolichoectatic vertebral arteries. Am J Otol 1995;16:377–81.

240. Baker PC, Price TR, Allen CD. Brain stem and cerebellar dysfunction with Legionnaires' disease. J Neurol Neurosurg Psychiatry 1981;44:1054–6.

241. Wagner J, Lehnen N, Glasauer S, et al. Prognosis of idiopathic downbeat nystagmus. Ann N Y Acad Sci 2009;1164:479–81.

242. Munro NA, Gaymard B, Rivaud S, et al. Upbeat nystagmus in a patient with a small medullary infarct. J Neurol Neurosurg Psychiatry 1993;56:1126–8.

243. Hirose G, Ogasawara T, Shirakawa T, et al. Primary position upbeat nystagmus due to unilateral medial medullary infarction. Ann Neurol 1998;43:403–6.

244. Janssen JC, Larner AJ, Morris H, et al. Upbeat nystagmus: clinicoanatomical correlation. J Neurol Neurosurg Psychiatry 1998;65:380–1.

245. Ohkoshi N, Komatsu Y, Mizusawa H, et al. Primary position upbeat nystagmus increased on downgaze: clinicopathologic study of a patient with multiple sclerosis. Neurology 1998;50:551–3.

246. Kim JS, Yoon B, Choi KD, et al. Upbeat nystagmus: clinicoanatomical correlations in 15 patients. J Clin Neurol 2006;2:58–65.

247. Pierrot-Deseilligny C, Richeh W, Bolgert F. Upbeat nystagmus due to a caudal medullary lesion and influenced by gravity. J Neurol 2007;254:120–1.

248. Saito T, Aizawa H, Sawada H, et al. Lesion of the nucleus intercalates in primary position upbeat nystagmus. Arch Neurol 2010;67:1403–4.

249. Hirose G, Kawada J, Tsukada K, et al. Upbeat nystagmus: clinicopathological and pathophysiological considerations. J Neurol Sci 1991;105:159–67.

250. Tilikete C, Milea D, Pierrot-Deseilligny C. Upbeat nystagmus from a demyelinating lesion in the caudal pons. J Neuroophthalmol 2008;28:202–6.

251. Baloh RW, Yee RD. Spontaneous vertical nystagmus. Rev Neurol (Paris) 1989; 145:527–32.

252. Wray SH, Dalmau J, Chen A, et al. Paraneoplastic disorders of eye movements. Ann N Y Acad Sci 2011;1233:279–84.

253. Liao K, Walker MF, Joshi A, et al. Vestibulo-ocular responses to vertical translation in normal human subjects. Exp Brain Res 2008;185:553–62.

254. Fisher A, Gresty M, Chambers B, et al. Primary position upbeating nystagmus. A variety of central positional nystagmus. Brain 1983;106:949–64.

255. Mizuno M, Kudo Y, Yamane M. Upbeat nystagmus influenced by posture: report of two cases. Auris Nasus Larynx 1990;16:215–21.

256. Sakuma A, Kato I, Ogino S, et al. Primary position upbeat nystagmus with special reference to alteration to downbeat nystagmus. Acta Otolaryngol Suppl 1996;522:43–6.

257. Kim HA, Yi HA, Lee H. Can upbeat nystagmus increase in downward, but not upward, gaze? J Clin Neurosci 2012;19:600–1.

258. Sibony PA, Evinger C, Manning KA. Tobacco-induced primary-position upbeat nystagmus. Ann Neurol 1987;21:53–8.

259. Kim JI, Somers JT, Stahl JS, et al. Vertical nystagmus in normal subjects: effects of head position, nicotine and scopolamine. J Vestib Res 2000;10:291–300.

260. Pereira CB, Strupp M, Eggert T, et al. Nicotine-induced nystagmus: three-dimensional analysis and dependence on head position. Neurology 2000;55:1563–6.

261. Pereira CB, Strupp M, Holzleitner T, et al. Smoking and balance: correlation of nicotine-induced nystagmus and postural body sway. Neuroreport 2001;12:1223–6.

262. Cox TA, Corbett JJ, Thompson HS, et al. Upbeat nystagmus changing to downbeat nystagmus with convergence. Neurology 1981;31:891–2.

263. Petzold A, Plant GT. Optic flow induced nystagmus. J Neurol Neurosurg Psychiatry 2005;76:1173–4.

264. Jay WM, Marcus RW, Jay MS. Primary position upbeat nystagmus with organophosphate poisoning. J Pediatr Ophthalmol Strabismus 1982;19:318–9.

265. Osborne SF, Vivian AJ. Primary position upbeat nystagmus associated with amitriptyline use. Eye (Lond) 2004;18:106.

266. Nakamagoe K, Fujizuka N, Koganezawa T, et al. Residual central nervous system damage due to organoarsenic poisoning. Neurotoxicol Teratol 2013;37:33–8.

267. Vulliemoz S, Vanini G, Truffert A, et al. Epilepsy and cerebellar ataxia associated with anti-glutamic acid decarboxylase antibodies. J Neurol Neurosurg Psychiatry 2007;78:187–9.

268. Bruce BB, Newman NJ, Biousse V. Ophthalmoparesis in idiopathic intracranial hypertension. Am J Ophthalmol 2006;142:878–80.

269. Neugebauer H, Winkler T, Feddersen B, et al. Upbeat nystagmus as a clinical sign of physostigmine-induced right occipital non-convulsive status epilepticus. J Neurol 2012;259:773–4.

270. Zingler VC, Strupp M, Jahn K, et al. Upbeat nystagmus as the initial clinical sign of Creutzfeldt-Jakob disease. Ann Neurol 2005;57:607–8.

271. Keane JR. Cysticercosis: unusual neuro-ophthalmologic signs. J Clin Neuro-ophthalmol 1993;13:194–9.

272. Buttner U, Helmchen C, Brandt T. Diagnostic criteria for central versus peripheral positioning nystagmus and vertigo: a review. Acta Otolaryngol 1999;119:1–5.

273. Bertholon P, Tringali S, Faye MB, et al. Prospective study of positional nystagmus in 100 consecutive patients. Ann Otol Rhinol Laryngol 2006;115:587–94.

274. Shoman N, Longridge N. Cerebellar vermis lesions and tumors of the fourth ventricle in patients with positional and positioning vertigo and nystagmus. J Laryngol Otol 2007;121:166–9.

275. Brandt T. Positional and positioning vertigo and nystagmus. J Neurol Sci 1990;95:3–28.

276. Bertholon P, Bronstein AM, Davies RA, et al. Positional down beating nystagmus in 50 patients: cerebellar disorders and possible anterior semicircular canalithiasis. J Neurol Neurosurg Psychiatry 2002;72:366–72.

277. Fernandez C, Alzate R, Lindsay JR. Experimental observations on postural nystagmus. II. Lesions of the nodulus. Ann Otol Rhinol Laryngol 1960;69:94–114.

278. Kattah JC, Kolsky MP, Lusessenhof AJ. Positional vertigo and the cerebellar vermis. Neurology 1984;34:527–9.

279. Kattah JC, Gujrati M. Familial positional downbeat nystagmus and cerebellar ataxia: clinical and pathologic findings. Ann N Y Acad Sci 2005;1039:540–3.

280. Sander T, Sprenger S, Marti T, et al. Effect of 4-aminopyridine on gravity dependence and neural integrator function in patients with idiopathic downbeat nystagmus. J Neurol 2011;258:618–22.

281. Pedersen RA, Troost BT, Abel LA, et al. Intermittent downbeat nystagmus and oscillopsia reversed by suboccipital craniectomy. Neurology 1980;30:1239–42.

282. Yee RD, Baloh RW, Honrubia V. Episodic vertical oscillopsia and downbeat nystagmus in a Chiari malformation. Arch Ophthalmol 1984;102:723–5.

283. Chan T, Logan P, Eustace P. Intermittent downbeat nystagmus secondary to vermian arachnoid cyst with associated obstructive hydrocephalus. J Clin Neuro-ophthalmol 1991;11:293–6.

284. Sakata E, Ohtsu K, Shimura H, et al. Positional nystagmus of benign paroxysmal type (BPPN) due to cerebellar vermis lesions. Pseudo-BPPN. Auris Nasus Larynx 1987;14:17–21.

285. Barber HO. Positional nystagmus. Otolaryngol Head Neck Surg 1984;92:649–55.

286. Kremmyda O, Zwergal A, la Fougere C, et al. 4-Aminopyridine suppresses positional nystagmus caused by cerebellar vermis lesion. J Neurol 2013;260:321–3.

287. Anagnostou E, Mandellos D, Limbitaki G, et al. Positional nystagmus and vertigo due to a solitary brachium conjunctivum plaque. J Neurol Neurosurg Psychiatry 2006;77:790–2.

288. Sedenhizadeh S, Keogh M, Wills AJ. Reversible hypomagnesaemia-induced subacute cerebellar syndrome. Biol Trace Elem Res 2011;142:127–9.

289. Versino M, Franciotta D, Colnaghi S, et al. Cerebellar signs in celiac disease. Neurology 2009;72:2046–8.

290. Ogawa E, Sakakibara R, Kawashima K, et al. VGCC antibody-positive paraneoplastic cerebellar degeneration presenting with positioning vertigo. Neurol Sci 2011;32:1209–12.

291. Oh SY, Kim JS, Lee YH, et al. Downbeat, positional, and perverted head-shaking nystagmus associated with lamotrigine toxicity. J Clin Neurol 2006;2:283–5.

292. Choi JY, Park YM, Woo YS, et al. Perverted head-shaking and positional downbeat nystagmus in pregabalin intoxication. J Neurol Sci 2014;337:243–4.

293. Arbusow V, Strupp M, Brandt T. Amiodarone-induced severe prolonged head-positional vertigo and vomiting. Neurology 1998;51:917.

294. Chang MB, Bath AP, Rutka JA. Are all atypical positional nystagmus patterns reflective of central pathology? J Otolaryngol 2001;30:280–2.

295. Sorensen BF. Bow hunter's stroke. Neurosurgery 1978;2:259–61.

296. Kuether TA, Nesbit RM, Clark WM, et al. Rotational vertebral artery occlusion: a mechanism of vertebrobasilar insufficiency. Neurosurgery 1997;41:427–32.

297. Marti S, Hegemann S, von Budingen HC, et al. Rotational vertebral artery syndrome: 3D kinematics of nystagmus suggest bilateral labyrinthine dysfunction. J Neurol 2008;255:663–7.

298. Greiner HM, Abruzzo TA, Kabbouche M, et al. Rotational vertebral artery occlusion in a child with multiple strokes: a case-based update. Childs Nerv Syst 2010;26:1669–74.

299. Taylor WB 3rd, Vandergriss CL, Opatowsky MJ, et al. Bowhunter's syndrome diagnosed with provocative digital subtraction cerebral angiography. Proc (Bayl Univ Med Cent) 2012;25:26–7.

300. Ogawa Y, Itani S, Otsuka K, et al. Intermittent positional downbeat nystagmus of cervical origin. Auris Nasus Larynx 2014;41:234–7.
301. Rosengart A, Hedges TR 3rd, Teal PA, et al. Intermittent downbeat nystagmus due to vertebral artery compression. Neurology 1993;43:216–8.
302. Vannucchi P, Pecci R, Giannoni B. Posterior semicircular canal benign paroxysmal positional vertigo presenting with torsional downbeating nystagmus: an apogeotropic variant. Int J Otolaryngol 2012;413603. http://dx.doi.org/10.1155/2012/413603.
303. Korres S, Riga M, Balatsouras D, et al. Benign paroxysmal positional vertigo of the anterior semicircular canal: atypical clinical findings and possible underlying mechanisms. Int J Audiol 2008;47:276–82.
304. Lopez LI, Bronstein AM, Gresty MA, et al. Clinical and MRI correlates in 27 patients with acquired pendular nystagmus. Brain 1996;119:465–72.
305. Deuschl G, Toro C, Valls-Solo J, et al. Symptomatic and essential palatal tremor. 1. Clinical, physiological and MRI analysis. Brain 1994;117:775–88.
306. Trobe JD, Sharpe JA, Hirsh DK, et al. Nystagmus of Pelizaeus-Merzbacher disease. A magnetic search-coil study. Arch Neurol 1991;48:87–91.
307. Kori AA, Robin NH, Jacobs JB, et al. Pendular nystagmus in patients with peroxisomal assembly disorder. Arch Neurol 1998;55:554–8.
308. Tilikete C, Jasse L, Pelisson D, et al. Acquired pendular nystagmus in multiple sclerosis and oculopalatal tremor. Neurology 2011;76:1650–7.
309. Aschoff JC, Conrad B, Kornhuber HH. Acquired pendular nystagmus with oscillopsia in multiple sclerosis: a sign of cerebellar nuclei disease. J Neurol Neurosurg Psychiatry 1974;37:570–7.
310. Gresty MA, Ell JJ, Findley LJ. Acquired pendular nystagmus: its characteristics, localising value and pathophysiology. J Neurol Neurosurg Psychiatry 1982;45:431–9.
311. Das VE, Oruganti P, Kramer PD, et al. Experimental tests of a neural-network model for ocular oscillations caused by disease of central myelin. Exp Brain Res 2000;133:189–97.
312. Shaikh AG, Thurtell MJ, Optican LM, et al. Pharmacological tests of hypotheses for acquired pendular nystagmus. Ann N Y Acad Sci 2011;1233:320–6.
313. Barton JJ, Cox TA. Acquired pendular nystagmus in multiple sclerosis: clinical observations and the role of optic neuropathy. J Neurol Neurosurg Psychiatry 1993;56:262–7.
314. Samuel M, Torun N, Tuite PJ, et al. Progressive ataxa and palatal tremor (PAPT): clinical and MRI assessment with review of palatal tremors. Brain 2004;127:1252–68.
315. Shaikh AG, Hong S, Liao K, et al. Oculopalatal tremor explained by a model of inferior olivary hypertrophy and cerebellar plasticity. Brain 2010;133:923–40.
316. De Zeeuw CI, Simpson JI, Hoogenraad CC, et al. Microcircuitry and function of the inferior olive. Trends Neurosci 1998;21:391–400.
317. Nagaoka M, Narabayashi H. Palatal myoclonus—its remote influence. J Neurol Neurosurg Psychiatry 1984;47:921–6.
318. Goyal M, Versnick E, Tuite P, et al. Hypertrophic olivary degeneration: metaanalysis of the temporal evolution of MR findings. AJNR Am J Neuroradiol 2000;21:1073–7.
319. Duffy CJ. MST neurons respond to optic flow and translational movement. J Neurophysiol 1998;80:1816–27.
320. Gu Y, Watkins PV, Angelaki DE, et al. Visual and nonvisual contributions to three-dimensional heading selectivity in the medial superior temporal area. J Neurosci 2006;26:73–85.

321. Schlack A, Hoffmann KP, Bremmer F. Interaction of linear vestibular and visual stimulation in the macaque ventral intraparietal area (VIP). Eur J Neurosci 2002;16:1877–86.
322. Chen A, DeAngelis GC, Angelaki DE. Convergence of vestibular and visual self-motion signals in an area of the posterior sylvian fissure. J Neurosci 2011;31: 11617–27.
323. Chen A, DeAngelis GC, Angelaki DE. Representation of vestibular and visual cues to self-motion in ventral intraparietal cortex. J Neurosci 2011;31:12036–52.
324. Yakusheva TA, Blazquez PM, Chen A, et al. Spatiotemporal properties of optic flow and vestibular tuning in the cerebellar nodulus and uvula. J Neurosci 2013;33:15145–60.
325. Brodal A. The olivocerebellar projection in the cat as studied with the method of retrograde axonal transport of horseradish peroxidase. II. The projection to the uvula. J Comp Neurol 1976;166:417–26.
326. Hoddevik GH, Brodal A. The olivocerebellar projection studied with the method of retrograde axonal transport of horseradish peroxidase. V. The projections to the flocculonodular lobe and the paraflocculus in the rabbit. J Comp Neurol 1977;176:269–80.
327. Korte GE, Mugnaini E. The cerebellar projection of the vestibular nerve in the cat. J Comp Neurol 1979;184:265–77.
328. Takeda T, Maekawa K. Collateralized projection of visual climbing fibers to the flocculus and nodulus of the rabbit. Neurosci Res 1984;2:125–32.
329. Brodal A, Brodal P. Observations on the secondary vestibulocerebellar projections in the macaque monkey. Exp Brain Res 1985;58:62–74.
330. Kevetter GA, Perachio AA. Distribution of vestibular afferents that innervate the sacculus and posterior canal in the gerbil. J Comp Neurol 1986;254:410–24.
331. Bernard JF. Topographical organization of olivocerebellar and corticonuclear connections in the rat-an WGA-HRP study: I. Lobules IX, X, and the flocculus. J Comp Neurol 1987;263:241–58.
332. Gerrits NM, Epema AH, van Linge A, et al. The primary vestibulocerebellar projection in the rabbit: absence of primary afferents in the flocculus. Neurosci Lett 1989;105:27–33.
333. Takeda T, Maekawa K. Olivary branching projections to the flocculus, nodulus and uvula in the rabbit. II. Retrograde double labeling study with fluorescent dyes. Exp Brain Res 1989;76:323–32.
334. Sato Y, Kanda K, Ikarashi K, et al. Differential mossy fiber projections to the dorsal and ventral uvula in the cat. J Comp Neurol 1989;279:149–64.
335. Epema AH, Gerrits NM, Voogd J. Secondary vestibulocerebellar projections to the flocculus and uvulo-nodular lobule of the rabbit: a study using HRP and double fluorescent tracer techniques. Exp Brain Res 1990;80:72–82.
336. Shojaku H, Barmack NH, Mizukoshi K. Influence of vestibular and visual climbing fiber signals on Purkinje cell discharge in the cerebellar nodulus of the rabbit. Acta Otolaryngol Suppl 1991;481:242–6.
337. Tan HS, Gerrits NM. Laterality in the vestibulo-cerebellar mossy fiber projection to flocculus and caudal vermis in the rabbit: a retrograde fluorescent double-labeling study. Neuroscience 1992;349:448–63.
338. Barmack NH, Baughman RW, Eckenstein FP, et al. Secondary vestibular cholinergic projection to the cerebellum of rabbit and rat as revealed by choline acetyltransferase immunohistochemistry, retrograde, and orthograde tracers. J Comp Neurol 1992;317:250–70.

339. Barmack NH, Baughman RW, Errico P, et al. Vestibular primary afferent projection to the cerebellum of the rabbit. J Comp Neurol 1993;327:521–34.

340. Voogd J, Gerrits NM, Ruigrok TJ. Organization of the vestibulocerebellum. Ann N Y Acad Sci 1996;781:553–79.

341. Ono S, Kushiro K, Zakir M, et al. Properties of utricular and saccular nerve-activated vestibulocerebellar neurons in cats. Exp Brain Res 2000;134:1–8.

342. Maklad A, Fritzsch B. Partial segregation of posterior crista and saccular fibers to the nodulus and uvula of the cerebellum in mice, and its development. Brain Res Dev Brain Res 2003;140:223–36.

343. Newlands SD, Vrabec JT, Purcell IM, et al. Central projections of the saccular and utricular nerves in macaques. J Comp Neurol 2003;466:31–47.

344. Ruigrok TJ. Collateralization of climbing and mossy fibers projecting to the nodulus and flocculus of the rat cerebellum. J Comp Neurol 2003;466:278–98.

345. Kevetter GA, Leonard RB, Newlands SD, et al. Central distribution of vestibular afferents that innervate the anterior or lateral semicircular canal in the Mongolian gerbil. J Vestib Res 2004;14:1–15.

346. Walker M, Zee DS. Directional abnormalities of vestibular and optokinetic responses in cerebellar disease. Ann N Y Acad Sci 1999;871:205–20.

347. Walker MF, Zee DS. Cerebellar disease alters the axis of the high-acceleration vestibuloocular reflex. J Neurophysiol 2005;94:3417–29.

348. Rabbitt RD. Directional coding of three-dimensional movements by the vestibular semicircular canals. Biol Cybern 1999;80:417–31.

349. Haque A, Angelaki DE, Dickman JD. Spatial tuning and dynamics of vestibular semicircular canal afferents in rhesus monkeys. Exp Brain Res 2004;155:81–90.

350. Della Santina CC, Potyagaylo V, Migliaccio AA, et al. Orientation of human semicircular canals measured by three-dimensional multi-planar CT reconstruction. J Assoc Res Otolaryngol 2005;6:191–206.

351. Robinson DA. The use of matrices in analyzing the three-dimensional behavior of the vestibulo-ocular reflex. Biol Cybern 1982;46:53–66.

352. Lisberger SG, Miles FA, Zee DS. Signals used to compute errors in the money vestibuloocular reflex: possible role of the flocculus. J Neurophysiol 1984;52:1140–53.

353. Robinson DA. Adaptive gain control of vestibuloocular reflex by the cerebellum. J Neurophysiol 1976;39:954–69.

354. Lisberger SG, Pavelko TA. Vestibular signals carried by pathways subserving plasticity of the vestibulo-ocular reflex in monkeys. J Neurosci 1986;6:346–54.

355. Schultheis LW, Robinson DA. Directional plasticity of the vestibulo-ocular reflex in the cat. Ann N Y Acad Sci 1981;374:504–12.

356. Angelaki DE, Hess BJ. Inertial representation of angular motion in the vestibular system of rhesus monkeys. II. Otolith-controlled transformation that depends on an intact cerebellar nodulus. J Neurophysiol 1995;73:1729–51.

357. Blazquez PM, Hirata Y, Heiney SA, et al. Cerebellar signatures of vestibulo-ocular reflex motor learning. J Neurosci 2003;23:9742–51.

358. Nagao S, Kitazawa H. Effects of reversible shutdown of the monkey flocculus on the retention of adaptation of the horizontal vestibule-ocular reflex. Neuroscience 2003;118:563–70.

359. Choi KD, Kim JS. Head-shaking nystagmus in central vestibulopathies. Ann N Y Acad Sci 2009;1164:338–43.

360. Halmagyi GM, Curthoys IS. A clinical sign of canal paresis. Arch Neurol 1988;45:737–9.

361. Cremer PD, Halmagyi GM, Aw ST, et al. Semicircular canal plane head impulses detect absent function of individual semicircular canals. Brain 1998;121: 699–716.
362. Newman-Toker DE, Kattah JC, Alvernia JE, et al. Normal head impulse test differentiates acute cerebellar strokes from vestibular neuritis. Neurology 2008;70: 2378–85.
363. Moon IS, Kim JS, Choi KD, et al. Isolated nodular infarction. Stroke 2009;40: 487–91.
364. Kattah JC, Talkad AV, Wang DZ, et al. HINTS to diagnose stroke in the acute vestibular syndrome: three-step bedside oculomotor examination more sensitive than early MRI diffusion-weighted imaging. Stroke 2009;10:3504–10.
365. Cnyrim CD, Newman-Toker D, Karch C, et al. Bedside differentiation of vestibular neuritis from central "vestibular pseudoneuritis". J Neurol Neurosurg Psychiatry 2008;79:458–60.
366. Park HK, Kim JS, Strupp M, et al. Isolated floccular infarction: impaired vestibular responses to horizontal head impulse. J Neurol 2013;260: 1576–82.
367. Sato Y, Kawasaki T. Operational unit responsible for plane-specific control of eye movement by cerebellar flocculus in cat. J Neurophysiol 1990;64:551–64.
368. Cohen B, John P, Yakushin SB, et al. The nodulus and uvula: source of cerebellar control of spatial orientation of the angular vestibulo-ocular reflex. Ann N Y Acad Sci 2002;978:28–45.
369. Schwartz U, Busettini C, Miles FA. Ocular responses to linear motion are inversely proportional to viewing distance. Science 1989;245:1394–6.
370. Telford L, Seidman SH, Paige GD. Dynamics of squirrel monkey linear vestibuloocular reflex and interactions with fixation distance. J Neurophysiol 1997;78: 1775–90.
371. Paige GD, Telford L, Seidman SH, et al. Human vestibuloocular reflex and its interactions with vision and fixation distance during linear and angular head movement. J Neurophysiol 1998;80:2391–404.
372. Baloh RW, Yue Q, Demer JL. The linear vestibulo-ocular reflex in normal subjects and patients with vestibular and cerebellar lesions. J Vestib Res 1995;5: 349–61.
373. Gomez CM, Thompson RM, Gammack JT, et al. Spinocerebellar ataxia type 6: gaze-evoked and vertical nystagmus, Purkinje cell degeneration, and variable age of onset. Ann Neurol 1997;42:933–50.
374. Bertolini G, Ramat S, Bockisch CJ, et al. Is vestibular self-motion perception controlled by the velocity storage? Insights from patients with chronic degeneration of the vestibulo-cerebellum. PLoS One 2012;7:e36763.
375. Cohen B, Matsuo V, Raphan T. Quantitative analysis of the velocity characteristics of optokinetic nystagmus and optokinetic after-nystagmus. J Physiol 1977; 270:321–44.
376. Raphan T, Matsuo V, Cohen B. Velocity storage in the vestibulo-ocular reflex arc (vestibulo-ocular reflex). Exp Brain Res 1979;35:229–48.
377. Harris LR. Vestibular and optokinetic eye movements evoked in the cat by rotation about a tilted axis. Exp Brain Res 1987;66:522–32.
378. Raphan T, Cohen B. Organizational principles of velocity storage in three dimensions. The effect of gravity on cross-coupling of optokinetic after-nystagmus. Ann N Y Acad Sci 1988;545:74–92.
379. Raphan T, Dai M, Cohen B. Spatial orientation of the vestibular system. Ann N Y Acad Sci 1992;656:140–57.

380. Wearne S, Raphan T, Cohen B. Contribution of vestibular commissural pathways to spatial orientation of the angular vestibuloocular reflex. J Neurophysiol 1997; 78:1193–7.

381. Wiest G, Deecke L, Trattnig S, et al. Abolished tilt suppression of the vestibulo-ocular reflex caused by a selective uvulo-nodular lesion. Neurology 1999;52:417–9.

382. Jeong HS, Oh JY, Kim JS, et al. Periodic alternating nystagmus in isolated nodular infarction. Neurology 2007;68:956–7.

383. Waespe W, Cohen B, Raphan T. Dynamic modification of the vestibulo-ocular reflex by the nodulus and uvula. Science 1985;228:199–202.

384. Wearne S, Raphan T, Cohen B. Nodulo-uvular control of central vestibular dynamics determines spatial orientation of the angular vestibulo-ocular reflex. Ann N Y Acad Sci 1996;781:364–84.

385. Wearne S, Raphan T, Cohen B. Control of spatial orientation of the angular vestibuloocular reflex by the nodulus and uvula. J Neurophysiol 1998;79: 2690–715.

386. Wylie DR, De Zeeuw CI, DiGiorgi PL, et al. Projections of individual Purkinje cells of identified zones in the ventral nodulus to the vestibular and cerebellar nuclei in the rabbit. J Comp Neurol 1994;349:448–63.

387. Barmack NH, Qian Z, Yoshimura J. Regional and cellular distribution of protein kinase C in rat cerebellar Purkinje cells. J Comp Neurol 2000;427:235–54.

388. Cohen B, Helwig D, Raphan T. Baclofen and velocity storage: a model of the effects of the drug on the vestibule-ocular reflex in the rhesus monkey. J Physiol 1987;393:703–25.

389. Schrader V, Koenig E, Dichgans J. Direction and angle of active head tilts influencing the Purkinje effect and the inhibition of postrotatory nystagmus I and II. Acta Otolaryngol 1985;100:337–43.

390. Hain TC, Zee DS, Maria BL. Tilt suppression of vestibulo-ocular reflex in patients with cerebellar lesions. Acta Otolaryngol 1988;105:13–20.

391. Heide W, Schrader V, Koenig E, et al. Impaired discharge of the eye velocity storage mechanism in patients with lesions of the vestibulo-cerebellum. Adv Otorhinolaryngol 1988;41:44–8.

392. Han GC, Cha HE, Hwang SH. Head tilt suppression test as a differential diagnostic tool in vertiginous patients. Acta Otolaryngol Suppl 2001;545:94–6.

393. Takahashi S, Fetter M, Koenig E, et al. The clinical significance of head-shaking nystagmus in the dizzy patient. Acta Otolaryngol 1990;109:8–14.

394. Perez P, Llorente JL, Gomez JR, et al. Functional significance of peripheral head-shaking nystagmus. Laryngoscope 2004;114:1078–84.

395. Huh YE, Kim JS. Patterns of spontaneous and head-shaking nystagmus in cerebellar infarction: imaging correlations. Brain 2011;134:3662–71.

396. Hain TC, Fetter M, Zee DS. Head-shaking nystagmus in patients with unilateral peripheral vestibular lesions. Am J Otolaryngol 1987;8:36–47.

397. Minagar A, Sheremata WA, Tusa RJ. Perverted head-shaking nystagmus: a possible mechanism. Neurology 2001;57:887–9.

398. Huh YE, Koo JW, Lee H, et al. Head-shaking aids in the diagnosis of acute audiovestibular loss due to anterior inferior cerebellar artery infarction. Audiol Neurootol 2013;18:114–24.

399. Choi KD, Oh SY, Park SH, et al. Head-shaking nystagmus in lateral medullary infarction: patterns and possible mechanisms. Neurology 2007;68:1337–44.

400. Baier B, Bense S, Dieterich M. Are signs of ocular tilt reaction in patients with cerebellar lesions mediated by the dentate nucleus? Brain 2008;131: 1445–54.

401. Nashold BS Jr, Slaughter DG, Gills JP. Ocular reactions in man from deep cerebellar stimulation and lesions. Arch Ophthalmol 1969;81:538–43.
402. Shallo-Hoffmann J, Riordan-Eva P. Recognizing periodic alternating nystagmus. Strabismus 2001;9:203–15.
403. Furman JM, Wall C, Pang D. Vestibular function in periodic alternating nystagmus. Brain 1990;113:1425–39.
404. Baloh RW, Honrubia V, Konrad HR. Periodic alternating nystagmus. Brain 1976; 99:11–26.
405. Leigh RJ, Robinson DA, Zee DS. A hypothetical explanation for periodic alternating nystagmus: instability in the optokinetic-vestibular system. Ann N Y Acad Sci 1981;374:619–35.
406. Cross SA, Smith JL, Norton EW. Periodic alternating nystagmus clearing after vitrectomy. J Clin Neuroophthalmol 1982;2:5–11.
407. Jay WM, Williams BB, De Chicchis A. Periodic alternating nystagmus clearing after cataract surgery. J Clin Neuroophthalmol 1985;5:149–52.
408. Murofushi T, Chihara Y, Ushio M, et al. Periodic alternating nystagmus in Meniere's disease: the peripheral type? Acta Otolaryngol 2008;128: 824–7.
409. Towle PA, Romanul F. Periodic alternating nystagmus: first pathologically studied case. Neurology 1970;20:408.
410. Castillo IG, Reinecke RD, Sergott RC, et al. Surgical treatment of trauma-induced periodic alternating nystagmus. Ophthalmology 2004;111:180–3.
411. Grant MP, Cohen M, Petersen RB, et al. Abnormal eye movements in Creutzfeldt-Jakob disease. Ann Neurol 1993;34:192–7.
412. Averbuch-Heller L, Meiner Z. Reversible periodic alternating gaze deviation in hepatic encephalopathy. Neurology 1995;45:191–2.
413. Schwankhaus JD, Kattah JC, Lux WE, et al. Primidone/phenobarbital-induced periodic alternating nystagmus. Ann Ophthalmol 1989;21:230–2.
414. Campbell WW Jr. Periodic alternating nystagmus in phenytoin intoxication. Arch Neurol 1980;37:178–80.
415. Lee MS, Lessell S. Lithium-induced periodic alternating nystagmus. Neurology 2003;60:344.
416. Gorman WF, Brock S. Periodic alternating nystagmus in Friedreich's ataxia. Am J Ophthalmol 1950;33:860–4.
417. Jeong SH, Nam J, Kwon MJ, et al. Nystagmus and ataxia associated with anti-ganglioside antibodies. J Neuroophthalmol 2011;31:326–30.
418. Tilikete C, Vighetto A, Trouillas P, et al. Potential role of anti-GAD antibodies in abnormal eye movements. Ann N Y Acad Sci 2005;1039:446–54.
419. Rabinovitch HE, Sharpe JA, Sylvester TO. The ocular tilt reaction: a paroxysmal dyskinesia associated with elliptical nystagmus. Arch Ophthalmol 1977;95:1395–8.
420. Hedges TR III, Hoyt WF. Ocular tilt reaction due to an upper brainstem lesion: paroxysmal skew deviation, torsion, and oscillation of the eyes with head tilt. Ann Neurol 1982;11:537–40.
421. Lawden MC, Bronstein AM, Kennard C. Repetitive paroxysmal nystagmus and vertigo. Neurology 1995;45:276–80.
422. Radtke A, Bronstein AM, Gresty MA, et al. Paroxysmal alternating skew deviation and nystagmus after partial destruction of the uvula. J Neurol Neurosurg Psychiatry 2001;70:790–3.
423. Lewis JM, Kline LB. Periodic alternating nystagmus associated with periodic alternating skew deviation. J Clin Neuroophthalmol 1983;3:115–7.

424. Colen CB, Ketko A, George E, et al. Periodic alternating nystagmus and periodic alternating skew deviation in spinocerebellar ataxia type 6. J Neuroophthalmol 2008;28:287–8.

425. Kennard C, Barger G, Hoyt WF. The association of periodic alternating nystagmus with periodic alternating gaze. A case report. J Clin Neuroophthalmol 1981;1:191–3.

426. Kayan A, Hood JD. Neuro-otological manifestations of migraine. Brain 1984;107: 1123–42.

427. Kuritzky A, Toglia UJ, Thomas D. Vestibular function in migraine. Headache 1981;21:110–2.

428. Cass SP, Furman JM, Ankerstjerne K. Migraine-related vestibulopathy. Ann Otol Rhinol Laryngol 1997;106:182–9.

429. Dieterich M, Brandt T. Episodic vertigo related to migraine (90 cases): vestibular migraine? J Neurol 1999;246:883–92.

430. Neuhauser H, Leopold M, von Brevern M, et al. The interrelations of migraine, vertigo, and migrainous vertigo. Neurology 2001;56:436–41.

431. Ishizaki K, More N, Takeshima T, et al. Static stabilometry in patients with migraine and tension-type headache during a headache-free period. Psychiatry Clin Neurosci 2002;56:85–90.

432. Furman JM, Marcus DA, Balaban CD. Migrainous vertigo: development of a pathogenetic model and structured diagnostic interview. Curr Opin Neurol 2003;16:5–13.

433. Furman JM, Sparto PJ, Soso M, et al. Vestibular function in migraine-related dizziness: a pilot study. J Vestib Res 2005;15:327–32.

434. von Brevern M, Zeise D, Neuhauser H, et al. Acute migrainous vertigo: clinical and oculographic findings. Brain 2005;128:365–74.

435. Evans RW, Marcus D, Furman JM. Motion sickness and migraine. Headache 2007;47:607–10.

436. Cha YH, Baloh RW. Migraine associated vertigo. J Clin Neurol 2007;3:121–6.

437. Jeong SH, Oh SY, Kim HJ, et al. Vestibular dysfunction in migraine: effects of associated vertigo and motion sickness. J Neurol 2010;257:905–12.

438. Bos JE, Bles W, de Graaf B. Eye movements to yaw, pitch, and roll about vertical and horizontal axes: adaptation and motion sickness. Aviat Space Environ Med 2002;73:436–44.

439. Cohen B, Dai M, Raphan T. The critical role of velocity storage in production of motion sickness. Ann N Y Acad Sci 2003;1004:359–76.

440. Dai M, Kunin M, Raphan T, et al. The relation of motion sickness to the spatial-temporal properties of velocity storage. Exp Brain Res 2003;151:173–89.

441. Arriaga MA, Chen DA, Hillman TA, et al. Visually enhanced vestibulo-ocular reflex: a diagnostic tool for migraine vestibulopathy. Laryngoscope 2006;116:1577–9.

442. Masseck OA, Hoffmann KP. Comparative neurobiology of the optokinetic reflex. Ann N Y Acad Sci 2009;1164:430–9.

443. Kashou NH, Leguire LE, Roberts CJ, et al. Instruction dependent activation during optokinetic nystagmus (OKN) stimulation: an FMRI study at 3T. Brain Res 2010;1336:10–21.

444. Ter Braak JWG. Untersuchungen fiber optokinetischen Nystagmus. Arch Neer Physiol 1936;21:309–76.

445. Honrubia V, Downey WL, Mitchell DP, et al. Experimental studies on optokinetic nystagmus. II. Normal humans. Acta Otolaryngol 1968;65:441–8.

446. Leguire LE, Zaff BS, Freeman S, et al. Contrast sensitivity of optokinetic nystagmus. Vision Res 1991;31:89–97.

447. Bucher SF, Dieterich M, Seelos KC, et al. Sensorimotor cerebral activation during optokinetic nystagmus. A functional MRI study. Neurology 1997;49:1370–7.
448. Dieterich M, Bucher SF, Seelos KC, et al. Cerebellar activation during optokinetic stimulation and saccades. Neurology 2000;54:148–55.
449. Dieterich M, Muller-Schunk S, Stephan T, et al. Functional magnetic resonance imaging activations of cortical eye fields during saccades, smooth pursuit, and optokinetic nystagmus. Ann N Y Acad Sci 2009;1164:282–92.
450. Takagi M, Zee DS, Tamargo RJ. Effects of lesions of the oculomotor cerebellar vermis on eye movements in primate: smooth pursuit. J Neurophysiol 2000; 83:2047–62.
451. Nitta T, Akao T, Kurkin S, et al. Involvement of the cerebellar dorsal vermis in vergence eye movements in monkeys. Cereb Cortex 2008;18:1042–57.
452. Suzuki DA, Yamada T, Hoedema R, et al. Smooth-pursuit eye-movement deficits with chemical lesions in macaque nucleus reticularis tegmenti pontis. J Neurophysiol 1999;82:1178–86.
453. Gamlin PD, Yoon K, Zhang H. The role of cerebro-ponto-cerebellar pathways in the control of vergence eye movements. Eye (Lond) 1996;10:167–71.
454. Gamlin PD. Neural mechanisms for the control of vergence eye movements. Ann N Y Acad Sci 2002;956:264–72.
455. Mays LE, Porter JD, Gamlin PD, et al. Neural control of vergence eye movements: neurons encoding vergence velocity. J Neurophysiol 1986;56:1007–21.
456. Zhang H, Gamlin PD. Neurons in the posterior interposed nucleus of the cerebellum related to vergence and accommodation. I. Steady-state characteristics. J Neurophysiol 1998;79:1255–69.
457. Nagao S, Kitamura T, Nakamura N, et al. Location of efferent terminals of the primate flocculus and ventral paraflocculus revealed by anterograde axonal transport methods. Neurosci Res 1997;27:257–69.
458. Akman S, Dayanir V, Sanac AS, et al. Acquired esotropia as presenting sign of cranio-cervical junction anomalies. Neuroophthalmology 1995;15:311–4.
459. Lewis AR, Kline LB, Sharpe JA. Acquired esotropia due to Arnold-Chiari I malformation. J Neuroophthalmol 1996;16:49–54.
460. Watson AP, Fielder AR. Sudden-onset squint. Dev Med Child Neurol 1987;29: 207–11.
461. Williams AS, Hoyt CS. Acute comitant esotropia in children with brain tumors. Arch Ophthalmol 1989;107:376–8.
462. Astle WF, Miller SJ. Acute comitant esotropia: a sign of intracranial disease. Can J Ophthalmol 1994;29:151–4.
463. Simon JW, Waldman JB, Couture KC. Cerebellar astrocytoma manifesting as isolated, comitant esotropia in childhood. Am J Ophthalmol 1996;121:584–6.
464. Liu GT, Hertle RW, Quinn GE, et al. Comitant esodeviation resulting from neurologic insult in children. J AAPOS 1997;1:143–6.
465. Holmes G. Clinical symptoms of cerebellar disease and their interpretation. Lancet 1922;2:59–65.
466. Brude RM, Stroud MH, Roper-Hall G, et al. Ocular motor dysfunction in total and hemicerebellectomized monkeys. Br J Ophthalmol 1975;59:560–5.
467. Keane JR. Alternating skew deviation: 47 patients. Neurology 1985;35:725–8.
468. Moster ML, Schatz NJ, Savino PJ, et al. Alternating skew on lateral gaze (bilateral abducting hypertropia). Ann Neurol 1988;23:190–2.
469. Hamed LA, Maria BL, Quisling RG, et al. Alternating skew on lateral gaze: neuroanatomic pathway and relationship to superior oblique overaction. Ophthalmology 1993;100:281–6.

470. Zee DS. Considerations on the mechanisms of alternating skew deviation in patients with cerebellar lesions. J Vestib Res 1996;6:395–401.

471. Liesch A, Simonsz HJ. Up- and downshoot in adduction after monocular patching in normal volunteers. Strabismus 1993;1:25–36.

472. Neikter B. Effects of diagnostic occlusion on ocular alignment in normal subjects. Strabismus 1994;2:67–77.

473. Mossman S, Halmagyi GM. Partial ocular tilt reaction due to unilateral cerebellar lesion. Neurology 1997;49:491–3.

474. Kim HA, Lee H, Yi HA, et al. Pattern of otolith dysfunction in posterior inferior cerebellar artery territory cerebellar infarction. J Neurol Sci 2009;280:65–70.

475. Tarnutzer AA, Palla A, Marti S, et al. Hypertrophy of the inferior olivary nucleus impacts perception of gravity. Front Neurol 2012;3:79.

476. Benomar A, Krols L, Stevanin G, et al. The gene for autosomal dominant cerebellar ataxia with pigmentary macular dystrophy maps to chromosome 3p12-p21.1. Nat Genet 1995;10:84–8.

477. Gouw LG, Kaplan CD, Haines JH, et al. Retinal degeneration characterizes a spinocerebellar ataxia mapping to chromosome 3p. Nat Genet 1995;10: 89–93.

478. Holmberg M, Johansson J, Forsgren L, et al. Localization of autosomal dominant cerebellar ataxia associated with retinal degeneration and anticipation to chromosome 3p12-p12.1. Hum Mol Genet 1995;4:1441–5.

479. Enevoldson TP, Sanders MD, Harding AE. Autosomal dominant cerebellar ataxia with pigmentary macular dystrophy. A clinical and genetic study of eight families. Brain 1994;117:445–60.

480. Martin JJ. Spinocerebellar ataxia type 7. Handb Clin Neurol 2012;103:475–91.

481. David G, Durr A, Stevanin G, et al. Molecular and clinical correlations in autosomal dominant cerebellar ataxia with progressive macular dystrophy (SCA7). Hum Mol Genet 1998;7:165–70.

482. Gouw LG, Digre KB, Harris CP, et al. Autosomal dominant cerebellar ataxia with retinal degeneration. Neurology 1994;44:1441–7.

483. Jöbsis GJ, Weber JW, Barth PG, et al. Autosomal dominant cerebellar ataxia with retinal degeneration (ADCA II): clinical and neuropathological findings in two pedigrees and genetic linkage to 3p12–p21.1. J Neurol Neurosurg Psychiatry 1997;62:367–71.

484. Manrique RK, Noval S, Aguilar-Amat MJ, et al. Ophthalmic features of spinocerebellar ataxia type 7. J Neuroophthalmol 2009;29:174–9.

485. Abe T, Abe K, Aoki M, et al. Ocular changes in patients with spinocerebellar degeneration and repeated trinucleotide expansion of spinocerebellar ataxia type 1 gene. Arch Ophthalmol 1997;115:231–6.

486. Thurtell MJ, Biousse V, Newman NJ. Rod-cone dystrophy in spinocerebellar ataxia type 1. Arch Ophthalmol 2011;129:956–8.

487. Vaclavik V, Bourrat FX, Ambresin A, et al. Novel maculopathy in patients with spinocerebellar ataxia type 1 autofluorescence findings and functional characteristics. JAMA Ophthalmol 2013;131:536–8.

488. Rufa A, Dotti MT, Galli L, et al. Spinocerebellar ataxia type 2 (SCA2) associated with retinal pigmentary degeneration. Eur Neurol 2002;47:128–9.

489. Ragothaman M, Sarangmath N, Chaudhary S, et al. Complex phenotypes in an Indian family with homozygous SCA2 mutations. Ann Neurol 2004;55: 130–3.

490. Ragothaman M, Muthane U. Homozygous SCA2 mutations changes phenotype and hastens progression. Mov Disord 2008;23:770–1.

491. Paciorkowski AR, Shafrir Y, Hrivnak J, et al. Massive expansion of SCA2 with autonomic dysfunction, retinitis pigmentosa, and infantile spasms. Neurology 2011;77:1055–60.

492. Fukutake T, Kamitsukasa I, Arai K, et al. A patient homozygous for the SCA6 gene with retinitis pigmentosa. Clin Genet 2002;61:375–9.

493. Pula JH, Towle VL, Staszak VM, et al. Retinal nerve fiber layer and macular thinning in spinocerebellar ataxia and cerebellar multisystem atrophy. Neuroophthalmology 2011;35:108–14.

494. Aubourg P, Wanders R. Peroxisomal disorders. Handb Clin Neurol 2013;113: 1593–609.

495. Fiskerstrand T, H'mida-Ben Brahim D, Johansson S, et al. Mutations in ABHD12 cause the neurodegenerative disease PHARC: an inborn error of endocannabinoid metabolism. Am J Hum Genet 2010;87:410–7.

496. Okuma H, Kitagawa Y, Tokuoka K, et al. Cerebrotendinous xanthomatosis with cerebellar ataxia as the chief symptom. Intern Med 2007;46:1259–61.

497. Federico A, Dotti MT, Gallus GN. Cerebrotendinous xanthomatosis. In: Pagon RA, Adam MP, Bird TD, et al, editors. GeneReviews™ [Internet]. Seattle (WA): University of Washington, Seattle; 1993–2014. Available at: http://www.ncbi.nlm.nih. gov.foyer.swmed.edu/books/NBK1409. Accessed February 5, 2014.

498. Cruysberg JR, Wevers RA, van Engelen BG, et al. Ocular and systemic manifestations of cerebrotendinous xanthomatosis. Am J Ophthalmol 1995;120: 597–604.

499. Dotti MT, Rufa A, Federico A. Cerebrotendinous xanthomatosis: heterogeneity of clinical phenotype with evidence of previously undescribed ophthalmological findings. J Inherit Metab Dis 2001;24:696–706.

500. Huijgen R, Stork AD, Defesche JC, et al. Extreme xanthomatosis in patients with both familial hypercholesterolemia and cerebrotendinous xanthomatosis. Clin Genet 2012;81:24–8.

501. Lagarde J, Sedel F, Degos B. Blepharospasm as a new feature of cerebrotendinous xanthomatosis. Parkinsonism Relat Disord 2013;19:764–5.

502. Baets J, Deconinck T, Smets K, et al. Mutations in SACS cause atypical and late-onset forms of ARSACS. Neurology 2010;75:1181–8.

503. Pfeffer G, Blakely EL, Alston CL, et al. Adult-onset spinocerebellar ataxia syndromes due to MTATP6 mutations. J Neurol Neurosurg Psychiatry 2012;83:883–6.

504. Teive HA, Munhoz RP, Muzzio JA, et al. Cerebellar ataxia, myoclonus, cervical lipomas, and MERRF syndrome. Case report. Mov Disord 2008;23:1191–2.

505. Ito S, Shirai W, Asahina M, et al. Clinical and brain MR imaging features focusing on the brain stem and cerebellum in patients with myoclonic epilepsy with ragged-red fibers due to mitochondrial A8344G mutation. AJNR Am J Neuroradiol 2008;29:392–5.

506. Horvath R, Kley RA, Lochmüller H, et al. Parkinson syndrome, neuropathy, and myopathy caused by the mutation A8344G (MERRF) in tRNALys. Neurology 2007;68:56–8.

507. Funakawa I, Kato H, Terao A, et al. Cerebellar ataxia in patients with Leber's hereditary optic neuropathy. J Neurol 1995;242:75–7.

508. Murakami T, Mita S, Tokunaga M, et al. Hereditary cerebellar ataxia with Leber's hereditary optic neuropathy mitochondrial DNA 11778 mutation. J Neurol Sci 1996;142:111–3.

509. Debray FG, Lambert M, Lortie A, et al. Long-term outcome of Leigh syndrome caused by the NARP-T8993C mtDNA mutation. Am J Med Genet 2007;143A: 2046–51.

510. Riera AR, Kaiser E, Levine P, et al. Kearns-Sayre syndrome: electro-vectorcardiographic evolution for left septal fascicular block of the His bundle. J Electrocardiol 2008;41:675–8.
511. Naumann M, Kiefer R, Toyka KV, et al. Mitochondrial dysfunction with myoclonus epilepsy and ragged-red fibers point mutation in nerve, muscle, and adipose tissue of a patient with multiple symmetric lipomatosis. Muscle Nerve 1997;20: 833–9.
512. Mancuso M, Filosto M, Bellan M, et al. POLG mutations causing ophthalmoplegia, sensorimotor polyneuropathy, ataxia, and deafness. Neurology 2004;62:316–8.
513. Gago MF, Rosas MJ, Guimaraes J, et al. SANDO: two novel mutations in POLG1 gene. Neuromuscul Disord 2006;16:507–9.
514. Milone M, Brunetti-Pierri N, Tang LY, et al. Sensory ataxic neuropathy with ophthalmoparesis caused by POLG mutations. Neuromuscul Disord 2008;18: 626–32.
515. Debouverie M, Wagner M, Ducrocq X, et al. MNGIE syndrome in 2 siblings. Rev Neurol (Paris) 1997;153:547–53.
516. Amati-Bonneau P, Valentino ML, Reynier P, et al. OPA1 mutations induce mito-chondrial DNA instability and optic atrophy 'plus' phenotypes. Brain 2008;131: 338–51.
517. Barrett TG, Bundey SE, Macleod AF. Neurodegeneration and diabetes: UK nationwide study of Wolfram (DIDMOAD) syndrome. Lancet 1995;346: 1458–63.
518. Medlej R, Wasson J, Baz P, et al. Diabetes mellitus and optic atrophy: a study of Wolfram syndrome in the Lebanese population. J Clin Endocrinol Metab 2004; 89:1656–61.
519. Finsterer J. Mitochondrial ataxias. Can J Neurol Sci 2009;36:543–53.
520. Pfeiffer RF. Neurologic manifestations of malabsorption syndromes. Handb Clin Neurol 2014;120:621–32.
521. Owada K, Uchihara T, Ishida K, et al. Motor weakness and cerebellar ataxia in Sjögren syndrome - identification of antineuronal antibody: a case report. J Neurol Sci 2002;197:79–84.
522. Ichikawa H, Ishihara K, Fujimoto R, et al. An autopsied case of Sjogren's syndrome with massive necrotic and demyelinating lesions of the cerebellar white matter. J Neurol Sci 2004;225:143–8.
523. Wong S, Pollock AN, Burnham JM, et al. Acute cerebellar ataxia due to Sjögren syndrome. Neurology 2004;62:2332–3.
524. Tzarouchi LC, Tsifetaki N, Konitsiotis S, et al. CNS involvement in primary Sjogren syndrome: assessment of gray and white matter changes with MRI and voxel-based morphometry. AJR Am J Roentgenol 2011;197:1207–12.
525. Kim MJ, Lee MC, Lee JH, et al. Cerebellar degeneration associated with Sjogren's syndrome. J Clin Neurol 2012;8:155–9.
526. Golnik KC. Neuro-ophthalmologic manifestations of systemic disease: rheuma-tologic/inflammatory. Ophthalmol Clin North Am 2004;17:389–96.
527. Bremner FD, Smith SE. Pupil abnormalities in selected autonomic neuropathies. J Neuroophthalmol 2006;26:209–19.
528. Voss EV, Stangel M. Nervous system involvement of connective tissue disease: mechanisms and diagnostic approach. Curr Opin Neurol 2012;25:306–15.
529. de Seze J. Atypical forms of optic neuritis. Rev Neurol (Paris) 2012;168: 697–701.
530. Tehrani R, Ostrowski RA, Hariman R, et al. Ocular toxicity of hydroxychloroquine. Semin Ophthalmol 2008;23:201–9.

531. Heidenhain A. Klinische und anatomische Untersuchungen uber eine eigenartige organische Erkrankung des Zentralnervensystems im Praesenium. Z Ges Neurol Psychiatr 1929;118:49–114.
532. Kropp S, Schulz-Schaeffer WJ, Finjenstaedt M, et al. The Heidenhain variant of Creutzfeldt-Jakob disease. Arch Neurol 1999;56:55–61.
533. Jacobs DA, Lesser RL, Mourelatos Z, et al. The Heidenhain variant of Creutzfeldt-Jakob disease: clinical, pathologic and neuroimaging findings. J Neuroophthalmol 2001;21:99–102.
534. Appleby BS, Appleby KK, Crain BJ, et al. Characteristics of established and proposed sporadic Creutzfeldt-Jakob disease variants. Arch Neurol 2009;66: 208–15.
535. Josephs KA, Tsuboi Y, Dickson DW. Creutzfeldt-Jakob disease presenting as progressive supranuclear gaze palsy. Eur J Neurol 2004;11:343–6.
536. Helmchen C, Buttner U. Centripetal nystagmus in a case of Creutzfeldt-Jakob disease. Neuroophthalmology 1995;15:187–92.
537. Bronstein AM, Miller DH, Rudge P, et al. Down beating nystagmus: magnetic resonance imaging and neuro-otological findings. J Neurol Sci 1987;81:173–84.
538. Zimmerman CF, Roach ES, Troost BT. See-saw nystagmus associated with Chiari malformation. Arch Neurol 1986;43:299–300.
539. Al-Awami A, Flanders ME, Andermann F, et al. Resolution of periodic alternating nystagmus after decompression for Chiari malformation. Can J Ophthalmol 2005;40:778–80.
540. Pieh C, Gottlob I. Arnold-Chiari malformation and nystagmus of skew. J Neurol Neurosurg Psychiatry 2000;69:124–6.
541. Kumar A, Patni AH, Charbel F. The Chiari I malformation and the neurotologist. Otol Neurotol 2002;23:727–35.
542. Kowal L, Yahalom C, Shuey NH. Chiari 1 malformation presenting as strabismus. Binocul Vis Strabismus Q 2006;21:18–26.
543. Spooner JW, Baloh RW. Arnold-Chiari malformation: improvement in eye movements after surgical treatment. Brain 1981;104:51–60.
544. Rowlands A, Sgouros S, Williams B. Ocular manifestations of hindbrain-related syringomyelia and outcome following craniovertebral decompression. Eye (Lond) 2000;14:884–8.
545. Lennerstrand G, Gallo JE. Neuro-ophthalmological evaluation of patients with myelomeningocele and Chiari malformations. Dev Med Child Neurol 1990;32: 415–22.
546. Salman MS, Dennis M, Sharpe JA. The cerebellar dysplasia of Chiari II malformation as revealed by eye movements. Can J Neurol Sci 2009;36:713–24.
547. Salman MS, Sharpe JA, Lillakas L, et al. Smooth ocular pursuit in Chiari type II malformation. Dev Med Child Neurol 2007;49:289–93.
548. Salman MS, Sharpe JA, Lillakas L, et al. The vestibulo-ocular reflex during active head motion in Chiari II malformation. Can J Neurol Sci 2008;35:495–500.
549. Salman MS, Sharpe JA, Eizenman M, et al. Saccades in children with spina bifida and Chiari type II malformation. Neurology 2005;64:2098–101.
550. Nishizaki T, Tamaki N, Nishida Y, et al. Bilateral internuclear ophthalmoplegia due to hydrocephalus: a case report. Neurosurgery 1985;17:822–5.
551. Woody RC, Reynolds JD. Association of bilateral internuclear ophthalmoplegia and myelomeningocele with Arnold-Chiari malformation, type II. J Clin Neuroophthalmol 1985;5:124–6.
552. Arnold AC, Baloh RW, Yee RD, et al. Internuclear ophthalmoplegia in the Chiari type II malformation. Neurology 1990;40:1850–4.

553. Campuzano V, Montermini L, Molto MD, et al. Friedreich's ataxia: autosomal recessive disease caused by an intronic GAA triplet repeat expansion. Science 1996;271:1423–7.

554. Parkinson MH, Boesch S, Nachbauer W, et al. Clinical features of Friedreich's ataxia: classical and atypical phenotypes. J Neurochem 2013;126:103–17.

555. Furman JM, Perlman S, Baloh RW. Eye movements in Friedreich's ataxia. Arch Neurol 1983;40:343–6.

556. Moschner C, Perlman S, Baloh RW. Comparison of oculomotor findings in the progressive ataxia syndromes. Brain 1994;117:15–25.

557. Harding AE, Zilkha KJ. Pseudo-dominant inheritance in Friedreich's ataxia. J Med Genet 1981;18:285–7.

558. Durr A, Cossee M, Agid Y, et al. Clinical and genetic abnormalities in patients with Friedreich's ataxia. N Engl J Med 1996;335:1169–75.

559. Schols JB, Amoiridis G, Przuntek H, et al. Friedreich's ataxia: revision of the phenotype according to molecular genetics. Brain 1997;120:2131–40.

560. Filla A, De Michele G, Caruso G, et al. Genetic data and natural history of Friedreich's disease: a study of 80 Italian patients. J Neurol 1990;237:345–51.

561. Arnold P, Boulat O, Mairec R, et al. Expanding view of phenotype and oxidative stress in Friedreich's ataxia patients with and without idebenone. Schweiz Arch Neurol Psychiatr 2006;157:169–76.

562. Fortuna F, Barboni P, Liguori R, et al. Visual system involvement in patients with Friedreich's ataxia. Brain 2009;132:116–23.

563. Boder E, Sedgwick RP. Ataxia-telangiectasia: a familial syndrome of progressive cerebellar ataxia, oculocutaneous telangiectasias and frequent pulmonary infection. Pediatrics 1958;21:526–54.

564. Woods CG, Taylor AM. Ataxia telangiectasia in the British Isles: the clinical and laboratory features of 70 affected individuals. Q J Med 1992;82:169–79.

565. Stankovic T, Kidd AM, Sutcliffe A, et al. ATM mutations and phenotypes in ataxia-telangiectasia families in the British Isles: expression of mutant ATM and the risk of leukemia, lymphoma, and breast cancer. Am J Hum Genet 1998;62:334–45.

566. Watanabe M, Sugai Y, Concannon P, et al. Familial spinocerebellar ataxia with cerebellar atrophy, peripheral neuropathy, and elevated level of serum creatine kinase, gamma-globulin, and alpha-fetoprotein. Ann Neurol 1998; 44:265–9.

567. Perlman S, Becker-Catania S, Gatti RA. Ataxia-telangiectasia: diagnosis and treatment. Semin Pediatr Neurol 2003;10:173–82.

568. Farina L, Uggetti C, Ottolini A, et al. Ataxia-telangiectasia: MR and CT findings. J Comput Assist Tomogr 1994;18:724–7.

569. Sardanelli F, Parodi RC, Ottonello C, et al. Cranial MRI in ataxia-telangiectasia. Neuroradiology 1995;37:77–82.

570. Crawford TO. Ataxia-telangiectasia. Semin Pediatr Neurol 1998;5:287–94.

571. Tavani F, Zimmerman RA, Berry GT, et al. Ataxia-telangiectasia: the pattern of cerebellar atrophy on MRI. Neuroradiology 2003;45:315–9.

572. Firat AK, Karakas HM, Firat Y, et al. Quantitative evaluation of brain involvement in ataxia telangiectasia by diffusion weighted MR imaging. Eur J Radiol 2005;56: 192–6.

573. Verhagen MM, Martin JJ, van Deuren M, et al. Neuropathology in classical and variant ataxia-telangiectasia. Neuropathology 2012;32:234–44.

574. Farr AK, Shalev B, Crawford TO, et al. Ocular manifestations of ataxia-telangiectasia. Am J Ophthalmol 2002;134:891–6.

575. Baloh RW, Yee RD, Boder E. Eye movements in ataxia-telangiectasia. Neurology 1978;28:1099–104.
576. Zee DS, Yee RD, Singer HS. Congenital ocular motor apraxia. Brain 1977;100: 581–99.
577. Lewis RF, Crawford TO. Slow target-directed eye movements in ataxia-telangiectasia. Invest Ophthalmol Vis Sci 2002;43:686–91.
578. Hyams SW, Reisner SH, Neumann E. The eye signs in ataxia-telangiectasia. Am J Ophthalmol 1966;62:1118–24.
579. Stell R, Bronstein AM, Plant GT, et al. Ataxia telangiectasia: a reappraisal of the ocular motor features and their value in the diagnosis of atypical cases. Mov Disord 1989;4:320–9.
580. Lewis RF, Lederman HM, Crawford TO. Ocular motor abnormalities in ataxia telangiectasia. Ann Neurol 1999;46:287–95.
581. Sari A, Okuyaz C, Adiquzel U, et al. Uncommon associations with ataxia-telangiectasia: vitiligo and optic disc drusen. Ophthalmic Genet 2009;30:19–22.
582. Rub U, Schols L, Paulson H, et al. Clinical features, neurogenetics, and neuropathology of the polyglutamine spinocerebellar ataxias type 1, 2, 3, 6, and 7. Prog Neurobiol 2013;104:38–66.
583. Buttner N, Geschwind D, Jen JC, et al. Oculomotor phenotypes in autosomal dominant ataxias. Arch Neurol 1998;55:1353–7.
584. Burk K, Fetter M, Abele M, et al. Autosomal dominant cerebellar ataxia type 1: oculomotor abnormalities in families with SCA1, SCA2, and SCA3. J Neurol 1999;246:789–97.
585. Pula JH, Gomez CM, Kattah JC. Ophthalmologic features of the common spinocerebellar ataxias. Curr Opin Ophthalmol 2010;21:447–53.
586. Jacobi H, Hauser TK, Giunti P, et al. Spinocerebellar ataxia types 1, 2, 3 and 6: the clinical spectrum of ataxia and morphometric brainstem and cerebellar findings. Cerebellum 2012;11:155–66.
587. Kim JS, Kim JS, Youn J, et al. Ocular motor characteristics of different subtypes of spinocerebellar ataxia: distinguishing features. Mov Disord 2013;28: 1271–7.
588. Schols L, Amoiridis G, Buttner T, et al. Autosomal dominant cerebellar ataxia: phenotypic differences in genetically defined subtypes? Ann Neurol 1997;42: 924–32.
589. Moro A, Munhoz RP, Arruda WO, et al. Clinical relevance of the "bulging eyes" for the differential diagnosis of spinocerebellar ataxias. Arq Neuropsiquiatr 2013;71:428–30.
590. Yu-Wai-Man P, Gorman G, Bateman DE, et al. Vertigo and vestibular abnormalities in spinocerebellar ataxia type 6. J Neurol 2009;256:78–82.
591. Yabe I, Sasaki H, Takeichi N, et al. Positional vertigo and macroscopic downbeat positioning nystagmus in spinocerebellar ataxia type 6 (SCA6). J Neurol 2003; 250:440–3.
592. Schols L, Amoiridis G, Epplen JT, et al. Relations between genotype and phenotype in German patients with the Machado-Joseph disease mutation. J Neurol Neurosurg Psychiatry 1996;61:466–70.
593. Schols L, Kruger R, Amoiridis G, et al. Spinocerebellar ataxia type 6: genotype and phenotype in German kindreds. J Neurol Neurosurg Psychiatry 1998;64: 67–73.
594. Rivaud-Pechoux S, Dürr A, Gaymard B, et al. Eye movement abnormalities correlate with genotype in autosomal dominant cerebellar ataxia type I. Ann Neurol 1998;43:297–302.

595. Hoche F, Seidel K, Brunt ER, et al. Involvement of the auditory brainstem system in spinocerebellar ataxia type 2 (SCA2), type 3 (SCA3), and type 7 (SCA7). Neuropathol Appl Neurobiol 2008;34:479–91.

596. Migliaccio AA, Halmagyi GM, McGarvie LA, et al. Cerebellar ataxia with bilateral vestibulopathy: description of a syndrome and its characteristic clinical sign. Brain 2004;127:280–93.

597. Szmulewicz DJ, Waterston JA, MacDougall HG, et al. Cerebellar ataxia, neuropathy, vestibular areflexia syndrome (CANVAS): a review of clinical features and video-oculographic diagnosis. Ann N Y Acad Sci 2011;1233:139–47.

598. Spacey S. Episodic ataxia type 2. In: Pagon RA, Adam MP, Bird TD, et al, editors. GeneReviews™ [Internet]. Seattle (WA): University of Washington, Seattle; 1993–2014. Available at: http://www.ncbi.nlm.nih.gov/books/NBK1501. Accessed February 6, 2014.

599. Strupp M, Zwergal A, Brandt T. Episodic ataxia type 2. Neurotherapeutics 2007; 4:267–73.

600. Jen J, Kim GW, Baloh RW. Clinical spectrum of episodic ataxia type 2. Neurology 2004;62:17–22.

601. Sasaki O, Jen JC, Baloh RW, et al. Neurotological findings in a family with episodic ataxia. J Neurol 2003;250:373–5.

602. Rucker JC, Jen J, Stahl JS, et al. Internuclear ophthalmoparesis in episodic ataxia type 2. Ann N Y Acad Sci 2005;1039:571–4.

603. Griggs RC, Moxley RT, Lafrance RA, et al. Hereditary paroxysmal ataxia: response to acetazolamide. Neurology 1978;28:1259–64.

604. Bain PG, Larkin GB, Calver DM, et al. Persistent superior oblique paresis as a manifestation of familial periodic cerebellar ataxia. Br J Ophthalmol 1991;75: 619–21.

605. Denier C, Ducros A, Vahedi K, et al. High prevalence of CACNA1A truncations and broader clinical spectrum in episodic ataxia type 2. Neurology 1999;52: 1816–21.

606. Jen JC, Graves TD, Hess EJ, et al. Primary episodic ataxias: diagnosis, pathogenesis, and treatment. Brain 2007;130:2484–93.

607. Zasorin NL, Baloh RW, Myers LB. Acetazolamide-responsive episodic ataxia syndrome. Neurology 1983;22:1212–4.

608. Bertholon P, Chabrier S, Riant F, et al. Episodic ataxia type 2: unusual aspects in clinical and genetic presentation. Special emphasis in childhood. J Neurol Neurosurg Psychiatry 2009;80:1289–92.

609. Moreira MC, Klur S, Watanabe M, et al. Senataxin, the ortholog of a yeast RNA helicase, is mutant in ataxia-ocular apraxia 2. Nat Genet 2004;36:225–7.

610. Izatt L, Nemeth AH, Meesaq A, et al. Autosomal recessive spinocerebellar ataxia and peripheral neuropathy with raised alpha-fetoprotein. J Neurol 2004; 251:805–12.

611. Le Ber I, Bouslam N, Rivaud-Pechoux S, et al. Frequency and phenotypic spectrum of ataxia with oculomotor apraxia 2: a clinical and genetic study in 18 patients. Brain 2004;127:759–67.

612. Anheim M, Monga B, Fleury M, et al. Ataxia with oculomotor apraxia type 2: clinical, biological and genotype/phenotype correlation study of a cohort of 90 patients. Brain 2009;132:2688–98.

613. Ahmed Z, Asi YT, Sailer A, et al. The neuropathology, pathophysiology and genetics of multiple system atrophy. Neuropathol Appl Neurobiol 2012;38:4–24.

614. Arpa J, Sarria J, Cruz-Martinez A, et al. Electro-oculogram in multiple system and late onset cerebellar atrophies. Rev Neurol 1995;23:969–74.

615. Wessel K, Moschner C, Wandinger KP, et al. Oculomotor testing in the differential diagnosis of degenerative ataxic disorders. Arch Neurol 1998;55:949–56.
616. Smith SA, Smith SE. Bilateral Horner's syndrome: detection and occurrence. J Neurol Neurosurg Psychiatry 1999;66:48–51.
617. Sakakibara R, Ito T, Yamamoto T, et al. Vergence paresis in multiple system atrophy. Intern Med 2005;44:911–2.
618. Pinkhardt EH, Kassubek J, Sussmuth S, et al. Comparison of smooth pursuit eye movement deficits in multiple system atrophy and Parkinson's disease. J Neurol 2009;256:1438–46.
619. Rascol O, Sabatini U, Simonetta-Moreau M, et al. Square wave jerks in parkinsonian syndromes. J Neurol Neurosurg Psychiatry 1991;54:599–602.
620. Pinnock RA, McGivern RC, Forbes F, et al. An exploration of ocular fixation in Parkinson's disease, multiple system atrophy and progressive supranuclear palsy. J Neurol 2010;257:533–9.
621. Albrecht P, Muller AK, Sudmeyer M, et al. Optical coherence tomography in parkinsonian syndromes. PLoS One 2012;7:e64891.
622. Fischer MD, Synofzik M, Heidlauf R, et al. Retinal nerve fiber layer loss in multiple system atrophy. Mov Disord 2011;26:914–6.
623. Fischer MD, Synofzik M, Kernstock C, et al. Decreased retinal sensitivity and loss of retinal nerve fibers in multiple system atrophy. Graefes Arch Clin Exp Ophthalmol 2013;251:235–41.
624. Yamashita F, Hirayama M, Nakamura T, et al. Pupillary autonomic dysfunction in multiple system atrophy and Parkinson's disease: an assessment by eye-drop tests. Clin Auton Res 2010;20:191–7.
625. Beh SC, Frohman TC, Frohman EM. Isolated mammillary body involvement on MRI in Wernicke's encephalopathy. J Neurol Sci 2013;334:172–5.
626. Sechi G, Serra A. Wernicke's encephalopathy: new clinical settings and recent advances in diagnosis and management. Lancet Neurol 2007;6:442–55.
627. Victor M, Adams RD, Collins GH. The Wernicke-Korsakoff syndrome: a clinical and pathological study of 245 patients, 882 with post-mortem examinations. Contemp Neurol Ser 1971;7:1–206.
628. Cogan DG, Witt ED, Goldman-Rakic PS. Ocular signs in thiamine-deficient monkeys and in Wernicke's disease in humans. Arch Ophthalmol 1985;103:1212–20.
629. Cogan DG, Victor M. Ocular signs of Wernicke's disease. Arch Ophthalmol 1954;51:204–11.
630. Suzuki Y, Matsuda T, Washio N, et al. Transition from upbeat to downbeat nystagmus observed in a patient with Wernicke's encephalopathy. Jpn J Ophthalmol 2005;49:220–2.
631. Ghez C. Vestibular paresis: a clinical feature of Wernicke's disease. J Neurol Neurosurg Psychiatry 1969;32:134–9.
632. Furman JM, Becker JT. Vestibular responses in Wernicke's encephalopathy. Ann Neurol 1989;26:669–74.
633. Choi KD, Oh SY, Kim HJ, et al. The vestibulo-ocular reflexes during head impulse in Wernicke's encephalopathy. J Neurol Neurosurg Psychiatry 2007;78:1161–2.
634. Vogel RM, Lee RV. Bilateral ptosis in Wernicke's disease. Neurology 1967;17:85–6.
635. Varavithya W, Dhanamitta S, Valyasevi A. Bilateral ptosis as a sign of thiamine deficiency in childhood. Response to corrective therapy is rapid. Clin Pediatr (Phila) 1975;14:1063–5.
636. Thompson RA, Lynde RH. Convergence spasm associated with Wernicke's encephalopathy. Neurology 1969;19:711–2.

637. Harper CG, Giles M, Finlay-Jones R. Clinical signs in the Wernicke-Korsakoff complex: a retrospective analysis of 131 cases diagnosed at necropsy. J Neurol Neurosurg Psychiatry 1986;49:341–5.

638. Mumford CJ. Papilloedema delaying diagnosis of Wernicke's encephalopathy in a comatose patient. Postgrad Med J 1989;65:371–3.

639. Kramer LD, Locke GE. Wernicke's encephalopathy. Complication of gastric plication. J Clin Gastroenterol 1987;9:549–52.

640. Bleggi-Torres LF, de Medeiros BC, Ogasawara VS, et al. Iatrogenic Wernicke's encephalopathy in allogeneic bone marrow transplantation: a study of eight cases. Bone Marrow Transplant 1997;20:391–5.

641. Tesfaye S, Achari V, Tang YC, et al. Pregnant, vomiting, and going blind. Lancet 1998;352:1594.

642. Kulkarni S, Lee AG, Holstein SA, et al. You are what you eat. Surv Ophthalmol 2005;50:389–93.

643. Bohnsack BL, Patel SS. Peripapillary nerve fiber layer thickening, telangiectasia, and retinal hemorrhages in Wernicke encephalopathy. J Neuroophthalmol 2010; 30:54–8.

644. Surges R, Beck S, Niesen WD, et al. Sudden bilateral blindness in Wernicke's encephalopathy: case report and review of the literature. J Neurol Sci 2007; 260:261–4.

645. Zieve I. Influence of magnesium deficiency on the utilization of thiamine. Ann N Y Acad Sci 1969;162:732–43.

646. Traviesa DC. Magnesium deficiency: a possible cause of thiamine refractoriness in Wernicke-Korsakoff encephalopathy. J Neurol Neurosurg Psychiatry 1974;37: 959–62.

647. McLean J, Manchip S. Wernicke's encephalopathy induced by magnesium depletion. Lancet 1999;353:1768.

648. Wilson SA. Progressive lenticular degeneration. A familial nervous disease associated with cirrhosis of the liver. Brain 1912;34:295–307.

649. Das SK, Ray K. Wilson's disease: an update. Nat Clin Pract Neurol 2006;2:482–93.

650. Harry J, Tripathi R. Kayser-Fleischer ring: a pathological study. Br J Ophthalmol 1970;54:794–800.

651. Kim HB, Kim JC, Byan YJ. Kayser Fleischer ring in Wilson's disease. J Korean Ophthal Soc 1979;20:129–31.

652. Innes JR, Strachan IM, Triger DR. Unilateral Kayser-Fleischer ring. Br J Ophthalmol 1986;70:469–70.

653. Rodman R, Burnstine M, Esmaeli B, et al. Wilson's disease: presymptomatic patients and Kayser-Fleischer rings. Ophthalmic Genet 1997;18:79–85.

654. Walshe JM. The eye in Wilson disease. QJM 2011;104:451–3.

655. Cairns JE, Parry Williams H, Walshe JM. 'Sunflower cataract' in Wilson's disease. Br Med J 1969;3:95–6.

656. Wiebers DO, Hollenhorst RW, Goldstein NP. The ophthalmologic manifestations of Wilson's disease. Mayo Clin Proc 1977;52:409–16.

657. Satishchandra P, Ravishankar Naik K. Visual pathway abnormalities Wilson's disease: an electrophysiological study using electroretinography and visual evoked potentials. J Neurol Sci 2000;176:13–20.

658. Arendt G, Hefter H, Stremmel W, et al. The diagnostic value of multi-modality evoked potentials in Wilson's disease. Electromyogr Clin Neurophysiol 1994; 34:137–48.

659. Hsu YS, Chang YC, Lee WT, et al. The diagnostic value of sensory evoked potentials in pediatric Wilson disease. Pediatr Neurol 2003;29:42–5.

660. Das M, Misra UK, Kalita J. A study of clinical, MRI and multimodality evoked potentials in neurologic Wilson disease. Eur J Neurol 2007;14:498–504.
661. Albrecht P, Muller AK, Ringelstein M, et al. Retinal neurodegeneration in Wilson's disease revealed by spectral domain optical coherence tomography. PLoS One 2012;7:e49825.
662. Lennox G, Jones R. Gaze distractibility in Wilson's disease. Ann Neurol 1989;25: 415–7.
663. Ingster-Moati I, Quoc EB, Pless M, et al. Ocular motility and Wilson's disease: a study of 34 patients. J Neurol Neurosurg Psychiatry 2007;78:1199–201.
664. Lesniak M, Czionkowska A, Seniow J. Abnormal antisaccades and smooth pursuit eye movements in patients with Wilson's disease. Mov Disord 2008;23: 2067–73.
665. Jung HK, Choi SY, Kim JM, et al. Selective slowing of downward saccades in Wilson's disease. Parkinsonism Relat Disord 2013;19:134–5.
666. Kirkham TH, Kamin DF. Slow saccadic eye movements in Wilson's disease. J Neurol Neurosurg Psychiatry 1974;37:191–4.
667. Hyman NM, Phuapradit P. Reading difficulty as a presenting symptom in Wilson's disease. J Neurol Neurosurg Psychiatry 1979;42:478–80.
668. Klingele TG, Newman SA, Burde RM. Accommodation defect in Wilson's disease. Am J Ophthalmol 1980;90:22–4.
669. Curran RE, Hedges T, Boger WP. Loss of accommodation and the near response in Wilson's disease. J Pediatr Ophthalmol Strabismus 1982;19:157–60.
670. Keane JD. Lid-opening apraxia in Wilson's disease. J Clin Neuroophthalmol 1988;8:31–3.
671. Lee MS, Kim YD, Lyoo CH. Oculogyric crisis as an initial manifestation of Wilson's disease. Neurology 1999;52:1714–5.
672. Whipple GH. A hitherto undescribed disease characterized anatomically by deposits of fat and fatty acids in the intestinal and mesenteric lymphatic tissues. Johns Hopkins Hosp Bull 1907;18:382–91.
673. Raoult D, Birg ML, Scola BL, et al. Cultivation of the bacillus of Whipple's disease. N Engl J Med 2000;342:620–5.
674. Fenollar F, Puechal X, Raoult D. Whipple's disease. N Engl J Med 2007;356: 55–66.
675. Matthews BR, Jones LK, Saad DA, et al. Cerebellar ataxia and central nervous system Whipple disease. Arch Neurol 2005;62:618–20.
676. Rickman LS, Freeman WR, Green WR, et al. Uveitis caused by *Tropheryma whippelii* (Whipple's bacillus). N Engl J Med 1995;332:363–6.
677. Chan RY, Yanuzzi LA, Foster CS. Ocular Whipple's disease: earlier definitive diagnosis. Ophthalmology 2001;108:2225–31.
678. Drancourt M, Raoult D, Lepidi H, et al. Culture of *Tropheryma whippelii* from the vitreous fluid of a patient presenting with unilateral uveitis. Ann Intern Med 2003; 139:1046–7.
679. Touitou V, Fenollar F, Cassoux N, et al. Ocular Whipple's disease: therapeutic strategy and long-term follow-up. Ophthalmology 2012;119:1465–9.
680. Lieger O, Otto S, Clemetson IA, et al. Orbital manifestation of Whipple's disease: an atypical case. J Craniomaxillofac Surg 2007;35:393–6.
681. Gerard A, Sarrot-Reynauld F, Liozon E, et al. Neurologic presentation of Whipple disease: report of 12 cases and review of the literature. Medicine (Baltimore) 2002;81:443–57.
682. Louis ED, Lynch T, Kaufmann P, et al. Diagnostic guidelines in central nervous system Whipple's disease. Ann Neurol 1996;40:561–8.

683. Fleming JL, Wiesner RH, Shorter RG. Whipple's disease: clinical, biochemical, and histopathological features and assessment of treatment in 29 patients. Mayo Clin Proc 1988;63:539–51.

684. Burk K, Farecki ML, Lamprecht G, et al. Neurological symptoms in patients with biopsy proven celiac disease. Mov Disord 2009;24:2358–62.

685. Cooke WT, Smith WT. Neurological disorders associated with adult celiac disease. Brain 1966;89:683–722.

686. Hadjivassiliou M, Gibson A, Davies-Jones GA, et al. Does cryptic gluten sensitivity play a part in neurological illness? Lancet 1996;347:369–71.

687. Hadjivassiliou M, Sanders DS, Grunewald RA, et al. Gluten sensitivity: from gut to brain. Lancet 2010;9:318–30.

688. Brucke T, Kollegger H, Schmidbauer M, et al. Adult celiac disease and brain stem encephalitis. J Neurol Neurosurg Psychiatry 1988;51:456–7.

689. Hadjivassiliou M, Sanders DS, Woodroofe N, et al. Gluten ataxia. Cerebellum 2008;7:494–8.

690. Solimena M, Folli F, Aparisi R, et al. Autoantibodies to GABA-ergic neurons and pancreatic beta cells in stiff-man syndrome. N Engl J Med 1990;322:1555–60.

691. Giometto B, Miotto D, Faresin F, et al. Anti-gabaergic neuron autoantibodies in a patient with stiff-man syndrome and ataxia. J Neurol Sci 1996;143:57–9.

692. Dinkel K, Meinck HM, Jury KM, et al. Inhibition of gama-aminobutyric acid synthesis by glutamic acid decarboxylase autoantibodies in stiff-man syndrome. Ann Neurol 1998;44:194–201.

693. Meinck HM, Faber L, Margenthaler N, et al. Antibodies against glutamic acid decarboxylase: prevalence in neurological disease. J Neurol Neurosurg Psychiatry 2001;71:100–3.

694. Nemni R, Braghi S, Natali-Sora MG, et al. Autoantibodies to glutamic acid decarboxylase in palatal myoclonus and epilepsy. Ann Neurol 1994;36:665–7.

695. Abele M, Weller M, Mescheriakov S, et al. Cerebellar ataxia with glutamic acid decarboxylase autoantibodies. Neurology 1999;52:857–9.

696. Peltola J, Kulmala P, Isojarvi J, et al. Autoantibodies to glutamic acid decarboxylase in patients with therapy-resistant epilepsy. Neurology 2000;55:46–50.

697. Hannorat J, Saiz A, Giometto B, et al. Cerebellar ataxia with anti-glutamic acid decarboxylase antibodies. Arch Neurol 2001;58:225–30.

698. Takenoshita H, Shizuka-Ikeda M, Mitoma H, et al. Presynaptic inhibition of cerebellar GABAergic transmission by glutamate decarboxylase autoantibodies in progressive cerebellar ataxia. J Neurol Neurosurg Psychiatry 2001;70:386–9.

699. Saltik S, Turkes M, Tuzun E, et al. Peripheral neuropathy associated with antiglutamic acid decarboxylase antibodies. Pediatr Neurol 2013;48:403–6.

700. Economides JR, Horton JC. Eye movement abnormalities in stiff person syndrome. Neurology 2005;65:1462–4.

701. Antonini G, Nemni R, Giubilei F, et al. Antoantibodies to glutamic acid decarboxylase in downbeat nystagmus. J Neurol Neurosurg Psychiatry 2003;74:998–9.

702. Piccolo G, Martino G, Moglia A, et al. Autoimmune myasthenia gravis with thymoma following the spontaneous remission of stiff-man syndrome. Ital J Neurol Sci 1990;11:177–80.

703. Saravanan PK, Paul J, Sayeed ZA. Stiff person syndrome and myasthenia gravis. Neurol India 2002;50:98–100.

704. Thomas S, Critchley P, Lawden M, et al. Stiff person syndrome with eye movement abnormality, myasthenia gravis, and thymoma. J Neurol Neurosurg Psychiatry 2005;76:141–2.

705. Dalmau J, Rosenfeld MR. Paraneoplastic syndromes of the CNS. Lancet Neurol 2008;7:327–40.
706. Mason WP, Graus F, Lang B, et al. Small-cell lung cancer, paraneoplastic cerebellar degeneration and the Lambert-Eaton myasthenic syndrome. Brain 1997; 120:1279–300.
707. Shams'ili S, Grefkens J, de Leeuw B, et al. Paraneoplastic cerebellar degeneration associated with antineuronal antibodies: analysis of 50 patients. Brain 2003;126:1409–18.
708. Ogita S, Llaguna OH, Feldman SM, et al. Paraneoplastic cerebellar degeneration with anti-Yo antibody in a patient with HER2/neu overexpressing breast cancer: a case report with a current literature review. Breast J 2008;14:382–4.
709. Mathew RM, Cohen AB, Galetta SL, et al. Paraneoplastic cerebellar degeneration: Yo-expressing tumor revealed after a 5-year follow-up with FDG-PET. J Neurol Sci 2006;250:153–5.
710. Graus F, Lang B, Pozo-Rosich P, et al. P/Q type calcium-channel antibodies in paraneoplastic cerebellar degeneration with lung cancer. Neurology 2002;59: 764–6.
711. de la Sayette V, Bertran F, Honnorat J, et al. Paraneoplastic cerebellar syndrome and optic neuritis with anti-CV2 antibodies: clinical response to excision of the primary tumor. Arch Neurol 1998;55:405–8.
712. Antoine JC, Honnorat J, Vocanson C, et al. Posterior uveitis, paraneoplastic encephalomyelitis and auto-antibodies reacting with developmental protein of brain and retina. J Neurol Sci 1993;117:215–23.
713. Cross SA, Salomao DR, Parisi JE, et al. Paraneoplastic autoimmune optic neuritis with retinitis defined by CRMP-5-IgG. Ann Neurol 2003;54:38–50.
714. Sheorajpanday R, Slabbynck H, Van De Sompel W, et al. Small cell lung carcinoma presenting as collapsin response-mediating protein (CRMP) -5 paraneoplastic optic neuropathy. J Neuroophthalmol 2006;26:168–72.
715. Bernal F, Shams'ili S, Rojas I, et al. Anti-Tr antibodies as markers of paraneoplastic cerebellar degeneration and Hodgkin's disease. Neurology 2003;60:230–4.
716. Eggers SD, Pittock SJ, Shepard NT, et al. Positional periodic alternating vertical nystagmus with PCA-Tr antibodies in Hodgkin lymphoma. Neurology 2012;78: 1800–2.
717. Voltz R, Carpentier AF, Rosenfeld MR, et al. P/Q-type voltage-gated calcium channel antibodies in paraneoplastic disorders of the central nervous system. Muscle Nerve 1999;22:119–22.
718. Lorenzoni PJ, Scola RH, Lang B, et al. Cerebellar ataxia in non-paraneoplastic Lambert-Eaton myasthenic syndrome. J Neurol Sci 2008;270:194–6.
719. Hoftberger R, Titulaer MJ, Sabater L, et al. Encephalitis and GABAB receptor antibodies: novel findings in a new case series of 20 patients. Neurology 2013;81:1500–6.
720. Barnett M, Prosser J, Sutton I, et al. Paraneoplastic brain stem encephalitis in a woman with anti-Ma2 antibody. J Neurol Neurosurg Psychiatry 2001;70:222–5.
721. Bennett JL, Galetta SL, Frohman LP, et al. Neuro-ophthalmologic manifestations of a paraneoplastic syndrome and testicular carcinoma. Neurology 1999;52: 864–7.
722. Castle J, Sakonju A, Dalmau J, et al. Anti-Ma2-associated encephalitis with normal FDG-PET: a case of pseudo-Whipple's disease. Nat Clin Pract Neurol 2006;2:566–72.
723. Wagner J, Schankin C, Birnbaum T, et al. Ocular motor and lid apraxia as initial symptom of anti-Ma1/Ma2-associated encephalitis. Neurology 2009;72:466–7.

724. Bruno MK, Winterkorn JM, Edgar MA, et al. Unilateral Adie pupil as sole ophthalmic sign of anti-Hu paraneoplastic syndrome. J Neuroophthalmol 2000;20:248–9.

725. Graus F, Keime-Guibert F, Rene R, et al. Anti-Hu-associated paraneoplastic encephalomyelitis: analysis of 200 patients. Brain 2001;124:1138–44.

726. Fujimoto S, Kumamoto T, Ito T, et al. A clinicopathological study of a patient with anti-Hu-associated paraneoplastic sensory neuronopathy with multiple cranial nerve palsies. Clin Neurol Neurosurg 2002;104:98–102.

727. Wabbels BK, Elflein H, Lorenz B, et al. Bilateral tonic pupils with evidence of anti-hu antibodies as a paraneoplastic manifestation of small cell lung cancer. Ophthalmologica 2004;218:141–3.

728. Saiz A, Bruna J, Stourac P, et al. Anti-Hu-associated brainstem encephalitis. J Neurol Neurosurg Psychiatry 2009;80:404–7.

729. Choe CH, Gausas RE. Blepharospasm and apraxia of eyelid opening associated with anti-Hu paraneoplastic antibodies: a case report. Ophthalmology 2012;119:865–8.

730. Sutton IJ, Barnett MH, Watson JD, et al. Paraneoplastic brainstem encephalitis and anti-Ri antibodies. J Neurol 2002;249:1597–8.

731. Pittock SJ, Parisi JE, McKeon A, et al. Paraneoplastic jaw dystonia and laryngospasm with antineuronal nuclear autoantibody type 2 (anti-Ri). Arch Neurol 2010;67:1109–15.

732. Luque FA, Furneaux HM, Ferziger R, et al. Anti-Ri: an antibody associated with paraneoplastic opsoclonus and breast cancer. Ann Neurol 1991;29:241–51.

733. Wirtz PW, Sillevis Smitt PA, Hoff JI, et al. Anti-Ri antibody positive opsoclonus-myoclonus in a male patient with breast carcinoma. J Neurol 2002;249:1710–2.

734. Strupp M, Schuler O, Krafczyk S, et al. Treatment of downbeat nystagmus with 3,4-diaminopyridine: a placebo-controlled study. Neurology 2003;61:165–70.

735. Kalla R, Glasauer S, Schautzer F, et al. 4-Aminopyridine improves downbeat nystagmus, smooth pursuit, and VOR gain. Neurology 2004;62:1228–9.

736. Kalla R, Glasauer S, Buttner U, et al. 4-Aminopyridine restores vertical and horizontal neural integrator function in downbeat nystagmus. Brain 2007;130:2441–51.

737. Strupp M, Brandt T. Current treatment of vestibular, ocular motor disorders and nystagmus. Ther Adv Neurol Disord 2009;2:223–39.

738. Kalla R, Spiegel R, Claassen J, et al. Comparison of 10-mg doses of 4-aminopyridine and 3,4-diaminopyridine for the treatment of downbeat nystagmus. J Neuroophthalmol 2011;31:320–5.

739. Strupp M, Kalla R, Claassen J, et al. A randomized trial of 4-aminopyridine in EA2 and related familial episodic ataxias. Neurology 2011;77:269–75.

740. Claassen J, Spiegel R, Kalla R, et al. A randomized double-blind, cross-over trial of 4-aminopyridine for downbeat nystagmus – effects on slowphase eye velocity, postural stability, locomotion and symptoms. J Neurol Neurosurg Psychiatry 2013;84:1392–9.

741. Van Diemen HA, Polman CH, Koetsier JC, et al. 4-Aminopyridine in patients with multiple sclerosis: dosage and serum level related to efficacy and safety. Clin Neuropharmacol 1993;16:195–204.

742. Bever CT, Young D, Anderson PA, et al. The effects of 4-aminopyridine in multiple sclerosis patients: results of a randomized, placebo-controlled, double-blind, concentration-controlled, crossover trial. Neurology 1994;44:1054–9.

743. Vollmer T, Blight AR, Henney HR III. Steady-state pharmacokinetics and tolerability of orally administered fampridine sustained-release 10-mg tablets in

patients with multiple sclerosis: a 2-week, open-label, follow-up study. Clin Ther 2009;31:2215–23.

744. Serra A, Liao K, Martinez-Conde S, et al. Suppression of saccadic intrusions in hereditary ataxia by memantine. Neurology 2008;70:810–2.

745. Traccis S, Marras MA, Puliga MV, et al. Square-wave jerks and square-wave oscillations: treatment with valproic acid. Neuroophthalmology 1997;18:51–8.

746. Ashe J, Hain TC, Zee DS, et al. Microsaccadic flutter. Brain 1991;114:461–72.

747. Pranzatelli MR. The neurobiology of the opsoclonus-myoclonus syndrome. Clin Neuropharmacol 1992;15:186–228.

748. Fernandes TD, Bazan R, Betting LE, et al. Topiramate effect in opsoclonus-myoclonus-ataxia syndrome. Arch Neurol 2012;69:133.

749. Pless M, Ronthal M. Treatment of opsoclonus-myoclonus with high-dose intravenous immunoglobulin. Neurology 1996;46:583–4.

750. Pranzatelli MR, Tate ED, Travelstead AL, et al. Rituximab (anti-CD20) adjunctive therapy for opsoclonus-myoclonus syndrome. J Pediatr Hematol Oncol 2006;28: 585–93.

751. Pranzatelli MR, Tate ED, Swan JA, et al. B cell depletion therapy for new-onset opsoclonus-myoclonus. Mov Disord 2010;25:238–42.

752. Tate ED, Pranzatelli MR, Verhulst SJ, et al. Active comparator-controlled, rater-blinded study of corticotropin-based immunotherapies for opsoclonus-myoclonus syndrome. J Child Neurol 2012;27:875–84.

753. Pranzatelli MR, Tate ED, Shenoy S, et al. Ofatumumab for a rituximab-allergic child with chronic-relapsing paraneoplastic opsoclonus-myoclonus. Pediatr Blood Cancer 2012;58:988–91.

754. Currie J, Matsuo V. The use of clonazepam in the treatment of nystagmus induced oscillopsia. Ophthalmology 1986;93:924–32.

755. Dieterich M, Straube A, Brandt T, et al. The effects of baclofen and cholinergic drugs on upbeat and downbeat nystagmus. J Neurol Neurosurg Psychiatry 1991;54:627–32.

756. Averbuch-Heller L, Tusa RJ, Fuhry L, et al. A double-blind controlled study of gabapentin and baclofen as treatment for acquired nystagmus. Ann Neurol 1997;41:818–25.

757. Barton JJ, Huaman AG, Sharpe JA. Muscarinic antagonists in the treatment of acquired pendular and downbeat nystagmus: a double-blind, randomized trial of three intravenous drugs. Ann Neurol 1994;35:319–25.

758. Feil K, Claassen J, Bardins S, et al. Effect of chlorzoxazone in patients with downbeat nystagmus: a pilot trial. Neurology 2013;81:1152–8.

759. Spiegel R, Kalla R, Rettinger N, et al. Head position during resting modifies spontaneous daytime decrease of downbeat nystagmus. Neurology 2010;75: 1928–32.

760. Glasauer S, Kalla R, Buttner U, et al. 4-Aminopyridine restores visual ocular motor function in upbeat nystagmus. J Neurol Neurosurg Psychiatry 2005;76:451–3.

761. Halmagyi MG, Rudge P, Gresty MA. Treatment of periodic alternating nystagmus. Ann Neurol 1980;8:609–11.

762. Isago H, Tsuboya R, Kataura A. A case of periodic alternating nystagmus: with special reference to the efficacy of baclofen treatment. Auris Nasus Larynx 1985;12:15–21.

763. Nuti D, Ciacci G, Ginnini F, et al. Aperiodic alternating nystagmus: report of two cases and treatment with baclofen. Ital J Neurol Sci 1986;7:452–9.

764. Comer RM, Dawson EL, Lee JP. Baclofen for patients with congenital periodic alternating nystagmus. Strabismus 2006;14:205–9.

765. Kumar A, Thomas S, McLean R, et al. Treatment of acquired periodic alternating nystagmus with memantine: a case report. Clin Neuropharmacol 2009;32:109–10.

766. Beh SC, Tehrani AS, Kheradmand A, et al. Damping of monocular pendular nystagmus with vibration in a patient with multiple sclerosis. Neurology 2014; 82(15):1380–1.

767. Starck M, Albrecht H, Pollmann W, et al. Drug therapy for acquired pendular nystagmus in multiple sclerosis. J Neurol 1997;244:9–16.

768. Bandini F, Castello E, Mazzella L, et al. Gabapentin but not vigabatrin is effective in the treatment of acquired nystagmus in multiple sclerosis: how valid is the GABAergic hypothesis? J Neurol Neurosurg Psychiatry 2001;71:107–10.

769. Shery T, Proudlock FA, Sarvananthan N, et al. The effects of gabapentin and memantine in acquired and congenital nystagmus: a retrospective study. Br J Ophthalmol 2006;90:839–43.

770. Thurtell MJ, Joshi AC, Leone AC, et al. Crossover trial of gabapentin and memantine as treatment for acquired nystagmus. Ann Neurol 2010;67:676–80.

771. Starck M, Albrecht H, Pollmann W, et al. Acquired pendular nystagmus in multiple sclerosis: an examiner-blind cross-over treatment of memantine and gabapentin. J Neurol 2010;257:322–7.

772. Jabbari B, Rosenberg M, Scherokman B. Effectiveness of trihexyphenidyl against pendular nystagmus and palatal myoclonus: evidence of cholinergic dysfunction. Mov Disord 1987;2:93–8.

773. Schon F, Hart PE, Hodgson TL, et al. Suppression of pendular nystagmus by smoking cannabis in a patient with multiple sclerosis. Neurology 1999;53:2209–10.

774. Dell'Osso LF. Suppression of pendular nystagmus by smoking cannabis in a patient with multiple sclerosis. Neurology 2000;13:2190–1.

The Role of the Cerebellum in Cognition

Beyond Coordination in the Central Nervous System

Maryam Noroozian, MD

KEYWORDS

- Cerebellum • Cognition • Executive function • Nonmotor • Memory • Language

KEY POINTS

- The cerebellum is involved not only in movement, but also intellect and emotion.
- Different parts of cerebellum regulate different functions.
- Damage to the anterior lobe results in dysmetria of movement, causing ataxia.
- Damage to the posterior lobe results in dysmetria of thought and emotion, causing Cerebellar Cognitive Affective Syndrome and the dysmetria of thought .
- Damage to the cerebellum can result in 4 broad categories of cognitive deficit: language (including speech perception, lexical retrieval, and working memory), temporal ordering and timing, implicit learning and memory, and visuospatial attention.

INTRODUCTION

Historically, research interest in cerebellar coordination of motor control has overshadowed investigation for the possible role of the cerebellum in the mediation of cognitive processes (**Box 1**).[1–3] Hence, less attention has been directed to the observation that cerebellar disorders are also associated with nonmotor abnormalities.[4–11] Consistent with this view, most cerebellar lesion studies reported throughout the twentieth century have largely focused on investigations into the nature of associated motor impairments, excluding the cerebellum's broader capabilities.

Recent advances in our understanding of the neuroanatomy of the cerebellum, combined with evidence from functional neuroimaging, and neurophysiological and neuropsychological research, have extended our view of the cerebellum from that of a simple coordinator of autonomic and somatic motor function, and discoveries have converged to suggest that most of the human cerebellum is connected to

The author has nothing to disclose.

Conflict of Interest: None.

Memory and Behavioral Neurology Division, Department of Psychiatry, Tehran University of Medical Sciences, Roozbeh Hospital, 606 South Kargar Avenue, Tehran 1333795914, Iran

E-mail address: mnoroozi@tums.ac.ir

> **Box 1**
> **Etymology**
>
> Although the nomenclature of cerebellum in many Indo-European languages, Persian included, in which the name ascribed to this organ literally translates as "small cerebrum": mokhche = mokh (brain) + che (diminutive suffix), denotes its resemblance to the cerebrum and addresses its size, scientific findings in recent decades have demonstrated that cerebellum has been essentially so developed as to play a significant role in nonmotor functions in the field of cognition, and have gradually unraveled cerebellum's significant connections with cerebral hemispheres contributing to executive functions, language, memory, and emotion; the organ's name is only now beginning to make sense.

cerebral association networks. It is now more widely accepted that the cerebellum, and in particular the right cerebellar hemisphere, participates in modulation of cognitive functioning, especially in relation to those parts of the brain to which it is reciprocally connected.

Currently, our understanding of roles the cerebellum plays has been expanded from its function in coordination of voluntary movements, orientation of the body and head in space, regulation and integration of sensory information for reflex organization, and regulating vestibulo-ocular movements and posture of the head, to its essential role in learning conditioned responses and last, and most currently, regulation of linguistic, cognitive, and affective functions.

The particular role of the cerebellum in language and cognition has been shown to be modulation rather than generation, the latter function (ie, cognition) being considered to be specific to supratentorial structures, particularly the cerebral cortex.[12] Based on anatomic, physiologic, and clinical information, investigators such as Snider and Maiti,[13] Dow,[14] and Heath,[15] suggested that the cerebellum is a great modulator of neurologic function, and that whatever it does for motor control, it also does for other kinds of behaviors. The concept of cerebellum as incorporated into the distributed cortico-subcortical neural system subserving cognition was more formally developed by the Leiners with Dow,[16] based on the expansion of the neocerebellum and dentate nucleus along with the cerebral association areas by Schmahmann and Pandya[10,17] and Middleton and Strick.[18]

Our understanding of the contribution of the cerebellum to neurocognition is still in a nascent stage, the current status quo being essentially due to the historical negligence of the nonmotor role of the cerebellum. But it, furthermore, is the result of the fact that the cerebellum acts primarily as a rather subtle modulator of neurocognitive processes. If this modulating function is impaired, deficits arise that are quantitatively and qualitatively different from the deficits produced by lesions of the supratentorial structures. Therefore, standard psychometric test batteries, which are designed to detect well-delineated neurocognitive impairments, are often not sensitive enough to pinpoint the "subclinical" deficits that may follow cerebellar damage. It is required to further refine the present neurocognitive test methodologies and develop specifically adapted clinical investigation tools to capture the rich spectrum of neurocognitive dysfunctions induced by cerebellar impairments. In addition, because neurocognitive impairment after cerebellar damage often evolves rapidly and is often transient in the case of stroke, the possibility of inadequate assessment increases even further.

This article reviews in further detail the current understanding of cognitive deficits associated with cerebellar impairments and unravels its modulating role in cognitive and behavioral processes.[19]

HISTORY

Around the time cerebellum was recognized as a motor control device, and long before the notion of cerebellum as a motor apparatus was affirmed through works of behaviorists and clinicians, investigators (perhaps starting with Combettes as early as 1831)[4] began to report associations between cerebellar pathology and clinical manifestations outside of the motor domain. Hence, the reports of the effects of ablation of the cerebellum in animals and the first clinical reports of patients with cerebellar pathology by Babinski (1913)[20] and Holmes (1917, 1922)[21,22] began to modify the traditional concept of cerebellum as a part of the brain entirely dedicated to the regulation and coordination of motor function. Accordingly, behavioral abnormalities and intellectual dysfunction were reported in patients with cerebellar agenesis and familial cerebellar degeneration as early as the nineteenth century; however, these findings did not leave deep impressions in the minds of neuroscientists. The association between cerebellum and cognition began to attract attention in the last century and dysmetria of movement, as first described by Babinski, was equated with "Dysmetria or Ataxia of Thought".[10,23,24]

Today, there are anatomic, clinical, and functional imaging studies providing crucial evidence in support of the hypothesis of cerebellar involvement in cognitive functions.

EVOLUTIONARY ASPECTS IN THE DEVELOPMENT OF CEREBELLUM

All vertebrate brains have a cerebellum, and most of them have one or more additional structures that are histologically similar to the cerebellum.[25,26] The cerebellar hemispheres in humans, as well as in the old world primates and great apes, are very large.[27] The neocortex has expanded during the course of phylogeny; the cerebellum has also, compared with other species, expanded 3 to 4 times in sapiens.[16] For those still skeptical about the involvement of cerebellum in cognition, it is useful to refer to the article by Leiner and colleagues,[28] in which it has been argued that the cerebellum has undergone functionally significant changes during the course of hominid evolution, increasing both in size and number of reciprocal connections with various regions of the cerebral cortex. Importantly, the cerebellum's expansion in size has not occurred in accordance with the cerebral cortex as a whole, but rather specifically in parallel with the cerebral association areas.[16] As the cerebellar cortex has selectively expanded,[29] there has been a dramatic increase in the size of the dentate nucleus of the cerebellum. Also, reciprocal connections have been identified between the prefrontal cortex and the dentate nucleus in humans, which are absent in other species.[30–32]

From an anatomic standpoint, considering that the cerebellum contains more than half of all the neurons in the brain, the probability that it may play a role in nonmotor brain functioning should not come as a surprise.[10] Specifically, Leiner and colleagues[16] drew attention to long-neglected role of the lateral portion of the cerebellar hemispheres and dentate nuclei. The hemispheres project to the dentate nucleus, which is the largest of the cerebellar nuclei in human and higher primates. Particularly, during the phylogenetic evolution of the human brain, the ventrolateral phylogenetically newer part, referred to as the neodentate, has enlarged significantly greater than any other part of the brain, the cerebral cortex excluded.[33–35] Another article[36] has shown that the link to the prefrontal cortex is part of a pathway through which, in monkeys, the cerebellum influences cognitive functions. Circuitry within the cerebellum, shaped by natural selection as part of the motor system, may have been well suited to perform cognitive tasks that were in need of similar neural architecture. It seems that during the long process of natural selection, cognitive operations, rather than replacing the prior motor functions, have been added to them. The case of cerebellum may be an example of an evolutionary process by which mechanisms that have originally evolved for one function (in this case, motor control) are adapted to other functions (cognition).[37]

EVIDENCE FROM NEUROANATOMICAL STUDIES

The cerebellum has several surprising anatomic and functional features; these include the following: there are more neurons in the cerebellum than any other part of the human nervous system, the cerebral cortex included; the speed of its operation enables rapid response to received information; it also has massive neural connections with the cerebral cortex, which sends more fibers to the cerebellum than any other part of the nervous system; and its output fibers have extensive connections, passing to many other sections of the nervous system, including areas of the cerebral cortex even beyond motor areas. Each cerebellar hemisphere sends information to, and receives it from, the contralateral cerebral hemisphere. Therefore, the right cerebellar hemisphere is connected to the left cerebral hemisphere and conversely. It has suggested that the cerebellar cortex is arranged in a medio-lateral organization.[38] The midline vermis, he proposed, controls proximal muscles, and the hemispheres, distal muscles. The cerebellum connects, mainly via the thalamus, to many brain areas relevant to cognition and behavior, including the dorsolateral prefrontal cortex, the medial frontal cortex, the parietal and superior temporal areas, the anterior cingulate, and the posterior hypothalamus.[39,40] There are also noradrenergic, serotonergic, and dopaminergic inputs to the cerebellum from brainstem nuclei.[39] Considering these connections, a role for the cerebellum in nonmotor functioning would seem likely. The microscopic anatomy of the cerebellar cortex is quite uniform.[41] Anatomic tract tracing studies indicate that there are pathways linking the cerebellum with autonomic,[42,43] limbic,[44] and associative regions of the cerebral cortex,[45,46] as well as with sensorimotor cortices. These links allow the cerebellum to communicate with brain areas involved in instinctive behaviors, mood, and the higher levels of cognition and reasoning.

Of particular relevance to enabling the cerebellum to contribute to cognitive/linguistic processes, these newly formed links between the neocerebellum and the frontal lobe included not only the frontal motor areas (Brodmann areas 4 and 6) but also other areas of the frontal cortex, including Broca's area (Brodmann areas 44 and 45), which in turn send back new connections to the cerebellum. A diagrammatic representation of major fronto-cerebellar loops in the human brain is shown in **Fig. 1**, which illustrates how the cerebellum is extensively interconnected with cerebral hemispheres both in feed-forward and feed-backward directions.

In summary, there are circuits, or anatomic loops, that link in a bidirectional manner higher-order areas of the brain with the cerebellum. These reciprocal neuroanatomical pathways provide a neural substrate and structural basis for putative functional roles of cerebellum in organization of motor and cognitive functions. These connections, which are proposed to mediate cerebellar input into cognitive linguistic functions, have a number of parallel features to equivalent pathways involved in the coordination and modulation of motor function.[47]

EVIDENCE FROM CLINICAL STUDIES

Subjects with cerebellar diseases have been often found to have "frontal-like" cognitive impairments with many variable manifestations in the areas of visuospatial dysfunction, language, and memory. Functional role of cerebellum in each cognitive domain is classified in **Table 1**, along with exemplary studies.

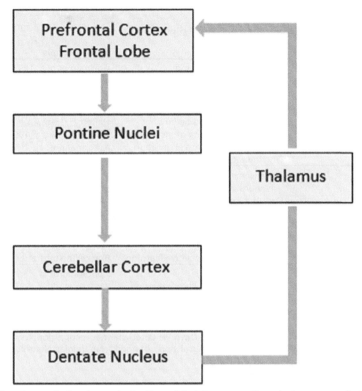

Fig. 1. Fronto-cerebellar loops indicating rich interconnections between cerebellum and frontal, prefrontal lobes, and subcortical structures.

It should be kept in mind that the current neuropsychological assessments indicating cognitive deficits in patients with cerebellar lesions may not be sufficient to account for the role of cerebellum in cognitive functions. To understand the impact of cerebellar lesions on cognitive and behavioral functions, it is essential to select more sophisticated assessments.

Cognitive Impairment in Hereditary Cerebellar Ataxia

Cognitive impairment is mentioned in clinical descriptions of hereditary ataxia to a variable extent. There is a body of evidence indicating a broad spectrum of cognitive dysfunctions in different types of spinocerebellar atrophy types 1, 2, 3 (Machado-Joseph disease), 13, 17, and 21. Regarding the neuropathological pattern in this spectrum, cognitive deficits in hereditary ataxia are probably not dependent on cerebellar degeneration, but result from disruption of cerebrocerebellar circuitries at several levels in the central nervous system.[48] Similarly, multiple deficits in intellect, memory, attention, language, and visuospatial and executive functions are reported in olivopontocerebellar atrophy. However, results regarding the nature and consistency of cognitive deficit in Friedreich's ataxia are conflicting.[49]

DIASCHISIS

A unilateral supratentorial lesion may cause hypometabolism in the contralateral cerebellar hemisphere (crossed cerebellar diaschisis). On the other side, "reversed

| Table 1 |
| Cerebellar involvement in neurocognitive functions |

Cognitive Domain	Function	Study Example
Executive planning	Frontal problem solving	Grafman et al,[70] 1992
	Cognitive planning	Grafman et al,[70] 1992
	Sequencing of plans	Hallett & Grafman,[129] 1997
Temporal sequencing	Judgment of time duration	Ivery & Keele,[125] 1989
	Timing of plans and actions	Hallett & Grafman,[129] 1997
	Judgment of velocity of movement	Ivery & Diener,[120] 1991
	Discrimination of vowel duration	Ackermann et al,[143] 1997
	Discrimination of VOT	Ackermann et al,[143] 1997
Attention	Enhancement in neural responsiveness	Yeo et al,[144] 1985
	Direction of selective attention	Akshoomoff et al,[145] 1997
Visuo-perception	Visuo-spatial processing	Silveri et al,[146] 1997
	Visuo-construction	Botez-Marquard et al,[115] 1994
Learning	Motor skill learning	Marr,[100] 1969; Tach,[147] 1997
	Procedural and associative learning	Bracke-Tolkmitt et al,[118] 1989
Memory	Long-term memory	Appolonio et al,[148] 1993
	Phonological short-term memory	Paulesu et al,[149] 1993
Imagery	Visuo-motor imagery	Decety et al,[150] 1990

Abbreviation: VOT, voice-onset time.
Adapted from Marien P, Engelborghs S, De Deyn PP. Cerebellar neurocognition: a new avenue. Acta Neurol Belg 2001;101(2):97. Copyright permission obtained from Belgian Neurologic Society, Belgium.

cerebellar diaschisis" is a term indicating regional hypoperfusion in cerebral association areas during positron emission tomography (PET)/single-photon emission computed tomography studies in patients with acute cerebellar lesions implicating the mechanism commonly suggested for the cognitive disturbances following acute cerebellar lesions.[50]

THE CEREBELLUM IN AGING AND DEMENTIA

The cerebellum also appears to have relevance to mechanisms in aging and dementia. It has been reported that a 10% to 40% decrease in Purkinje cell layer[51] and a reduction in the area of the dorsal vermis[52] is evident in aging. Alcoholic dementia is one of the classic dementias associated with cerebellar atrophy. Although alcoholic dementia is usually complicated because of medical comorbidity, patients with this condition may manifest more ataxia and stereotypic behavior changes, but less overt cortical dysfunction (eg, less anomia, less deterioration in cognitive status) than those with Alzheimer disease (AD) do.[53]

Although the cerebellum is not considered to be of primary pathologic focus in AD, diffuse amyloid plaques and increased microglia (but an absence of neurofibrillary tangles) can be found in the cerebellum, usually later in the AD process. Purkinje cell density is decreased, especially in familial AD.[54] Ishii and colleagues[55] reported decreased cerebellar metabolism in severe AD, which was correlated with cognitive decline. In one autopsy study,[56] gross cerebellar atrophy on brain computed tomography has been cautiously suggested as a marker for mixed dementia; an observation that might be most helpful clinically if replicable. Affective liability and emotional incontinence in dementia are associated with cerebellar atrophy, third ventricular width, and interhemispheric fissure width, but not with other measures of cortical atrophy; therefore, the cerebellum may be implicated in the behavioral aspects of dementia.[57]

EVIDENCE FORM NEUROIMAGING STUDIES

Apart from the neuroanatomical and clinical evidence outlined previously, data in support of participation of the cerebellum in cognition has also come from a number of functional neuroimaging studies that have used techniques such as PET and functional magnetic resonance imaging (fMRI)[49] to evaluate cerebellar activation by a large number of cognitive tasks in which no movement is present.[49]

Petersen and colleagues[58,59] were among the first to report changes in cerebellar blood flow as measured by PET during a word-generation task. Activation of the right lateral cerebellum during word-generation tasks has been consistently reproduced in different studies.[60–62] Leiner and colleagues[34] interpreted simultaneous activation of the right lateral cerebellum and Broca area during word generation to be a reflection of accelerated transmission of signals between these two centers.

Based on observations in one study,[63] it has been suggested that the left frontal cortex, left thalamus, and right cerebellum may form a circuit in certain language tasks. Later, using PET activation study of naming-related brain activity, rearchers[64] also implicated the cerebellum in a left-lateralized network that also included the left-dominant frontotemporal areas that is recruited during naming of newly learned objects. Interestingly, the right dorsolateral prefrontal cortex and the right cerebellum have also been suggested to form part of the syntactic analysis network involved in prosodic segmentation and pitch processing.[65]

However, in contrast to the previously discussed findings, Ackermann and colleagues[66] reported that during continuous silent automatic speech (recitation of names of the months of the year), right cerebellar activation appeared to be related to the articulatory level of speech rather than cognitive operation.

Using fMRI, Desmond and Fiez[67] argued that the cerebellum is involved in basic cognitive processes, such as working memory, implicit and explicit learning and memory, and language. Additionally, they showed that cerebellum may play a role in the search for valid responses from semantic memory; a role that possibly forms the basis for improved performance evident with repeated exposure of the same items. Further studies have demonstrated cerebellar role in shifting attention[68,69] and planning time.[70,71]

THE CEREBELLAR COGNITIVE AFFECTIVE SYNDROME

To deal with the persistent uncertainty about cognitive dysfunction associated with cerebellar lesions, Schmahmann and Sherman[72] conveyed a study on 20 patients with heterogeneous diseases confined to the cerebellum prospectively over a span of 7 years and evaluated the nature and severity of the changes in neurologic and mental function. Although lesions of the anterior lobe of the cerebellum brought about only minor changes in executive and visual-spatial functions, behavioral changes were clinically prominent in patients with lesions involving the posterior lobe of the cerebellum and the vermis, and in some cases they were the most noticeable aspects of the presentation. Additionally, they showed that abnormalities of the posterior cerebellum, especially if bilateral, were particularly associated with these cognitive difficulties. They called this defined clinical entity the cerebellar cognitive affective syndrome (CCAS). The characteristics of this syndrome are summarized in **Box 2**.

The term CCAS has been coined by Schmahmann and Sherman[72] to describe a syndrome typically characterized by impaired executive function, spatial cognition,

---

Box 2
Cerebellar cognitive affective syndrome

Cerebellar cognitive affective syndrome (CCAS) is characterized by impairment in

- Executive function: planning, set-shifting, verbal fluency, abstract reasoning, working memory;
- Spatial cognition: visual spatial organization, and memory;
- Language deficits: agrammatism, aprosody, and mild anomia;
- Personality change: blunting of affect, disinhibited and inappropriate behavior.

Adapted from Schmahmann JD. Disorders of the cerebellum: ataxia, dysmetria of thought, and the cerebellar cognitive affective syndrome. J Neuropsychiatry Clin Neurosci 2004;16(3):371. Copyright permission obtained from American Psychiatric Press Inc.

---

linguistic processing, and affective regulation. This syndrome is suggestive of disturbance in the cerebellar modulation of neural circuits that link prefrontal, posterior parietal, superior temporal, and limbic cortices with the cerebellum, indicating cerebellum as an essential node in the distributed neural circuitry subserving higher-order behaviors. In their study, the net effect of CCAS in cognitive functioning was presented as a general decrease in overall intellectual function. Difficulties with motor control could not explain the impairment in cognitive and personality profile because in many cases the motor incoordination was mild. In those with bilateral or large unilateral infarctions in the posterior lobes in the territory of the posterior inferior cerebellar arteries, and in those with subacute onset of pancerebellar disorders, such as occurs with postinfectious cerebellitis, the neurobehavioral presentation was more pronounced and generalized. In patients with more slowly progressive cerebellar degenerations, in the recovery phase (3–4 months) after acute stroke and in those with restricted cerebellar pathology due to smaller strokes, the neurobehavioral presentation was less evident. The vermis was consistently involved in patients with pronounced affective presentations. Subsequent reports of adults with cerebellar strokes have replicated the clinical relevance of the CCAS. Malm and colleagues[73] demonstrated deficits in attention, working memory, visuospatial skills, and cognitive flexibility in patients with cerebellar strokes.

Cerebellar Cognitive Affective Syndrome in Children

Levisohn and colleagues[74] investigated the behavioral consequences of tumor resection in 19 children who underwent resection of cerebellar tumors and who did receive either cranial irradiation or chemotherapy. Impairments were noted in executive function, including planning and sequencing, perseveration, and difficulty in maintaining set as well as prominent deficits in visual-spatial function and verbal memory. In children with right hemispheric damage, impairment in language function, which included impaired verbal fluency and word-finding difficulties, were observed. Lesions of the vermis in particular were associated with dysregulation of affect. Similar study[75] showed impairment in verbal intelligence and complex language tasks following right cerebellar hemisphere lesions, and deficient nonverbal tasks and prosody after left cerebellar hemisphere lesions. In contrast to previous studies, cognitive and behavioral problems have been observed either in complete or partial cerebellar agenesis, as well as nonprogressive cerebellar ataxia, what used to be called ataxic cerebral palsy.[76] In those with more pronounced agenesis, the amount and spectrum of motor, cognitive, and psychiatric impairments were greater.[77] Impaired executive impairments included perseveration, disinhibition, and poor abstract reasoning, working memory and verbal fluency, spatial cognition was evident in these patients. Some children presented expressive language delay as the principal manifestation; in 2 instances the delay being so severe that they required instruction in sign language. Interestingly, in longitudinal follow-up, extensive rehabilitation enhanced motor, linguistic, and cognitive performance. Allin and colleagues[78] found that, in children born very preterm, the cerebellum is significantly smaller, and this is correlated with impaired executive and visual-spatial functions, as well as impaired language skills; all being the principal features of the CCAS.

DYSMETRIA OF THOUGHT THEORY

Consideration the neuroanatomical basis of cerebellum and its connections with the cerebral hemispheres and the brain stem can facilitate understanding of the main role of the cerebellum and provides evidence to develop the conceptual approach to the hypothesis known as "Dysmetria of Thought."[10,24,79] This theory was described by Schmahmann in 1991[10] for the first time when he proposed that " *in the same way that the cerebellum regulates the rate, force, rhythm, and accuracy of movements, so does it regulate the speed, capacity, consistency, and appropriateness of mental or cognitive processes.*"[10,23,80]

Within this hypothesis, the components of the CCAS, together with the ataxic motor disability of cerebellar disorders, are conceptualized. The universal cerebellar impairment manifests itself as ataxia, when the sensorimotor cerebellum is involved, and as the CCAS, when pathology is in the lateral hemisphere of the posterior cerebellum (involved in cognitive processing) or in the vermis (limbic cerebellum).[77]

In relation to cognition, the intact cerebellum has been described as capable of detecting, preventing, and correcting mismatches between the intended outcomes and the perceived outcomes of an organism's interaction with the environment (Schmahmann, 1998[72]). Analogous to the overshooting and undershooting of ataxic limb movements, "dysmetria of thought" has been hypothesized to involve either inadequate or exaggerated planning or misinterpretation of stimuli. The cerebellum, as a modulator of behavior, serves as an oscillation dampener that keeps function automatically around a homeostatic baseline and smooths out performance in all domains. The functional topography of cerebellum is classified in **Table 2**.[10,24,79]

Table 2
Postulated topography of function in the human cerebellum

Organization and Function	Topography
Anterior-posterior organization	
Sensorimotor	Anterior lobe (lobules I–V) "Secondary" representation (lobules VIII/IX)
Cognitive, affective	Neocerebellum (lobules VI, VII–vermis and hemispheres)
Medial-lateral organization	
Autonomic regulation, affect, emotionally important memory	Vermis and fastigial nucleus
Executive, visual-spatial, linguistic, learning and memory	Cerebellar hemispheres and dentate nucleus

Adapted from Schmahmann JD. Disorders of the cerebellum: ataxia, dysmetria of thought, and the cerebellar cognitive affective syndrome. J Neuropsychiatry Clin Neurosci 2004;16(3):375. Copyright permission obtained from American Psychiatric Press Inc.

CEREBELLUM AND LANGUAGE

Among the reciprocal connections linking the cerebellum with cerebral cortex, neuro-anatomical and functional neuroimaging studies have demonstrated inclusion of areas crucially involved in high-level linguistic functions[81] and cerebellar activation during a range of linguistic tasks that require no motor response.[58,81,82] Several theories have been proposed to explain the possible mechanisms involved in the occurrence of language disorders subsequent to cerebellar lesions.

First, it has been suggested that crossed cerebello-cerebrocortical diaschisis, which reflects a functional depression of supratentorial language areas due to reduced input to the cerebral cortex via cerebello-cerebrocortical pathways, may represent the neuro-pathological mechanism responsible for linguistic deficits associated with cerebellar pathology.[83,84] In support of this suggestion, functional neuroimaging studies have consistently revealed regions of contralateral cortical hypoperfusion in relation to the orientation of the cerebellar lesion.[85,86] According to the cerebello-cerebrocortical dia-schisis model, therefore, the cerebellum is not involved in the generation of language (which remains a supratentorial activity) but rather modulates language function.

A second theory is the timing hypothesis, which proposes that although the cere-bellum has no direct influence on linguistic processes, it plays an important role in the timing of linguistic functions represented on a supratentorial level.[85-87]

A third hypothesis proposes a direct cerebellar contribution via the topographically organized reciprocal connections with the cerebral cortex. According to this theory, the cerebellum does not have a mere modulatory role with regard to language, but is actively involved in the organization, construction, and execution of linguistic processes.

Overall findings provide evidence in support of a functional role for the cerebellum in language and suggest strong associations, first, between damage to the lateral cere-bellum, especially the right cerebellar hemisphere, and verbal fluency deficits, and second, between medial cerebellar lesions and the prevalence of motor deficits. These findings were later confirmed by Leggio and colleagues,[88] who also demon-strated that the observed deficits in verbal fluency were not the outcome of motor speech impairment.

One of the most interesting findings in patients with cerebellar lesions is agrammatic speech. This condition is characterized by simplification of the syntactic structures, shortening of sentences, and omission and substitution of grammatical mor-phemes.[12,86] Several other researchers have also reported agrammatism in association with right cerebellar lesions.[89-91] Silveri and colleagues[86] proposed that the cerebellum has an important role in the timing of linguistic functions represented at the level of the cerebral cortex. According to this "timing hypothesis," patients with cerebellar damage experience trouble in temporal modulation, which is required for several linguistic pro-cesses, of which phonological processing, sentence construction, and comprehension and application of syntactic rules can be named as examples. Therefore, language def-icits brought about by right cerebellar lesions are not in fact aphasic disorders but occur because some cognitive components (eg, working memory) that are involved in lan-guage processing are impaired. In addition, the role of cerebellum has been known in other aspects of linguistic domains and disorders, including verb generation, ataxic dysarthria, inner speech, apraxia of speech, agrammatism, transient cerebellar mutism syndrome, and cerebellar induced aphasia (**Table 3**).

DYSLEXIA

Although most children do master fluent reading skills, 5% to 10% of the population develops dyslexia. Apart from unexpected low reading achievement despite adequate

Table 3
Cerebellar involvement in speech and language functions

Linguistic Level	Function	Disturbance	Studies
Articulation	Muscular speech control	Ataxic dysarthria	Holmes,[21] 1917; Darley et al,[151] 1975; Ackermann et al,[152] 1992
Speech perception	Covert articulation Articulatory planning Discrimination of VOT and vowel duration	Speech apraxia	Fiez & Rachle,[153] 1997; Marien et al,[19] 2001; Ackermann et al,[126] 1997
Spelling	Visuospatial organization	Afferent dysgraphia	Silveri et al,[146,154] 1997;1999
Linguistic processing	Verbal associations	Lexical retrieval defects	Petersen et al,[58,59] 1988;1989
	Semantic associations	Lexical retrieval defects	Fiez et al,[155] 1992
	Phonological generation	Verbal fluency defects	Leggio et al,[156] 1995
	Expressive grammar	Expressive agrammatism	Silveri et al,[86] 1994; Zettin et al,[89] 1997
	Syntactic knowledge	Agrammatism	Marien et al,[157,158] 1996; 2000; Riva,[160] 1998; Gasparini et al,[90] 1999; Fabbro et al,[159] 2000; Riva and Giorgi,[75] 2000
	Language dynamics	Dynamic aphasia	Marien et al,[157,158]1996; 2000; Riva,[160] 1998; Gasparini et al,[90] 1999; Fabbro et al,[159] 2000; Riva and Giorgi,[75] 2000

Adapted from Marien P, Engelborghs S, De Deyn PP. Cerebellar neurocognition: a new avenue. Acta Neurol Belg 2001;101(2):97. Copyright permission obtained from Belgian Neurologic Society, Belgium.

intelligence, education, and motivation,[92] some dyslexic individuals also have impairments in attention, short-term memory, sequencing (letters, word sounds, and motor acts), eye movements, and balance, and suffer from general clumsiness. The presence of "cerebellar" motor and fluency symptoms has led to the proposal that cerebellar dysfunction contributes to the etiology of dyslexia. In support of the proposal, functional imaging studies suggest that the cerebellum is part of the neural network supporting reading in typically developing readers, and reading difficulties have been reported in patients with cerebellar damage. Compared with good readers, differences in both cerebellar asymmetry and gray matter volume are two of the most consistent structural brain findings in dyslexic individuals. Furthermore, cerebellar functional activation patterns during reading and motor learning can differ in dyslexic readers. Concerning behavior, some children and adults with dyslexia show poorer performance in cerebellar motor tasks, including eye movement control, postural stability, and implicit motor learning. It is important to note that many dyslexic individuals do not manifest cerebellar signs, many cerebellar patients do not have reading problems, and differences in dyslexic brains are found throughout the whole reading network, and are not isolated to the cerebellum. Therefore, cerebellar dysfunction is probably not the underlying cause of dyslexia, but rather a more fundamental neurodevelopmental abnormality that leads to differences throughout the reading network.

Fernandez and colleagues[93] suggested that cerebellar deficits and subsequent impairment in procedural learning may contribute to both motor difficulties and reading impairment in dyslexia. Another study[94] postulated that dyslexia results from a phonological deficit, whereas another hypothesized[95] that these phonological problems stem from more fundamental speech perception problems. A plausible anatomic counterpart for the observed functional disconnection in dyslexic readers could be deficits seen in white matter tract, because these tracts guarantee an efficient signal transmission between distant cortical regions.

To explore the anatomic basis of anomalous connections underlying reading impairments, Vandermosten and colleagues[96] conveyed a study by diffusion tensor imaging (DTI) and tracked neural pathways and linked them to reading-related skills. They argued that adults with dyslexia show reduced white matter integrity in the left arcuate fasciculus, particularly in the section that directly links the Wernicke to the Broca area, and suggested that the integrity of white matter in the left arcuate fasciculus, and to a certain extent also in the left arcuate fasciculus-posterior, is related to phonological processes, whereas the integrity of white matter in the left inferior fronto-occipital fasciculus is related to orthographic processes. One theory explaining the pathophysiology of dyslexia is that cerebellar abnormalities prevent normal eye movements and interfere with the acquisition of lexical information.[78] This theory has been further supported by the study of Nicolson and colleagues,[97] which used brain PET scan.

MEMORY AND LEARNING

Experimental and clinical studies have demonstrated that the cerebellum is involved in many different aspects of memory, such as procedural and associative learning, classical conditioning of the eye blink response, sequential learning (motor skill learning), and conceptual stimulus response tasks (paired associate learning).[98,99] Apart from being involved in conditioned responses, it has been shown that the cerebellum plays an essential role in the acquisition of complex motor sequences. Marr[100] first identified cerebellar involvement in motor learning. Brindley[101] proposed that the acquisition of skilled performance is guided only by higher cerebral control in the initial learning phase. He speculated that once the movement is practiced, it is given over to the cerebellum for the execution of automatic motor control.

Implicit and Procedural Memory

Clinical and neuroimaging studies on patients with cerebellar damage and on healthy subjects have confirmed that the cerebellum (together with the prefrontal and subcortical structures) is involved in procedural and associative learning.[102–105] That cerebellar patients show impairment in eye-blink conditioning for the eye ipsilateral to their cerebellar lesion supports the link between the cerebellum and eye-blink classical conditioning (unconscious) learning in humans.[106–108] Additionally, elderly participants manifest slower acquisition rates, which is correlated with a decrease in Purkinje cell volume.[109] Other forms of implicit learning may be mediated by the cerebellum, not because they have temporal properties but because many forms of unconscious knowledge are procedural and are rooted in motor representations.

The role of the cerebellum in procedural learning is well established,[103] and it may be the case that the cerebellum is recruited in other forms of implicit learning as well.

Classical conditioning of the eye-blink response (motor adaptation learning), sequential learning (motor skill learning), and conceptual stimulus response tasks (paired associate learning) have been used in many experimental studies to demonstrate the role of the cerebellum in associative learning and procedural learning tasks and habits.[98,99]

Declarative Memory, Explicit Memory

Interestingly, cerebellum also contributes to declarative memory. Deficits in verbal memory have been observed in patients with acute cerebellar infarcts.[74,110] Additionally, survivors of acute cerebellar lesions have manifested deficits in visual memory in neuropsychological testing.[72,111]

Long-Term Memory

In a study, patients without dementia with cerebellar neurodegenerative disorders manifested impairment in free delayed recall but not in recognition memory or in implicit learning. This resembles the pattern found in patients with amnesia with prefrontal lesions and contrasts with the pattern found in patients with amnesia with temporal lobe lesions; in the latter group, both recall and recognition are deficient.[112]

Verbal Working Memory

Verbal working memory system is divided in 2 separate components: (1) the phonological short-term memory subserves the retention of verbal information for a brief period of time, which allows verbal repetition and sentence comprehension, implying a crucial importance in language learning; and (2) the rehearsal system, which recirculates stored verbal information to prevent rapid decay,[112] in which the right cerebellar hemisphere is involved as well. Both neuroimaging and neuropsychological studies have shown the role of cerebellum in working memory.[86]

VISUOSPATIAL PROCESSING

Cerebellum is engaged in visuospatial processing and visuospatial attention. In a patient with chronic phenytoin intoxication, Botez and colleagues[113] encountered reversible cerebellar ataxia and mild frontal-like and parietal-like symptoms. They speculated that the possible anatomo-physiological substrate for these symptoms was the dysfunction of cerebello-frontal and cerebello-parietal associative loops. Many of the subsequent studies in the patients with focal and neurodegenerative disorders of the cerebellum (especially olivopontocerebellar ataxia, Friedreich ataxia, and cerebellar cortical atrophy), have explored the role of the cerebellum in visuospatial procedures and shown the link between right hemisphere deficits of visuospatial organization to left cerebellar hemisphere damage.[50,114,115] Even though visuospatial deficits also have been observed in a heterogeneous group of patients with cerebellar disorders,[111,115,116] standard neuropsychological tests of visuospatial ability may not provide strong support in the cerebellum's role in this cognitive domain.[117,118] One study has suggested[119] that the initial impairment was restricted to patients with atrophy extending into the brainstem, whereas another[120] has shown that cerebellar patients would have difficulty in performing any visual task requiring precise timing.

CEREBELLUM AND INTELLIGENCE QUOTIENT

Only a few studies have emphasized the global intellectual capacity of the patients with cerebellar damage with conflicting results.[121] Frangou and colleagues[122] addressed the question of whether the relationship between general intellectual quotient (IQ) and gray matter morphometry reflects differential involvement of particular brain areas. According to this study, there were 7 Gy matter regions that were positively correlated with IQ, including (1) cerebellum and (2) thalamus (both bilaterally), (3) inferior frontal cortex, including middle and superior frontal gyri bilaterally, (4) anterior cingulate gyrus, (5) medial frontal gyrus, (6) posterior cingulate, and (7) paracentral lobule and precuneus (**Fig. 2**).

PATHOLOGIC LAUGHTER AND CRYING

In patients with pathologic laughter and crying (PLC), the relatively uncontrollable episodes of laughter, crying, or both occur either without an apparent triggering stimulus or after a stimulus that would not have led the subject to laugh or cry before the onset of the condition. Rather than being a primary disturbance of feelings, PLC is a disorder of emotional expression, and is thus distinct from mood disorders in which laughter and crying are associated with feelings of happiness or sadness. It has been hypothesized that PLC is caused by a loss of voluntary inhibition of a presumed center for laughter and crying located in the upper brainstem[123]; the loss having been brought about by lesions of the voluntary paths from the motor areas of the cerebral cortex or by any state in which these areas exercise imperfect control over the laughter and crying center. This interpretation is identified in the literature as the "disinhibition" or "release phenomenon" hypothesis.

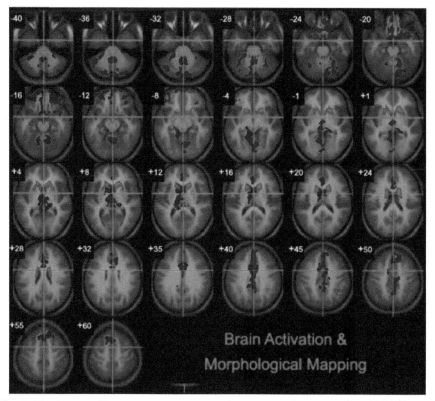

Fig. 2. Distribution of brain regions positively (*blue*) and negatively (*red*) correlated with IQ. (Cerebellar involvement is shown in the upper images.) (*Adapted from* Frangou S, Chitins X, Williams SC. Mapping IQ and gray matter density in healthy young people. Neuroimage 2004;23(3):803; with permission. Copyright permission obtained from NeuroImage/Elsevier.)

Parvizi and colleagues[124] proposed an alternative hypothesis for this phenomena based on the new knowledge on the neurobiology of emotion and the neuroanatomical findings in a case of PLC, indicating that the critical PLC lesions occur in the cerebro-ponto-cerebellar pathways, and consequently the cerebellar structures that serve to automatically adjust the execution of laughter or crying to the cognitive and situational context of a potential stimulus operate based on incomplete information about that context, resulting in inadequate and even chaotic behavior.

TIMING AND TEMPORAL SEQUENCING IMPAIRMENT

Perception of time is one of the cognitive domains in which the role of cerebellum has been studied[87,125] indicating the cerebellum's role as a general timing device in perception and action. It has been demonstrated that, in patients with cerebellar atrophy, both motor programming and perceptual timing show impairment. It seems the cerebellum acts as an "internal clock" during any condition requiring temporal computations. Consonant with this view are the results of clinical studies that reveal that patients with cerebellar lesions show impaired judgment in the relative duration of time intervals or the velocity of moving visual stimuli,[87,120,125] as well as severe distortions in the discrimination of onset time of voice and vowel durations.[126] Moreover, it has been shown that temporal processing deficits observed in these patients are distinct from those seen in frontal lobe lesion cases. Although cerebellar patients are impaired at discriminating intervals both in the 400 milliseconds and 4 seconds ranges, frontal patients are impaired only at the latter,[127] which suggests that frontal impairment may be related to increased working memory demands that arise for the longer interval.[128] It also has been postulated that *"lesions of the prefrontal cortex would hypothetically affect the activation of plans and actions, subcortical structures might allow for their automatic execution, and the cerebellum would ensure their correct sequencing and timing."*[129]

MUSIC

Musicians are skilled in performing complex physical and mental operations, such as translation of visually presented musical symbols into complex, sequential finger movements, improvisation, memorization of long musical phrases, and identification of tones without the use of a reference tone. To play a musical instrument, it is typically required to simultaneously combine multimodal sensory and motor information with multimodal sensory feedback mechanisms to monitor performance.[130] Hutchinson and colleagues[131] investigated whether professional keyboard players, who learn specialized motor skills early in life and practice them intensely throughout, have larger cerebellar volumes than corresponding nonmusicians. Their studies on 120 subjects using magnetic resonance images showed that the male musicians had significantly greater cerebellar volumes and that there was a positive correlation between relative cerebellar volume and lifelong intensity of practice. The finding represents structural adaptation to long-term motor and cognitive functional demands in the human cerebellum.

BALLET DANCE

Integration of rhythm, spatial pattern, synchronization to external stimuli, and coordination of the whole body are involved in many natural, complex sensorimotor activities. Such activities include old evolutionary adaptations, such as hunting, fighting, and playing, as well as more recent ones, such as group physical labor, sport, marching, musical performance, and dance. Dance is a universal human behavior, one associated with group rituals.[132,133] Although depictions of it are found in cave arts from more than 20,000 years ago,[134] dance may be much more ancient than that. Dance may in fact be as old as the human capacities for bipedal walking and running, which date back 2 to 5 million years.[135,136]

One of the principal properties of dance is that body movements are organized into spatial patterns and synchronization of movements with timekeepers, such as musical beats; a capacity that is apparently specific to humans. Indeed, it is striking how human bodies can spontaneously move to a musical beat. Almost all dancing is done to musical rhythms, a feature that permits temporal synchronization among dancers. Neuroimaging studies have examined some components of the complex actions involved in such properties as the entrainment of movement to musical beat and spatial positioning of bodily movement.

Dance moves generally mirror the ordered arrangement of strong and weak beats found in musical rhythm patterns. In waltz music, for example, the first beat is stressed and the second and third beats are weaker; likewise in waltz movements, the first step is the broadest and most forceful, the second and third steps being shorter and weaker. Thus, the relationship of dance to music not only involves synchronization in time but a spatial element related to equating hierarchies in the motor pattern with those in the musical rhythm.

Therefore dance, like numerous natural, complex sensorimotor activities (eg, sport, group physical labor, and musical performance), requires the integration of spatial pattern, rhythm, synchronization to external stimuli, and whole-body coordination. Researchers have observed, using brain PET, greater variety and number of anterior cerebellar activations during the more unfamiliar conditions, suggesting a role in adjusting fine, complex sensorimotor coordination to relatively novel entrainment signals.[137–139]

Another aspect of brain mechanisms manifest in dancing is adaptation to repeated whole-body rotations; in ballet, for example, training is known to reduce vestibular responses. Nigmatullina and colleagues[140] showed that in dancers' vestibular cerebellum, a selective gray matter reduction was evident in correlation with ballet experience. They suggested that this relatively attenuated white matter cortical network that mediates vestibular perception may have resulted from vestibular cerebellar gating of ascending vestibular signals, then cerebellar gating may allow dancers to perform pirouettes at ease with little dizziness.

MANAGEMENT AND TREATMENT

Patients with cerebellar dysfunction may struggle with restrictions in cognitive ability and flexibility, slowed reaction times, and impaired attentional modulation, as well as less ability to do "multitasking" automatically.[141] Impairment in these important aspects of higher-order behavior have an adverse impact on quality of life and employment and need to be recognized by both the medical profession and the patients and their families. By recognition of cerebellar role in cognitive function,[77] patients with cerebellar disorders could potentially benefit from optimal therapeutic and novel cognitive rehabilitation strategies. Considering the regulatory role of cerebellum in cognition, it is clinically sensible to be alert for signs of cognitive, affective, and behavioral disturbance in neuropsychological assessment before planning the treatment and rehabilitation of patients with cerebellar illness.

It seems that there is still a long way to recognition of definitive treatment approaches for cognitive dysfunctions in patients with cerebellar disorders. The most beneficial approach for now would be to apply cognitive behavioral therapies to help patients bring actions to conscious awareness and focus on one task at a time. Also, in the management plan, appropriate symptomatic treatment and physical rehabilitation strategies influencing motor control, as well as mood and cognition and neuropsychiatric diagnosis and care, should be included.[142]

SUMMARY

The functional role of the cerebellum has been traditionally defined as a mere coordinator of automatic and somatic motor functions. And, in fact, the cerebellar role in motor functioning has overshadowed the development of insights in the causal relationship between cerebellar pathology and a variety of neurocognitive deficits. However, during the past decades a substantial modification of the traditional view of the cerebellum has been brought about through collaborations across contemporary neuroscience disciplines.

In the late 1970s and early 1980s, new neuroimaging techniques resulted in increased interest in the nonmotor functions of the cerebellum. Functional neuroimaging studies demonstrated that the cerebellum is activated, even in the complete absence of any motor activity, while performing various cognitive and linguistic tasks. In a similar way, at the end of the 1980s, the long-held view that the cerebellum participates solely in motor speech started to change. Neuro-anatomical connections that were newly traced between the lateral part of the right cerebellum and the frontal areas of the language dominant hemisphere (Brodmann areas 6, 44, and 45) were suggestive of the possibility that, beyond the pure motor processes of articulation and phonation, cerebellar signals to these areas contribute to linguistic skills. Soon thereafter, neuroimaging and clinical studies provided evidence in support of the role of the cerebellum in modulating the dynamics of language and even led to the concept of aphasia induced by cerebellar impairment.

Based on neural evidence and information processing theory,[16] it has been shown that the phylogenetically newest part of the cerebellum (particularly the lateral portions of the cerebellar hemispheres and dentate nuclei) might interact with the frontal association cortex to make skilled manipulation of information or ideas possible. Further research[28] proposed that, during the course of hominid evolution, the cerebellum has undergone functionally significant changes, increasing both in size and in the number of reciprocal connections with various regions of the cerebral cortex.[46] Circuitry within the cerebellum shaped by natural selection may be well suited to perform cognitive tasks in need of similar neural constructs. Additionally, the increase in size and the expansion of connections to the cerebral hemispheres may have resulted in the cognitive operations of the cerebellum. Moreover, cognitive operations are added to the already present motor functions of cerebellum rather than replacing them.[19] Several studies have provided evidence of the modulatory role of the cerebellum through reciprocal cerebello-cerebral pathways in cognitive domains. Hence, the concept of cerebellar neurocognition has evolved to an exciting new multifaceted area of contemporary neuroscientific investigation. Now, it might be crucial to address the possibility of cerebellar disease in patients manifesting changes in higher cognitive or behavioral domains. From a research perspective, the use of the cerebellum as a control or reference region in functional neuroimaging studies may need to be reconsidered, or at least adopted cautiously in subjects with psychiatric disturbances. Furthermore, it is important for imaging studies of mood, behavior, and cognitive disorders to take the cerebellum into account. Clearly, much more is yet to be learned about the cerebellum's role in both healthy individuals and patient populations.

ACKNOWLEDGMENTS

The author is grateful to Dr Shahrzad Irannejad for her valuable comments and Parisa Azadfar for her timely assistance in organizing the literature.

REFERENCES

1. Holmes G. A form of familial degeneration of the cerebellum. Brain 1907;30:23.
2. Roses AD, Lutz MW, Amrine-Madsen H, et al. A TOMM40 variable-length polymorphism predicts the age of late-onset Alzheimer's disease. Pharmacogenomics J 2010;10(5):375–84.
3. Reznik-Wolf H, Treves TA, Davidson M, et al. A novel mutation of presenilin 1 in familial Alzheimer's disease in Israel detected by denaturing gradient gel electrophoresis. Hum Genet 1996;98(6):700–2.
4. Combettes M. Absence compléte du cervelet, des pédoncules postérieurs et de la protubérance cérébrale chez une jeune fille morte dans sa onziéme anneé. Bull Soc Anat Paris 1831;5:10.
5. Andral G. 4th edition. Clinique médicale, vol. 5. Paris (France): Fortin, Masson et Cie; 1848.
6. Knoepfel HK, Macken J. Le syndrome psycho-organique dans les hérédo-ataxies. J Belge Neurol Psychiatr 1947;47:10.
7. Dow RS, Moruzzi G. The physiology and pathology of the cerebellum. Minneapolis (MN): University of Minnesota Press; 1958.
8. Watson PJ. Nonmotor functions of the cerebellum. Psychol Bull 1978;85:24.
9. Heath RG, Franklin DE, Shraberg D. Gross pathology of the cerebellum in patients diagnosed and treated as functional psychiatric disorders. J Nerv Ment Dis 1979;167(10):585–92.
10. Schmahmann JD. An emerging concept. The cerebellar contribution to higher function. Arch Neurol 1991;48(11):1178–87.
11. Schmahmann JD. Rediscovery of an early concept. Int Rev Neurobiol 1997;41:23.
12. Silveri MC, Misciagna S. Language, memory, and the cerebellum. J Neurol 2000;13(2):129–43.
13. Snider RS, Maiti A. Cerebellar contributions to the Papez circuit. J Neurosci Res 1976;2(2):133–46.
14. Dow RS. Some novel concepts of cerebellar physiology. Mt Sinai J Med 1974; 41(1):103–19.
15. Heath RG. Modulation of emotion with a brain pacemamer. Treatment for intractable psychiatric illness. J Nerv Ment Dis 1977;165(5):300–17.
16. Leiner HC, Leiner AL, Dow RS. Does the cerebellum contribute to mental skills? Behav Neurosci 1986;100(4):443–54.
17. Schmahmann JD, Pandya DN. Anatomical investigation of projections to the basis pontis from posterior parietal association cortices in rhesus monkey. J Comp Neurol 1989;289(1):53–73.
18. Middleton FA, Strick PL. Anatomical evidence for cerebellar and basal ganglia involvement in higher cognitive function. Science 1994;266(5184):458–61.
19. Marien P, Engelborghs S, De Deyn PP. Cerebellar neurocognition: a new avenue. Acta Neurol Belg 2001;101(2):96–109.
20. Babinski J. Exposé des travaux scientifiques. Paris: Masson; 1913.
21. Holmes G. The symptoms of acute cerebellar injuries due to gunshot injuries. Brain Dev 1917;40:34.
22. Holmes G. The Croonian lectures on the clinical symptoms of cerebellar disease and their interpretation. Lancet 1922;1(8):1177–82.

23. Schmahmann JD. Dysmetria of thought: correlations and conundrums in the relationship between the cerebellum, learning, and cognitive processing. Behav Brain Sci 1996;19(03):472–3.
24. Schmahmann JD. The role of the cerebellum in affect and psychosis. J Neurol 2000;13(2):189–214.
25. Nieuwenhuys R. Comparative anatomy of the cerebellum. Prog Brain Res 1967; 25:1–93.
26. Larsell O, Jansen J. Comparative anatomy and histology of the cerebellum: from myxinoids through birds. 1st edition. Minneapolis (MN): University of Minnesota Press; 1967.
27. Matano S, Baron G, Stephan H, et al. Volume comparisons in the cerebellar complex of primates. II. Cerebellar nuclei. Folia Primatol (Basel) 1985;44(3–4):182–203.
28. Leiner HC, Leiner AL, Dow RS. Cognitive and language functions of the human cerebellum. Trends Neurosci 1993;16(11):444–7.
29. Balsters JH, Cussans E, Diedrichsen J, et al. Evolution of the cerebellar cortex: the selective expansion of prefrontal-projecting cerebellar lobules. Neuroimage 2010;49(3):2045–52.
30. Middleton FA, Strick PL. Basal ganglia and cerebellar loops: motor and cognitive circuits. Brain Res Brain Res Rev 2000;31(2–3):236–50.
31. Middleton FA, Strick PL. Cerebellar projections to the prefrontal cortex of the primate. J Neurosci 2001;21(2):700–12.
32. Ramnani N. The primate cortico-cerebellar system: anatomy and function. Nature reviews. Neuroscience 2006;7(7):511–22.
33. Leiner HC, Leiner AL, Dow RS. Cerebro-cerebellar learning loops in apes and humans. Ital J Neurol Sci 1987;8(5):425–36.
34. Leiner HC, Leiner AL, Dow RS. Reappraising the cerebellum: what does the hindbrain contribute to the forebrain? Behav Neurosci 1989;103(5):998–1008.
35. Leiner HC, Leiner AL, Dow RS. The human cerebro-cerebellar system: its computing, cognitive, and language skills. Behav Brain Res 1991;44(2):113–28.
36. Kelly RM, Strick PL. Cerebellar loops with motor cortex and prefrontal cortex of a nonhuman primate. J Neurosci 2003;23(23):8432–44.
37. Justus TC, Ivry RB. The cognitive neuropsychology of the cerebellum. Int Rev Psychiatry 2001;13(4):276–82.
38. Bolk L. Das Cerebellum der Säugetiere. Jena (Thuringia): Fiches; 1906.
39. Dolan RJ. A cognitive affective role for the cerebellum. Brain 1998;121(Pt 4):545–6.
40. Middleton FA, Strick PL. Cerebellar output channels. Int Rev Neurobiol 1997;41: 61–82.
41. Voogd J, Glickstein M. The anatomy of the cerebellum. Trends Neurosci 1998; 21(9):370–5.
42. Andrezik JA, Dormer KJ, Foreman RD, et al. Fastigial nucleus projections to the brain stem in beagles: pathways for autonomic regulation. Neuroscience 1984; 11(2):497–507.
43. Haines DE, Dietrichs E. An HRP study of hypothalamo-cerebellar and cerebello-hypothalamic connections in squirrel monkey (*Saimiri sciureus*). J Comp Neurol 1984;229(4):559–75.
44. Heath RG. Fastigial nucleus connections to the septal region in monkey and cat: a demonstration with evoked potentials of a bilateral pathway. Biol Psychiatry 1973;6(2):193–6.
45. Schmahmann JD, Pandya DN. Anatomic organization of the basilar pontine projections from prefrontal cortices in rhesus monkey. J Neurosci 1997;17(1): 438–58.

46. Schmahmann JD, Pandya DN. The cerebrocerebellar system. Int Rev Neurobiol 1997;41:31–60.
47. Murdoch BE. The cerebellum and language: historical perspective and review. Cortex 2010;46(7):858–68.
48. Burk K. Cognition in hereditary ataxia. Cerebellum 2007;6(3):280–6.
49. Roy MK, Dutt A. The cerebellum in cognitive function. Neurosciences Today 2003;VII(1):7.
50. Botez MI, Leveille J, Lambert R, et al. Single photon emission computed tomography (SPECT) in cerebellar disease: cerebello-cerebral diaschisis. Eur Neurol 1991;31(6):405–12.
51. Hall TC, Miller AK, Corsellis JA. Variations in the human Purkinje cell population according to age and sex. Neuropathol Appl Neurobiol 1975;1(3):267–92.
52. Raz N, Torres IJ, Spencer WD, et al. Age-related regional differences in cerebellar vermis observed in vivo. Arch Neurol 1992;49(4):412–6.
53. Atkinson RM, Ganzini L. Substance abuse. In: Coffey CE, Cummings J, editors. The American psychiatric press textbook of geriatric neuropsychiatry. Washington, DC: American Psychiatric Press; 1994. p. 297–321.
54. Fukutani Y, Cairns NJ, Rossor MN, et al. Purkinje cell loss and astrocytosis in the cerebellum in familial and sporadic Alzheimer's disease. Neurosci Lett 1996; 214(1):33–6.
55. Ishii K, Sasaki M, Kitagaki H, et al. Reduction of cerebellar glucose metabolism in advanced Alzheimer's disease. J Nucl Med 1997;38(6):925–8.
56. Barclay LL, Brady PA. Cerebellar atrophy as a CT marker for mixed dementia. Biol Psychiatry 1992;31(5):520–4.
57. Gutzmann H, Kuhl KP. Emotion control and cerebellar atrophy in senile dementia. Arch Gerontol Geriatr 1987;6(1):61–71.
58. Petersen SE, Fox PT, Posner MI, et al. Positron emission tomographic studies of the cortical anatomy of single-word processing. Nature 1988;331(6157):585–9.
59. Petersen SE, Fox PT, Posner MI, et al. Positron emission tomographic studies of the processing of singe words. J Cogn Neurosci 1989;1(2):153–70.
60. Grabowski TJ, Frank RJ, Brown CK, et al. Reliability of PET activation across statistical methods, subject groups, and sample sizes. Hum Brain Mapp 1996;4(1): 23–46.
61. Martin A, Haxby JV, Lalonde FM, et al. Discrete cortical regions associated with knowledge of color and knowledge of action. Science 1995;270(5233):102–5.
62. Raichle ME, Fiez JA, Videen TO, et al. Practice-related changes in human brain functional anatomy during nonmotor learning. Cereb Cortex 1994;4(1):8–26.
63. Shulman GL, Corbetta M, Buckner RL, et al. Common blood flow changes across visual tasks: I. Increases in subcortical structures and cerebellum but not in nonvisual cortex. J Cogn Neurosci 1997;9(5):624–47.
64. Gronholm P, Rinne JO, Vorobyev V, et al. Naming of newly learned objects: a PET activation study. Brain Res Cogn Brain Res 2005;25(1):359–71.
65. Strelnikov KN, Vorobyev VA, Chernigovskaya TV, et al. Prosodic clues to syntactic processing—a PET and ERP study. Neuroimage 2006;29(4):1127–34.
66. Ackermann H, Wildgruber D, Daum I, et al. Does the cerebellum contribute to cognitive aspects of speech production? A functional magnetic resonance imaging (fMRI) study in humans. Neurosci Lett 1998;247(2–3):187–90.
67. Desmond JE, Fiez JA. Neuroimaging studies of the cerebellum: language, learning and memory. Trends Cogn Sci 1998;2(9):355–62.
68. Akshoomoff NA, Courchesne E. A new role for the cerebellum in cognitive operations. Behav Neurosci 1992;106(5):731–8.

69. Townsend J, Courchesne E, Covington J, et al. Spatial attention deficits in pa-
    tients with acquired or developmental cerebellar abnormality. J Neurosci
    1999;19(13):5632–43.
70. Grafman J, Litvan I, Massaquoi S, et al. Cognitive planning deficit in patients
    with cerebellar atrophy. Neurology 1992;42(8):1493–6.
71. Kim SG, Ugurbil K, Strick PL. Activation of a cerebellar output nucleus during
    cognitive processing. Science 1994;265(5174):949–51.
72. Schmahmann JD, Sherman JC. The cerebellar cognitive affective syndrome.
    Brain 1998;121(Pt 4):561–79.
73. Malm J, Kristensen B, Karlsson T, et al. Cognitive impairment in young adults
    with infratentorial infarcts. Neurology 1998;51(2):433–40.
74. Levisohn L, Cronin-Golomb A, Schmahmann JD. Neuropsychological conse-
    quences of cerebellar tumour resection in children: cerebellar cognitive affec-
    tive syndrome in a paediatric population. Brain 2000;123(Pt 5):1041–50.
75. Riva D, Giorgi C. The cerebellum contributes to higher functions during devel-
    opment: evidence from a series of children surgically treated for posterior fossa
    tumours. Brain 2000;123(Pt 5):1051–61.
76. Glickstein M. Cerebellar agenesis. Brain 1994;117(Pt 5):1209–12.
77. Schmahmann JD. Disorders of the cerebellum: ataxia, dysmetria of thought, and
    the cerebellar cognitive affective syndrome. J Nerv Ment Dis 2004;16(3):367–78.
78. Allin M, Matsumoto H, Santhouse AM, et al. Cognitive and motor function and the
    size of the cerebellum in adolescents born very pre-term. Brain 2001;124(Pt 1):
    60–6.
79. Schmahmann JD. From movement to thought: anatomic substrates of the cere-
    bellar contribution to cognitive processing. Hum Brain Mapp 1996;4(3):174–98.
80. Gottwald B, Wilde B, Mihajlovic Z, et al. Evidence for distinct cognitive deficits after
    focal cerebellar lesions. J Neurol Neurosurg Psychiatry 2004;75(11):1524–31.
81. Middleton FA, Strick PL. Basal ganglia output and cognition: evidence from
    anatomical, behavioral, and clinical studies. Brain Cogn 2000;42(2):183–200.
82. Murdoch BE, Whelan BM. Language disorders subsequent to left cerebellar le-
    sions: a case for bilateral cerebellar involvement in language? Folia Phoniatr
    Logop 2007;59(4):184–9.
83. Broich K, Hartmann A, Biersack HJ, et al. Crossed cerebello-cerebral diaschisis
    in a patient with cerebellar infarction. Neurosci Lett 1987;83(1–2):7–12.
84. Marien P, Engelborghs S, Fabbro F, et al. The lateralized linguistic cerebellum: a
    review and a new hypothesis. Brain Lang 2001;79(3):580–600.
85. Gomez Beldarrain M, Garcia-Monco JC, Quintana JM, et al. Diaschisis and neu-
    ropsychological performance after cerebellar stroke. Eur Neurol 1997;37(2):82–9.
86. Silveri MC, Leggio MG, Molinari M. The cerebellum contributes to linguistic pro-
    duction: a case of agrammatic speech following a right cerebellar lesion.
    Neurology 1994;44(11):2047–50.
87. Keele SW, Ivry R. Does the cerebellum provide a common computation for
    diverse tasks? A timing hypothesis. Ann N Y Acad Sci 1990;608:179–207 [dis-
    cussion: 207–11].
88. Leggio MG, Silveri MC, Petrosini L, et al. Phonological grouping is specifically
    affected in cerebellar patients: a verbal fluency study. J Neurol Neurosurg Psy-
    chiatry 2000;69(1):102–6.
89. Zettin M, Cappa SF, D'Amico A, et al. Agrammatic speech production after a
    right cerebellar haemorrhage. Neurocase 1997;3(5):375–80.
90. Gasparini M, Piero VD, Ciccarelli O, et al. Linguistic impairment after right cere-
    bellar stroke: a case report. Eur J Neurol 1999;6(3):353–6.

91. Justus T. The cerebellum and English grammatical morphology: evidence from production, comprehension, and grammaticality judgments. J Cogn Neurosci 2004;16(7):1115–30.
92. Shaywitz SE. Dyslexia. N Engl J Med 1998;338(5):307–12.
93. Fernandez VG, Stuebing K, Juranek J, et al. Volumetric analysis of regional variability in the cerebellum of children with dyslexia. Cerebellum 2013;12(6):906–15.
94. Snowling MJ. Dyslexia. 2nd edition. Oxford (England): Blackwell; 2000.
95. Boets B, Vandermosten M, Poelmans H, et al. Preschool impairments in auditory processing and speech perception uniquely predict future reading problems. Res Dev Disabil 2011;32(2):560–70.
96. Vandermosten M, Boets B, Luts H, et al. Impairments in speech and nonspeech sound categorization in children with dyslexia are driven by temporal processing difficulties. Res Dev Disabil 2011;32(2):593–603.
97. Nicolson RI, Fawcett AJ, Dean P. Developmental dyslexia: the cerebellar deficit hypothesis. Trends Neurosci 2001;24(9):508–11.
98. McCormick DA, Lavond DG, Clark GA, et al. The engram found? Role of the cerebellum in classical conditioning of nictitating membrane and eyelid responses. Bull Psychon Soc 1981;18(3):103–5.
99. Thompson RF, Bao S, Chen L, et al. Associative learning. Int Rev Neurobiol 1997;41:151–89.
100. Marr D. A theory of cerebellar cortex. J Physiol 1969;202(2):437–70.
101. Brindley G. The use made by the cerebellum of the information that it receives from sense organs. IBRO Bull 1964;3(3):80.
102. Grafton S, Hazeltine E, Ivry R. Localization of independent cortical systems in human motor learning. J Cogn Neurosci 1995;7:497–510.
103. Molinari M, Leggio MG, Solida A, et al. Cerebellum and procedural learning: evidence from focal cerebellar lesions. Brain 1997;120(Pt 10):1753–62.
104. Pascual-Leone A, Grafman J, Clark K, et al. Procedural learning in Parkinson's disease and cerebellar degeneration. Ann Neurol 1993;34(4):594–602.
105. Jenkins IH, Brooks DJ, Nixon PD, et al. Motor sequence learning: a study with positron emission tomography. J Neurosci 1994;14(6):3775–90.
106. Topka H, Valls-Solé J, Massaquoi SG, et al. Deficit in classical conditioning in patients with cerebellar degeneration. Brain 1993;116(4):961–9.
107. Woodruff-Pak DS, Papka M, Ivry RB. Cerebellar involvement in eyeblink classical conditioning in humans. Neuropsychology 1996;10(4):443.
108. Daum I, Schugens MM, Ackermann H, et al. Classical conditioning after cerebellar lesions in humans. Behav Neurosci 1993;107(5):748.
109. Woodruff-Pak DS, Cronholm JF, Sheffield JB. Purkinje cell number related to rate of classical conditioning. Neuroreport 1990;1(2):165–8.
110. Chafetz MD, Friedman AL, Kevorkian CG, et al. The cerebellum and cognitive function: implications for rehabilitation. Arch Phys Med Rehabil 1996;77(12):1303–8.
111. Ciesielski KT, Yanofsky R, Ludwig RN, et al. Hypoplasia of the cerebellar vermis and cognitive deficits in survivors of childhood leukemia. Arch Neurol 1994;51(10):985–93.
112. Salame P, Baddeley A. Disruption of short-term memory by unattended speech: implications for the structure of working memory. J Verbal Learning Verbal Behav 1982;21(2):150–64.
113. Botez MI, Gravel J, Attig E, et al. Reversible chronic cerebellar ataxia after phenytoin intoxication: possible role of cerebellum in cognitive thought. Neurology 1985;35(8):1152–7.

114. Botez-Marquard T, Botez MI. Cognitive behavior in heredodegenerative ataxias. Eur Neurol 1993;33(5):351–7.
115. Botez-Marquard T, Leveille J, Botez MI. Neuropsychological functioning in unilateral cerebellar damage. Can J Neurol Sci 1994;21(4):353–7.
116. Wallesch CW, Horn A. Long-term effects of cerebellar pathology on cognitive functions. Brain Cogn 1990;14(1):19–25.
117. Burk K, Globas C, Bosch S, et al. Cognitive deficits in spinocerebellar ataxia 2. Brain 1999;122(Pt 4):769–77.
118. Bracke-Tolkmitt R, Linden A, Canavan AG, et al. The cerebellum contributes to mental skills. Behav Neurosci 1989;103(2):442.
119. Daum I, Ackermann H, Schugens MM, et al. The cerebellum and cognitive functions in humans. Behav Neurosci 1993;107(3):411–9.
120. Ivry RB, Diener HC. Impaired velocity perception in patients with lesions of the cerebellum. J Cogn Neurosci 1991;3(4):355–66.
121. Malm J, Kristensen B, Karlsson T, et al. Cognitive impairment in young adults with infratentorial infarcts. Neurology 1998;51(2):433–40.
122. Frangou S, Chitins X, Williams SC. Mapping IQ and gray matter density in healthy young people. Neuroimage 2004;23(3):800–5.
123. Wilson SA. Some problems in neurology. II: pathological laughing and crying. J Neurol Psychopathol 1924;IV(16):36.
124. Parvizi J, Anderson SW, Martin CO, et al. Pathological laughter and crying: a link to the cerebellum. Brain 2001;124(Pt 9):1708–19.
125. Ivry RB, Keele SW. Timing functions of the cerebellum. J Cogn Neurosci 1989;1(2):136–52.
126. Ackermann H, Hertrich I. Voice onset time in ataxic dysarthria. Brain Lang 1997;56(3):321–33.
127. Mangels JA, Ivry RB, Shimizu N. Dissociable contributions of the prefrontal and neocerebellar cortex to time perception. Brain Res Cogn Brain Res 1998;7(1):15–39.
128. Casini L, Ivry RB. Effects of divided attention on temporal processing in patients with lesions of the cerebellum or frontal lobe. Neuropsychology 1999;13(1):10–21.
129. Hallett M, Grafman J. Executive function and motor skill learning. Int Rev Neurobiol 1997;41:297–323.
130. Gaser C, Schlaug G. Brain structures differ between musicians and non-musicians. J Neurosci 2003;23(27):9240–5.
131. Hutchinson S, Lee LH, Gaab N, et al. Cerebellar volume of musicians. Cereb Cortex 2003;13(9):943–9.
132. Farnell B. Moving bodies, acting selves. Annu Rev Anthropol 1999;28:33.
133. Sachs C. World history of the dance. New York: Norton; 1937.
134. Appenzeller T. Evolution or revolution. Science 1998;282(5393):1451–4.
135. Bramble DM, Lieberman DE. Endurance running and the evolution of Homo. Nature 2004;432(7015):345–52.
136. Ward CV. Interpreting the posture and locomotion of *Australopithecus afarensis*: where do we stand? Am J Phys Anthropol 2002;(Suppl 35):185–215.
137. Ivry R. Cerebellar timing systems. In: Schahmmann JD, editor. The cerebellum and cognition. Waltham (MA): Academic Press; 1997. p. 556–73.
138. Bower JM, Parsons LM. Rethinking the "lesser brain". Sci Am 2003;289(2):50–7.
139. Wolpert DM, Miall RC, Kawato M. Internal models in the cerebellum. Trends Cogn Sci 1998;2(9):338–47.

140. Nigmatullina Y, Hellyer PJ, Nachev P, et al. The neuroanatomical correlates of training-related perceptuo-reflex uncoupling in dancers. Cereb Cortex 2013. [Epub ahead of print].

141. Schmahmann JD, Caplan D. Cognition, emotion and the cerebellum. Brain 2006;129(Pt 2):290–2.

142. Rapoport M, van Reekum R, Mayberg H. The role of the cerebellum in cognition and behavior: a selective review. J Nerv Ment Dis 2000;12(2):193–8.

143. Ackermann H, Gräber S, Hertrich I, et al. Categorical speech perception in cerebellar disorders. Brain Lang 1997;60:323–31.

144. Yeo C, Hardiman M, Glickstein M. Classical conditioning of nictitating membrane response of the rabbit. II. Lesions of the cerebellar cortex. Exp Brain Res 1985;60:99–113.

145. Akshoomoff NA, Courchesne E, Townsend J. Attention coordination and anticipatory control. In: Schmahmann JD, editor. The cerebellum and cognition (International Review of Neurobiology, vol. 41. San Diego (CA): Academic Press; 1997. p. 575–98.

146. Silveri MC, Misciagna S, Leggio MG, et al. Spatial dysgraphia and cerebellar lesion: a case report. Neurology 1997;48:1529–32.

147. Tach WT. Context-response linkage. In: Schmahmann JD, editor. The cerebellum and cognition (International Review of Neurobiology, vol. 41. San Diego (CA): Academic Press; 1997. p. 599–611.

148. Appollonio IM, Grafman J, Schwartz V, et al. Memory in patients with cerebellar degeneration. Neurology 1993;43:1536–44.

149. Paulesu E, Frith CD, Frackowiak RS. The neural correlates of the verbal component of working memory. Nature 1993;362:342–5.

150. Decety J, Sjoholm H, Ryding E, et al. The cerebellum participates in mental activity: tomographic measurements of regional cerebral blood flow. Brain Res 1990;535:313–7.

151. Darley FL, Aronson AE, Brown JR. Motor speech disorders. Philadelphia: WB Saunders; 1975.

152. Ackermann H, Vogel M, Petersen D, et al. Speech deficits in ischaemic cerebellar lesions. J Neurol 1992;239:223–7.

153. Fiez JA, Raichle ME. Linguistic processing. In: Schmahmann JD, editor. The cerebellum and cognition (International Review of Neurobiology, vol. 41. San Diego (CA): Academic Press; 1997. p. 233–54.

154. Silveri MC, Misciagna S, Leggio MG, et al. Cerebellar spatial dysgraphia: further evidence. J. Neurol 1999;246:321–3.

155. Fiez JA, Peterson SE, Cheney MK, et al. Impaired non-motor learning and error detection associated with cerebellar damage. A single case study. Brain 1992; 115:155–78.

156. Leggio MG, Solida A, Silveri MC, et al. Verbal fluency impairments in patients with cerebellar lesions. Soc Neurosci Abstr 1995;21:917.

157. Mariën P, Saerens J, Nanhoe R, et al. Cerebellar induced aphasia: case report of cerebellar induced prefrontal aphasic language phenomena supported by SPECT findings. J Neurol Sci 1996;144:34–43.

158. Mariën P, Engelborghs S, Pickut BA, et al. Aphasia following cerebellar damage: fact of fallacy? J Neurolinguistics 2000;13:145–71.

159. Fabbro F, Moretti R, Bava A. Language impairments in patients with cerebellar lesions. J Neurolinguistics 2000;13:173–88.

160. Riva D. The cerebellar contribution to language and sequential functions: evidence from a child with cerebellitis. Cortex 1998;24:279–87.

The Role of the Cerebellum in Neurobiology of Psychiatric Disorders

Alia Shakiba, MD

KEYWORDS

- Cerebellum • Mood disorders • Schizophrenia • Attention deficit • Autism

KEY POINTS

- The cerebellum, not only literally but also functionally, can be expounded as the *diminutive of cerebrum*.
- The cerebellum primarily, by itself, does not generate any motor, emotive, or cognitive outputs; but it plays a modulatory, rather than generative, role in nearly all human cerebrum functions.
- Just like an *equalizer* device in sound recording, the cerebellum, by its close interconnections with supratentorial structures, serves as a device to adjust our cerebrum tones and maintain the balance in our performance in all domains.

INTRODUCTION

For a long time, the cerebellum was only known for its role in movement coordination. Although the emotional and behavioral disturbances were described in patients with cerebellar diseases as early as 1831, until recently, the role of cerebellum in nonmotor aspects of the brain function was largely ignored.[1] In fact, the discovery of the involvement of cerebellum in emotion processing goes back to the eighteenth century, when Gall, the Swiss founder of phrenology, mentioned the cerebellum as the primary anatomic locus of love.[2]

After a long period of latency, by the mid twentieth century, Snider and colleagues hypothesized the role of the cerebellum on the *non-motor centers of cerebrum*.[3] Later in 1970, it was shown that chronic stimulation of cerebellum not only improves seizure control but also improves emotional symptoms, such as aggression, anxiety, and depression, in the affected patients. In 1998, Schmahmann and Sherman[4] discussed the possibility of a cerebellar contribution to emotions and behaviors, publishing the

The author has nothing to disclose.
Conflict of Interest: None.
Department of Psychiatry, Tehran University of Medical Sciences, Rouzbeh Hospital, 606 South Kargar Avenue, Tehran 1333795914, Iran
E-mail address: a_shakiba@razi.tums.ac.ir

Neurol Clin 32 (2014) 1105–1115
http://dx.doi.org/10.1016/j.ncl.2014.07.008
0733-8619/14/$ – see front matter © 2014 Elsevier Inc. All rights reserved.
neurologic.theclinics.com

first systematized work on the subject. They studied 20 patients with cerebellar lesions and described their psychiatric symptoms. The newly delineated clinical entity was called cerebellar cognitive affective syndrome (CCAS). Schmahmann is now a research pioneer in this field; he categorized the affective part of the CCAS into 5 axes: attentional control, emotional control, autism spectrum disorders, psychosis spectrum disorders, and social skills set.[5]

This article aims to review the current evidences supporting the role of cerebellum in the pathophysiology of psychiatric disorders, including studies using volumetric and/or functional imaging techniques, genetic and molecular studies, and clinical reports. The implication of these findings, their potential use, and future directions are also discussed.

CEREBELLUM AND EMOTIONAL CONTROL
Bipolar Mood Disorder and Major Depressive Disorder

Mood disorders are among the most frequent psychiatric illnesses. The lifetime prevalence of major depressive disorder is about 12%, and approximately 2.5% of the population has bipolar mood disorder. Mood disorders are characterized by pervasive dysregulation of mood that is accompanied by cognitive, biorhythmic, and psychomotor activity disturbances.[6,7] Unfortunately, our knowledge about the cause and pathophysiological basis of bipolar disorder is very limited. The neural system involved in mood regulation is very complex, and extensive interconnecting neural networks are involved.

Current theories in the pathophysiology of mood disorders mainly focus on 3 cortical-striatal-limbic circuits:

1. Orbital frontal circuit
2. Ventromedial emotion circuit
3. Dorsal cognitive circuit

The last circuit includes dorsolateral and dorsomedial frontal cortices. There are several neuroanatomical, electrophysiological, functional neuroimaging, and clinical evidences that indicate the role of the cerebellum in emotion regulation and affective disorders.

Limbic system including the Papez circuit is the neural substrate for emotional experience and expression. The cerebellum influences various substructures in the Papez circuit. Specifically, cerebellum nuclei and vermis are closely interconnected with midbrain substructures.[8,9] The fastigial nucleus has projections to the ventral tegmental area. Cerebellum is not only directly interconnected to the septum, hippocampus, amygdala, and hypothalamus but is also indirectly connected to the nucleus accumbence, the mesolimbic center for reward. The cingulate cortex, which plays a crucial role in motivation and drives, is also interconnected with the cerebellum. Electrophysiological studies corroborate these interconnections.[10] As mentioned before, those brainstem areas are concerned with motivation, emotions, and drives. Even neocortical areas implicated in higher-order emotional processing, including prefrontal cortex, posterior parietal lobe, superior temporal lobe, and parahippocampus, are closely connected to the cerebellum.[8] Considering these closed cerebrocerebellar circuits, cerebellar vermis is appropriately named "limbic cerebellum"[10] and "emotional pacemaker."[11]

Cerebellar volume

There are many volumetric studies on people who suffer affective disorders. Reduced cerebellar volume has been reported in several studies and case reports in both bipolar mood disorder and unipolar depression. The probable mediating factors include an age of 50 years and older, alcohol consumption, greater number of previous manic episodes, and greater number of previous depressive episodes.[12] Contrary to this finding, a study on women affected by premenstrual dysphoric disorder (PMDD), a periodic mood disturbance of luteal phase closely related to major depressive disorder, has revealed an elevated gray matter volume of the emotional cerebellum among the affected women.[13]

Cerebellum topographic organization

Defining topographic organization of the human cerebellum using functional imaging methods on either the healthy subjects or those affected by various mood disorders has revealed the activation of various regions of the cerebellum during affective processing.[14] In one study aimed to define the neuroanatomy of grief (which is the prototype of reactive depression), cerebellar vermis was significantly activated while a photograph of the deceased loved one was shown to the subjects.[15] Some other studies using the International Affective Picture Scale showed that viewing emotional pictures, either positive or negative, leads to activation of the cerebellum, from the middle into medial regions of left hemisphere, along with the activation of the prefrontal cortex and midbrain structures.[16] The cerebellar hemisphere showed increased activation during sessions of emotion-evoking movies in a group of healthy volunteers.[17] Another similar study showed activation of anterior cerebellum when subjects watched a movie that evoked sadness.[18] One study on patients with bipolar mood disorder reported reduced regional cerebral blood flow in the cerebellum[3]; in another one, the largest reduction was in the cerebellar vermis, the so-called *limbic vermis*.[19] Reduced cerebellar activity in patients with major depressive disorder is correlated with cognitive deficits.[12] Another study using a positron emission tomography scan to map functional brain abnormalities associated with negative mood states in PMDD in the absence of explicit provocation showed greater increase in cerebellar activity from the follicular phase to the symptomatic late luteal phase in the affected group. Elevated brain activity was localized primarily to the midline vermis and fastigial cerebellar nuclei, the so-called *limbic cerebellum*; the increase in cerebellar activity paralleled with the worsening of mood.[20]

Cerebellum lesions

Emotional disturbances in patients with lesions localized to the cerebellum provide clinical evidence for the role of the cerebellum in emotion regulation. Schmahmann and Sherman,[4] in their case series published in 1998, reported a range of emotional disturbances from flattening of affect to disinhibition in patients with cerebellar lesions, especially lesions confined to the vermis and paravermian regions.[4] In another case series, Levisohn and colleagues[21] reported affective changes, including irritability, impulsivity, agitation, and apathy, among children after cerebellar tumor resection.

Anxiety Disorders

Anxiety disorders are the most prevalent mental disorder among the general population and affect nearly 1 in 5 adults. Anxiety is a core negative emotion and refers to brain states elicited by signals that predict impending danger. Anxiety disorders include cognitive, emotive, and physical symptoms.[22]

Current concepts on anxiety disorders mainly focus on monosynaptic projections from the sensory thalamus to the amygdala for rapid responses to simple perceptual elements of potentially threatening stimuli and projections from the sensory association cortices, hippocampus, and related mesiotemporal areas to the amygdala for processing more complex stimuli.[23]

Posttraumatic stress disorder

Posttraumatic stress disorder (PTSD) is characterized by symptoms of re-experience, avoidance, and hyperarousal following exposure to a traumatic event. Structural imaging studies using the magnetic resonance imaging technique have revealed smaller cerebellar volume in patients with PTSD. Decreased cerebellar volume was more prominent in the left hemisphere and vermis and was correlated with symptoms of anxiety and depression.[24] It has been argued that diminished cerebellum size is in fact the consequence of trauma in the early life and is a predictor of developing PTSD after trauma exposure later. A volumetric study has shown smaller cerebellum as an indicator of neuroticism; neuroticism can be defined as impaired coping under stress and is a risk factor for psychopathology, in particular, anxiety and depressive disorders.[25] Increased cerebellar perfusion in PTSD has been shown in one study and may be associated with the delay in habituation observed in the disorder.[26]

Cerebellum in fear conditioning

Many studies on either human or animal models have shown the role of the cerebellum in fear conditioning. Fear conditioning can contribute to phobias, PTSD, and panic disorder. These studies specifically localize aversive conditioning in the vermis and in associating unconditioned stimulus with the conditioned one. The cerebellum is also involved in both motor and emotional aspects of eye-blink conditioning.[27] Moreover, activation of the cerebellum is documented in functional imaging studies during tasks that require recall of emotional personal episodes, painful stimulus, and pain-anticipating stimulus and studies that expose subjects to fear-relevant cues in people with a specific phobia[28] and social anxiety disorder.[29]

Congenital lesions of cerebellum

Anxiety as a symptom has been reported in patients with either congenital lesions of the cerebellum (ie, agenesis, hypoplasia, and dysplasia of cerebellum) or acquired ones (ie, cerebellar tumors, stroke, traumatic injuries, and degenerative disorders).[30]

Cerebellum as modulator of emotional processing

All the evidences mentioned earlier corroborate the role of the cerebellum in developing anxiety disorders. The role of the cerebellum can be hypothesized as the modulator of emotional processing. It does its modulatory role with both an excitatory and GABAergic inhibitory tone[27] and via its direct connections to ventral tegmental area.

Cerebellum not only plays a role in the cognitive and emotive aspects of anxiety but also in its somatic manifestations. The medial cerebellum contains nuclei that serve as functional complements to the hypothalamus in the modulation of autonomic responses.[23]

CEREBELLUM AND ATTENTIONAL CONTROL AND TIME PERCEPTION
Attention-Deficit/Hyperactivity Disorder

Attention-deficit/hyperactivity disorder (ADHD), the most common childhood behavioral disorder diagnosed in outpatient settings, affects approximately 5% of children and 4% of the adult population. ADHD is a behavioral and neurocognitive condition characterized by motor overactivity, inattention, and impulsivity.[31] Current theories suggest that impairment in the fronto-striatal circuit is the core of ADHD.[32] Dysfunction of the attention network, including the prefrontal, superior temporal and external parietal cortices, corpus striatal, hippocampus, and thalamus, is related to inattention symptoms of the disorder. The cerebellum is involved in most aspects of attention, such as shifting attention.[33] Another point of view formulates ADHD as the disease of deficient inhibitory control. Inhibitory control function relies on the fronto-striatal network, including the cerebellum.[34]

Cerebellum volume in ADHD

Many volumetric studies have revealed decrease cerebellar volume along with other brain regions in children with ADHD. This volume reduction is mainly in the posterior vermis.[35–37] One longitudinal study has found that smaller vermal volume persists regardless of the clinical outcome[37]; however, another study has found normalization of the vermal volume if treated with stimulant drugs.[36]

Cerebellum function in ADHD

Diffusion tensor imaging studies have found reduced fractional anisotropy in the cerebellum parallel to the prefrontal cortex.[38,39] Evidence from functional studies also corroborates the role of cerebellum dysfunction in patients with ADHD. Both reduced resting activity that normalizes with stimulant therapy and altered cerebellar activity while doing cognitive tasks, related to time perception in particular, have been reported in patients with ADHD.[40] Aberrant cerebellar activity has been reported in cognitive tasks needing prediction of temporal occurrence of events or in subsecond motor timing tasks.

Timing theory

Time blindness is one of the most common and problematic symptoms of ADHD. It is suggested that timing problems play a key role in the clinical behavioral profile of ADHD. *Dedicated theory of timing* presumes that there are specific brain regions dedicated or specialized in time processing. These regions include the cerebellum, basal ganglia, and right prefrontal cortex.[41]

CEREBELLUM AND AUTISM SPECTRUM DISORDERS

Autism is an early onset condition characterized by delay and deviance in the development of social, communicative, and other skills. Marked and sustained impairment in social interaction is evident along with delays in acquisition of language. Approximately 1 in every 1000 children may have autism, with many exhibiting some features of the condition (ie, autism spectrum disorders [ASD]).

Disturbance in nearly every neural network in the brain has been proposed to be a fundamental mechanism causing ASD. Of the disturbed neural networks, one can refer to limbic system dysfunction related to emotional deficits, and underactivation of fusiform gyrus associated with face perception.[42]

Cerebellum Volume in Autism Spectrum Disorders

Many volumetric studies have been performed on children and adults diagnosed with autism. The results are not consistent: smaller cerebellar volume, especially in lobule VI and VII[43]; reduced cerebellar volume but not specific to any anatomic site[44]; no difference in cerebellar volume among patients with autism and controls[45,46]; or even an increase in cerebellar volume among autistic ones.[47] Patients' age, IQ, and functional level are reported as mediators of cerebellar volume reduction among autistic patients.[44–46] Selective abnormalities of cerebellar vermis lobules VI to VII is reported in syndromic autism in fragile X syndrome as well as other syndromic disorders that have autistic features.

Cerebellum Function in Autism Spectrum Disorders

More recent studies using functional imaging techniques also reveal aberrant cerebellar activity during tasks that are related to domains that are dysfunctional in autistic patients. Among them, motor and attentional activity, emotional and auditory, and tactile sensory-activating tasks can be named.[48–51]

Cerebellum Histology

Histologic studies on the cerebellum of patients with autism have invariably reported decreased number of Purkinje cells primarily in the posterolateral neocerebellar cortex and also in archicerebellar cortex of the cerebellar hemispheres.[44,52] The role of altered immune responses in the pathogenesis of autism has been highlighted by several studies. Postmortem histologic studies have revealed marked activation of microglia and astrocytes in various brain regions, including the cerebellum.[53] Several studies have supported the role of the cerebellum in the pathogenesis of the disorder in the molecular level. It has been shown that glutamic acid decarboxylase enzymes 65 and 67 proteins are reduced in the cerebella of patients with autism.[52] Alterations in GABAergic,[54] glutamatergic, and cholinergic[55] neurotransmission are also reported.

CEREBELLUM AND SCHIZOPHRENIA

Schizophrenia, the prototype of psychotic disorders, is perhaps the most puzzling and tragic psychiatric illness and probably the most disabling one. It affects 1% of the population, and the prevalence is almost even worldwide. Schizophrenia is characterized by disordered cognition and emotion and severe loss of function.[56,57]

Although the psychopathology of schizophrenia was described many centuries ago and therapeutic modalities are currently available, the neurobiology and genetics underlying its manifestations remain unclear. Morphologic brain studies have revealed anatomic differences in the brains of affected individuals and healthy subjects involving both gray and white matter. These differences are mainly in the prefrontal cortex, hippocampus, thalamus, and basal ganglia; the last difference is perhaps caused by antipsychotic effects rather than the disorder itself. Nearly all neurotransmitter systems are altered in schizophrenia, but none can be named as the core of the disorder. Altered dopamine activity in mesocortical and mesolimbic circuits has been the main area of study and the target of conventional treatment modalities for a long time. But dysfunction of these circuits alone cannot explain many aspects of the disorder, such as cognitive and motor disturbances.[58]

Schizophrenia Unitary Model

In 1999, Andreasen[59] proposed a *unitary model* for schizophrenia. Through this model, schizophrenia is defined as a neurodevelopmental disorder, actually a *misconnection syndrome*, which is an equivalent of Bleuler's *fragmented phrene* concept. She explains the deficits in the *cortico-cerebello-thalamo-cortical circuit*. Cerebellum is involved in the pathophysiology of schizophrenia, not only in symptoms related to motor coordination deficits but also in cognitive and emotional deficits, the so-called *cognitive dysmetria* described by Schmahmann and Sherman[4] in 1998. Cognition refers to both the rational and emotional components of mental activity.[59] Cognitive impairment in patients with schizophrenia is clinically profound and is a separate domain of psychopathology.

Cerebellum Volume in Schizophrenia

Volumetric studies have shown decreased cerebellar volume in patients with schizophrenia. This decreased volume cannot be related to treatment, as it is seen in drug-naïve patients and in patients with first-episode psychosis. Cerebellar volume reduction, less severe than in patients, is seen in their nonaffected family members.[60–62]

Cerebellum Function in Schizophrenia

Nearly all studies on schizophrenia using functional imaging tools have found abnormalities in cerebellar function along with other brain region abnormalities. Dysfunction of the cerebellum has been seen especially in cerebellar vermis during emotional tasks that are related to limbic regions.[63,64]

On the cellular and synaptic level, which is the focus of recent studies, there is evidence for cerebellar involvement in the pathophysiology of schizophrenia. Alteration in the expression of synaptophysin, Complexin I, Complexin II, and GABA$_A$ receptor expression is shown in patients with schizophrenia and could underlie some of the cognitive, psychotic, and mood dysfunctions associated with the disorder.[63,65]

SUMMARY

The aim of this review is to put forth the new recognition that the cerebellum is not only the device of motor coordination but also has an essential role in the modulation of personality, mood, and intellect.

An evolving body of knowledge has revealed the role of the cerebellum in psychiatric disorders. Further studies on this issue will extend our current knowledge. Studies designed to differentiate subtypes of each disorder based on the differences in cerebellar activation during various series of cognitive and emotive tasks can be a novel area of research. Assembling data from clinical, structural and functional brain imaging, genetic, and molecular studies can provide a unique opportunity to better demonstrate the pathophysiology of psychiatric disorders.

Changes in cerebellar function during conventional pharmacologic and psychological therapeutic interventions for patients with psychiatric disorders, as well as anecdotal reports of successful management of their symptoms through cerebellar stimulation, can lead us to new therapeutic interventions.

ACKNOWLEDGMENTS

The author gratefully acknowledges the contribution of Dr Raheleh Rahimi Darabad, Masoumeh Taromi, and Mohammad Shakiba in helping her to locate and organize the relevant literature. Thanks are also due to Dr Maryam Shahri for her suggestions on preparing the article.

REFERENCES

1. Rapoport M, van Reekum R, Mayberg H. The role of the cerebellum in cognition and behavior: a selective review. J Neuropsychiatry Clin Neurosci 2000;12(2): 193–8.
2. Macklis RM, Macklis JD. Historical and phrenologic reflections on the nonmotor functions of the cerebellum: love under the tent? Neurology 1992;42(4):928–32.
3. Snider RS. Recent contributions to the anatomy and physiology of the cerebellum. Archives of neurology and psychiatry 1950;64(2):196–219.
4. Schmahmann JD, Sherman JC. The cerebellar cognitive affective syndrome. Brain 1998;121(Pt 4):561–79.
5. Schmahmann JD. Cerebellar non-motor functions: what it means for you. Annual Members' Meeting National Ataxia Foundation. San Antonio, March 18, 2012.
6. Akiskal HS. Mood disorders: clinical features. In: Sadock BJ, Sadock VA, Ruiz P, editors. Kaplan & Sadock's comprehensive textbook of psychiatry, vol. 1. Philadelphia: Lippincott Williams & Wilkins; 2009. p. 1693–733.

7. Zoltán Rihmer JA. Mood disorders: epidemiology. In: Sadock BJ, Virginia A, Ruiz P, editors. Kaplan & Sadock's comprehensive textbook of psychiatry, vol. 1, 9th edition. Philadelphia: Lippincott Williams & Wilkins; 2009. p. 1645–53.
8. Blatt GJ, Oblak AL, Schmahmann JD. Cerebellar connections with limbic circuits: anatomy and functional implications. In: Mario M, Schmahmann JD, Rossi F, et al, editors. Handbook of the cerebellum and cerebellar disorders. Houten (Netherlands): Springer; 2013. p. 479–96.
9. Snider RS, Maiti A. Cerebellar contributions to the Papez circuit. J Neurosci Res 1976;2(2):133–46.
10. Heath RG, Dempesy CW, Fontana CJ, et al. Cerebellar stimulation: effects on septal region, hippocampus, and amygdala of cats and rats. Biol Psychiatry 1978;13(5):501–29.
11. Heath RG. Modulation of emotion with a brain pacemamer. Treatment for intractable psychiatric illness. J Nerv Ment Dis 1977;165(5):300–17.
12. Baldacara L, Borgio JG, Lacerda AL, et al. Cerebellum and psychiatric disorders. Rev Bras Psiquiatr 2008;30(3):281–9.
13. Berman SM, London ED, Morgan M, et al. Elevated gray matter volume of the emotional cerebellum in women with premenstrual dysphoric disorder. J Affect Disord 2013;146(2):266–71.
14. Stoodley CJ, Schmahmann JD. Evidence for topographic organization in the cerebellum of motor control versus cognitive and affective processing. Cortex 2010;46(7):831–44.
15. Gundel H, O'Connor MF, Littrell L, et al. Functional neuroanatomy of grief: an FMRI study. Am J Psychiatry 2003;160(11):1946–53.
16. Stoodley CJ, Schmahmann JD. Functional topography in the human cerebellum: a meta-analysis of neuroimaging studies. Neuroimage 2009;44(2):489–501.
17. Reiman EM, Lane RD, Ahern GL, et al. Neuroanatomical correlates of externally and internally generated human emotion. Am J Psychiatry 1997;154(7):918–25.
18. Liotti M, Mayberg HS, McGinnis S, et al. Unmasking disease-specific cerebral blood flow abnormalities: mood challenge in patients with remitted unipolar depression. Am J Psychiatry 2002;159(11):1830–40.
19. Loeber RT, Sherwood AR, Renshaw PF, et al. Differences in cerebellar blood volume in schizophrenia and bipolar disorder. Schizophr Res 1999;37(1):81–9.
20. Rapkin AJ, Berman SM, Mandelkern MA, et al. Neuroimaging evidence of cerebellar involvement in premenstrual dysphoric disorder. Biol Psychiatry 2011; 69(4):374–80.
21. Levisohn L, Cronin-Golomb A, Schmahmann JD. Neuropsychological consequences of cerebellar tumour resection in children: cerebellar cognitive affective syndrome in a paediatric population. Brain 2000;123(Pt 5):1041–50.
22. Merikangas KR, Kalaydjian AE. Epidemiology of anxiety disorders. In: Sadock BJ, Virginia A, Ruiz P, editors. Kaplan & Sadock's comprehensive textbook of psychiatry, vol. 1, 9th edition. Philadelphia: Lippincott Williams & Wilkins; 2009. p. 1856–64.
23. Drevets WC, Charney DS, Rauch SL. Neuroimaging and the neuroanatomical circuits implicated in anxiety, fear, and stress-induced circuitry disorders. In: Sadock BJ, Virginia A, Ruiz P, editors. Kaplan & Sadock's comprehensive textbook of psychiatry, vol. 1, 9th edition. Philadelphia: Lippincott Williams & Wilkins; 2009. p. 1881–98.
24. Baldacara L, Jackowski AP, Schoedl A, et al. Reduced cerebellar left hemisphere and vermal volume in adults with PTSD from a community sample. J Psychiatr Res 2011;45(12):1627–33.

25. Schutter DJ, Koolschijn PC, Peper JS, et al. The cerebellum link to neuroticism: a volumetric MRI association study in healthy volunteers. PLoS One 2012;7(5): e37252.
26. Bonne O, Gilboa A, Louzoun Y, et al. Resting regional cerebral perfusion in recent posttraumatic stress disorder. Biol Psychiatry 2003;54(10):1077–86.
27. Sacchetti B, Scelfo B, Strata P. Cerebellum and emotional behavior. Neuroscience 2009;162(3):756–62.
28. Del Casale A, Ferracuti S, Rapinesi C, et al. Functional neuroimaging in specific phobia. Psychiatry Res 2012;202(3):181–97.
29. Gimenez M, Pujol J, Ortiz H, et al. Altered brain functional connectivity in relation to perception of scrutiny in social anxiety disorder. Psychiatry Res 2012;202(3): 214–23.
30. Schmahmann JD. The role of the cerebellum in cognition and emotion: personal reflections since 1982 on the dysmetria of thought hypothesis, and its historical evolution from theory to therapy. Neuropsychol Rev 2010;20(3):236–60.
31. Greenhill LL, Hechtman LI. Attention-deficit/hyperactivity disorder. In: Sadock BJ, Virginia A, Ruiz P, editors. Kaplan & Sadock's comprehensive textbook of psychiatry, vol. 2, 9th edition. Philadelphia: Lippincott Williams & Wilkins; 2009. p. 3560–71.
32. Emond V, Joyal C, Poissant H. Structural and functional neuroanatomy of attention-deficit hyperactivity disorder (ADHD). Encephale 2009;35(2):107–14 [in French].
33. Castellanos FX, Lee PP, Sharp W, et al. Developmental trajectories of brain volume abnormalities in children and adolescents with attention-deficit/hyperactivity disorder. JAMA 2002;288(14):1740–8.
34. Liston C, Malter Cohen M, Teslovich T, et al. Atypical prefrontal connectivity in attention-deficit/hyperactivity disorder: pathway to disease or pathological end point? Biol Psychiatry 2011;69(12):1168–77.
35. Berquin PC, Giedd JN, Jacobsen LK, et al. Cerebellum in attention-deficit hyperactivity disorder: a morphometric MRI study. Neurology 1998;50(4):1087–93.
36. Bledsoe J, Semrud-Clikeman M, Pliszka SR. A magnetic resonance imaging study of the cerebellar vermis in chronically treated and treatment-naive children with attention-deficit/hyperactivity disorder combined type. Biol Psychiatry 2009;65(7):620–4.
37. Mackie S, Shaw P, Lenroot R, et al. Cerebellar development and clinical outcome in attention deficit hyperactivity disorder. Am J Psychiatry 2007; 164(4):647–55.
38. Ashtari M, Kumra S, Bhaskar SL, et al. Attention-deficit/hyperactivity disorder: a preliminary diffusion tensor imaging study. Biol Psychiatry 2005;57(5): 448–55.
39. Pavuluri MN, Yang S, Kamineni K, et al. Diffusion tensor imaging study of white matter fiber tracts in pediatric bipolar disorder and attention-deficit/hyperactivity disorder. Biol Psychiatry 2009;65(7):586–93.
40. Cherkasova MV, Hechtman L. Neuroimaging in attention-deficit hyperactivity disorder: beyond the frontostriatal circuitry. Can J Psychiatry 2009;54(10): 651–64.
41. Noreika V, Falter CM, Rubia K. Timing deficits in attention-deficit/hyperactivity disorder (ADHD): evidence from neurocognitive and neuroimaging studies. Neuropsychologia 2013;51(2):235–66.
42. Volkmar FR, Schultz RT, State MW, et al. Pervasive developmental disorders. In: Sadock BJ, Virginia A, Ruiz P, editors. Kaplan & Sadock's comprehensive

textbook of psychiatry, vol. 2, 9th edition. Philadelphia: Lippincott Williams & Wilkins; 2009. p. 3540–59.

43. Courchesne E, Yeung-Courchesne R, Press GA, et al. Hypoplasia of cerebellar vermal lobules VI and VII in autism. N Engl J Med 1988;318(21):1349–54.

44. Scott JA, Schumann CM, Goodlin-Jones BL, et al. A comprehensive volumetric analysis of the cerebellum in children and adolescents with autism spectrum disorder. Autism Res 2009;2(5):246–57.

45. Holttum JR, Minshew NJ, Sanders RS, et al. Magnetic resonance imaging of the posterior fossa in autism. Biol Psychiatry 1992;32(12):1091–101.

46. Piven J, Nehme E, Simon J, et al. Magnetic resonance imaging in autism: measurement of the cerebellum, pons, and fourth ventricle. Biol Psychiatry 1992; 31(5):491–504.

47. Stanfield AC, McIntosh AM, Spencer MD, et al. Towards a neuroanatomy of autism: a systematic review and meta-analysis of structural magnetic resonance imaging studies. Eur Psychiatry 2008;23(4):289–99.

48. Allen G, Courchesne E. Differential effects of developmental cerebellar abnormality on cognitive and motor functions in the cerebellum: an fMRI study of autism. Am J Psychiatry 2003;160(2):262–73.

49. Padmanabhan A, Lynn A, Foran W, et al. Age related changes in striatal resting state functional connectivity in autism. Front Hum Neurosci 2013;7:814.

50. Philip RC, Dauvermann MR, Whalley HC, et al. A systematic review and meta-analysis of the fMRI investigation of autism spectrum disorders. Neurosci Biobehav Rev 2012;36(2):901–42.

51. Kern JK. Purkinje cell vulnerability and autism: a possible etiological connection. Brain Dev 2003;25(6):377–82.

52. Fatemi SH, Halt AR, Stary JM, et al. Glutamic acid decarboxylase 65 and 67 kDa proteins are reduced in autistic parietal and cerebellar cortices. Biol Psychiatry 2002;52(8):805–10.

53. Fatemi SH, Aldinger KA, Ashwood P, et al. Consensus paper: pathological role of the cerebellum in autism. Cerebellum 2012;11(3):777–807.

54. Fatemi SH, Reutiman TJ, Folsom TD, et al. mRNA and protein levels for GABAAalpha4, alpha5, beta1 and GABABR1 receptors are altered in brains from subjects with autism. J Autism Dev Disord 2010;40(6):743–50.

55. Lee M, Martin-Ruiz C, Graham A, et al. Nicotinic receptor abnormalities in the cerebellar cortex in autism. Brain 2002;125(Pt 7):1483–95.

56. Lewis S, Escalona PR, Keith SJ. Phenomenology of schizophrenia. In: Sadock BJ, Virginia A, Ruiz P, editors. Kaplan & Sadock's comprehensive textbook of psychiatry, vol. 1, 9th edition. Philadelphia: Lippincott Williams & Wilkins; 2009. p. 1434–50.

57. Tamminga CA. Introduction and overview. In: Sadock BJ, Virginia A, Ruiz P, editors. Kaplan & Sadock's comprehensive textbook of psychiatry, vol. 1, 9th edition. Philadelphia: Lippincott Williams & Wilkins; 2009. p. 1432–3.

58. Shenton ME, Kubicki M. Structural brain imaging in schizophrenia. In: Sadock BJ, Virginia A, Ruiz P, editors. Kaplan & Sadock's comprehensive textbook of psychiatry, vol. 1, 9th edition. Philadelphia: Lippincott Williams & Wilkins; 2009. p. 1494–507.

59. Andreasen NC. A unitary model of schizophrenia: Bleuler's "fragmented phrene" as schizencephaly. Arch Gen Psychiatry 1999;56(9):781–7.

60. Greenstein D, Lenroot R, Clausen L, et al. Cerebellar development in childhood onset schizophrenia and non-psychotic siblings. Psychiatry Res 2011;193(3): 131–7.

61. Watson DR, Anderson JM, Bai F, et al. A voxel based morphometry study investigating brain structural changes in first episode psychosis. Behav Brain Res 2012;227(1):91–9.
62. Roman-Urrestarazu A, Murray GK, Barnes A, et al. Brain structure in different psychosis risk groups in the Northern Finland 1986 Birth Cohort. Schizophr Res 2014;153(1):7.
63. Andreasen NC, Pierson R. The role of the cerebellum in schizophrenia. Biol Psychiatry 2008;64(2):81–8.
64. Picard H, Amado I, Mouchet-Mages S, et al. The role of the cerebellum in schizophrenia: an update of clinical, cognitive, and functional evidences. Schizophr Bull 2008;34(1):155–72.
65. Fatemi SH, Folsom TD, Rooney RJ, et al. Expression of GABAA alpha2-, beta1- and epsilon-receptors are altered significantly in the lateral cerebellum of subjects with schizophrenia, major depression and bipolar disorder. Transl Psychiatry 2013;3:e303.

Infections of the Cerebellum

Amy A. Pruitt, MD

KEYWORDS

- Autoimmune cerebellitis • CLIPPERS • Creutzfeldt-Jakob disease
- Epstein-Barr virus • Influenza • JC virus granule cell neuronopathy
- *Listeria* rhombencephalitis • Progressive multifocal leukoencephalopathy

KEY POINTS

- Infectious pathogens that frequently or preferentially affect the cerebellum include *Listeria monocytogenes*, varicella-zoster virus, JC virus, and Creutzfeldt-Jakob disease. Fever, headache, and brainstem signs and symptoms may accompany cerebellar signs. Magnetic resonance imaging (MRI) may show leptomeningeal enhancement and swelling.
- Acute postinfectious cerebellitis is more common in children and young adults. It is a pure cerebellar syndrome often with normal MRI at onset. Reported antecedent infections include Epstein-Barr virus, influenza A and B, mumps, varicella-zoster, Coxsackie virus, rotavirus, echovirus, *Mycoplasma*, and immunization.
- Acute ataxia caused by cerebellar disease must be distinguished from other anatomic sites whose dysfunction causes imbalance, including vestibular nuclei, and peripheral neuropathies, such as Guillain-Barré syndrome and Miller Fisher syndrome.
- Acute cerebellitis can result in significant cerebellar edema, and the resulting obstructive hydrocephalus can require surgical decompression.
- Some patients with acute postinfectious cerebellitis may benefit from immunologic modification with intravenous immunoglobulin or plasmapheresis.

INTRODUCTION: SUSPECTING AN INFECTIOUS CEREBELLITIS
Definitions and Terms

Acute cerebellitis (AC) can be caused by either primary infection or postinfectious immune-mediated processes. In this article, the term *acute* is defined as symptoms evolving over a few hours to 2 days. *AC* denotes an infection that directly affects the cerebellum often with abnormal magnetic resonance imaging (MRI) and with symptoms and signs beyond a pure cerebellar syndrome. AC may be unilateral or bilateral. The term *acute postinfectious cerebellar ataxia* (APCA) designates a postinfectious (mostly viral) cerebellitis that is usually a pure pan-cerebellar syndrome

Disclosures: The author has no relevant disclosures.
University of Pennsylvania, 3400 Spruce Street, Philadelphia, PA 19104, USA
E-mail address: pruitt@mail.med.upenn.edu

without other signs of central nervous system (CNS) infection often with an initially normal MRI scan. Although the 2 entities may represent a spectrum, the presentation, outcome, and therapeutic implications are often different.

Laboratory Investigations

Because the differential diagnosis of cerebellar infection is broad (**Box 1**), the clinician must consider concurrent drugs, patient immune status, and a limited range of distinguishing radiographic characteristics. Cerebrospinal fluid (CSF) may show a nonspecific lymphocytic pleocytosis of multiple possible causes. **Table 1** summarizes additional special studies. MRI, particularly diffusion-weighted imaging (DWI), can be helpful but often is nonspecific or normal in APCA. Transient cerebellar cortical swelling leptomeningeal enhancement, limited involvement of deep cerebellar nuclei, middle cerebellar peduncles, other brainstem structures, and splenial lesions can aid differential diagnostic considerations. Cerebellar atrophy may develop after the acute cerebellar infectious or parainfectious insult. Succinate peaks on MR spectroscopy (MRS) raise suspicion of infection.

Physical Examination

Article reviews cerebellar signs and symptoms. In the setting of acute presentations suggestive of infection, the examination should also be directed at sensory or vestibular dysfunction that can cause ataxia.[1] In most infections, motor dysfunction will predominant; but when dentate nuclei are preferentially involved, the cognitive-affective syndrome may color the clinical presentation.[2]

DIFFERENTIAL DIAGNOSIS: NONINFECTIOUS MIMES
Neoplasms

The cerebellum and its coverings can be sites of parenchymal metastatic disease, primary brain tumors, or leptomeningeal dissemination usually in the context of known malignancy. However, one recently described syndrome is predominantly seen in the posterior fossa and has diagnostic and therapeutic implications. The recently described definable disorder of chronic lymphocytic inflammation with pontine perivascular enhancement responsive to steroids (CLIPPERS) was reported in 2010 and could be confused with infection (**Fig. 1**).[5] Concern that it may not be a benign steroid-responsive condition but rather a sentinel lesion of primary CNS lymphoma has since arisen. Use of MRS may suggest the correct diagnosis with rising Cho:NAA ratios as well as lipid and lactate resonances.[6] CLIPPERS also may represent a form of immune reconstitution inflammatory syndrome in patients who have been withdrawn from natalizumab.[7]

Paraneoplastic Syndromes

Acute cerebellar symptoms evolving over hours to a few days can raise the possibility of antibody-associated disorders as an alternative to infection. The paraneoplastic disorders most likely to present with a predominantly cerebellar syndrome include the onconeural antibodies, such as anti-Hu, anti-Ri, anti-Tr, and anti-Yo. Nonparaneoplastic cerebellitis associated with antibodies can be seen with glutamic acid decarboxylase, metabotropic glutamate receptor type I,[8] and contactin-associated protein 2.[9] Homer 3 antibodies have been described in 2 adult patients without neoplasm who presented with a subacute pancerebellar syndrome.[10,11] The onset of paraneoplastic cerebellar degeneration can be extremely acute and accompanied by significant pleocytosis, thus, mimicking acute postinfectious cerebellitis.[12]

Box 1
Differential diagnosis of an acute cerebellar syndrome

Infections (details see **Table 1**)

  Viral

  Bacterial

  Fungal

  Prion

Postinfectious APCA

Other

  ADEM

  NMO

Paraneoplastic/autoimmune

  Opsoclonus-myoclonus syndrome

GAD, Tr, Caspr2, Homer 3, Yo, Hu, Ri, mGluR1

Neoplastic +/− hydrocephalus

Carcinomatous meningitis

Neurosarcoidosis

Drug related

  Heroin

  Metronidazole

  Vigabatrin

  Phenytoin

  Carbamazepine

  Barbiturates

  Gabapentin

  Oxycodone[3]

  Benzodiazepines

Vitamin deficiencies: thiamine, vitamin E

Inherited diseases with episodic ataxia

  Maple syrup urine[4] disease

EA-1, EA-2

Erdheim-Chester

Osmotic demyelination

Vascular vertebral dissection

AICA infarction

Heat stroke

Acute vestibular ataxia[a] (BPV, migraine)

Acute sensory ataxia[a] (GBS, Miller Fisher)

Psychogenic[a]

Abbreviations: ADEM, acute disseminated encephalomyelitis; AICA, anterior inferior cerebellar artery; BPV, benign positional vertigo; Caspr2, contactin-associated protein 2; EA, episodic ataxia; GAD, glutamic acid decarboxylase; GBS, Guillain-Barré syndrome; mGluR1, metabotropic glutamate receptor type I; NMO, neuromyelitis optica.
[a] Noncerebellar causes of ataxia (sensory or vestibular) to be distinguished on physical examination.

Table 1
Infectious pathogens frequently involving cerebellum

Pathogen	Affected Hosts (Competent, Immunocompromised)	Laboratory Testing
Viral		
Varicella-zoster	C, I	CSF IgG, PCR
JC virus (PML)	I	CSF PCR, biopsy
Dengue	C, I	Serum IgM, IgG
Epstein-Barr	C, I	CSF PCR
Influenza	C, I	For remaining entities in this
Enterovirus 71	C, I	column: Serum IgM, CSF PCR
Parvovirus B19	C	
Respiratory syncytial virus	C	
APCA-associated pathogens		
Measles	C	
Rubella	C	
Mumps	C	
Pertussis	C	
Rotavirus	C	
Coxsackie	C	
Bacterial		
Listeria monocytogenes	C (rhombencephalitis), I	Blood, CSF culture
Mycoplasma pneumoniae	C	Tissue biopsy, blood cultures
Sinus/otitis/septic phlebitis	C, I	Serum Western blot, serum:
Typhoid fever	C	CSF antibody ratio
Lyme disease	C	CSF PCR, small bowel biopsy
Whipple disease	C	
Fungal		
Aspergillus	I	CSF galactomannan, skin or
Histoplasmosis	C, I	lung biopsy
Exserohilum rostratum	C (epidural injections)	Sinus, lung biopsy; serology
		CSF culture
		CSF culture
Prion		
Creutzfeldt-Jakob disease	C	CSF 14-3-3 protein
		MRI (DWI sequence), EEG,
		brain biopsy

Abbreviations: DWI, diffusion-weighted imaging; EEG, electroencephalogram; IgG, immunoglobulin G; IgM, immunoglobulin M; PCR, polymerase chain reaction; PML, progressive multifocal leukoencephalopathy.

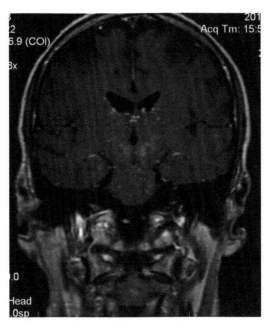

Fig. 1. Coronal T1-weighted gadolinium-enhanced MRI shows curvilinear and punctuate enhancement in brainstem, cerebral, and cerebellar peduncles and upper spinal cord of the newly described syndrome called CLIPPERS.

Considerations in Immunocompromised Patients

Acute cerebellar syndromes in immunocompromised patients can represent a broad spectrum of infectious and noninfectious causes. Autoimmune conditions preferentially affecting the cerebellum should be considered in patients with relevant systemic illness. Patients with myelodysplastic syndromes can develop recurring pseudotumoral mass lesions including a true cerebellitis with inflammatory infiltrates and sometimes with enough mass effect to require surgical intervention (**Fig. 2**).[13] Similar fulminant cerebellitis with recurrence has been reported in an adult patient with Crohn disease.[14] Sarcoidosis presenting in the brain parenchyma or leptomeninges can mimic acute cerebellar infection; the diagnosis is facilitated when the disease is steroid responsive and recurrent (**Fig. 3**).

Drug-Related Ataxia

Rapid evolution of ataxia and dysarthria in patients receiving metronidazole for *Clostridium difficile* reveals the specific pattern of dentate nuclei hyperintensities. Symptoms resolve quickly on discontinuation of the drug.[15] Another patient's symptoms were episodic ataxia and dysarthria while on the drug for ulcerative colitis. Both patients had been on the drug for more than 3 months when the symptoms developed.[16] A similar pattern of dentate involvement has been described with vigabatrin.[17]

Heat Stroke

A febrile cerebellar syndrome could also signal heat stroke. Cerebellar neurons are particularly susceptible to heat injury.[18] DWI abnormalities may evolve over a period of days in the dentate nuclei and superior cerebellar peduncles.[19]

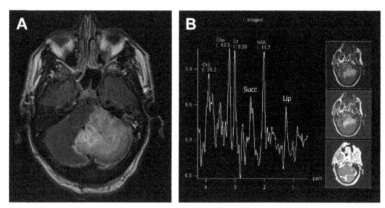

Fig. 2. T2-weighted fluid-attenuated inversion recovery MRI shows large left hemicerebellar mass with compression of fourth ventricle (*A*). MRS, although not definitive, suggests an inflammatory process with a slightly elevated Choline: Creatine ratio and succinate and lipid peaks (*B*). Patient had untreated systemic small lymphocytic lymphoma. At resection, pathology showed a perivascular inflammatory process. Ten months following the biopsy, patient had a right temporal recurrence with a similar-appearing mass lesion that responded to a trial of corticosteroids.

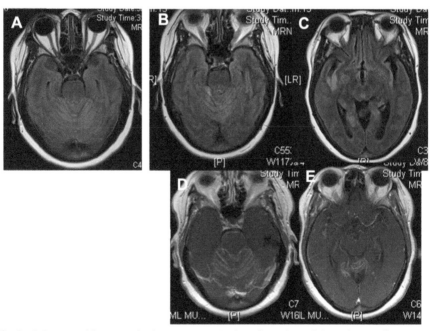

Fig. 3. A 52-year-old woman had recurrent episodes of ataxia and dysarthria with concomitant enhancement of the leptomeninges and cerebellar cortex. (*A*) Fluid-attenuated inversion recovery (FLAIR) abnormality in cerebellum at first presentation. Initial diagnostic consideration after the first episode was APCA; but when symptoms recurred both in the cerebellum (*B*, FLAIR) and supratentorially (*C*, FLAIR) 8 months later and now showed gadolinium enhancement (*D*, *E*), a biopsy was undertaken that revealed neurosarcoidosis.

ACUTE INFECTIOUS CEREBELLITIS

In this section, the author discusses the direct tropic effects of the pathogen causing cerebellar dysfunction in the form of encephalitis, meningitis, and parenchymal or extra-axial abscesses (as opposed to postinfectious immune-mediated mechanisms) and highlights particular syndromes suggestive of specific infectious causes.

VIRAL INFECTIONS
Varicella-Zoster Virus

Varicella-zoster virus (VZV) is a human neurotropic alphaherpesvirus that causes primary varicella. The virus then becomes latent. As people age or acquire illnesses that produce immunosuppression or require immunosuppressive therapies, cell mediated immunity declines and leads to a large variety of acute, subacute, and chronic manifestations of virus reactivation. These manifestations include cranial nerve palsies, paresis, meningoencephalitis, myelopathy, many kinds of eye disorders, and vasculopathy that produces strokes or mimics giant cell arteritis.[20] Those syndromes that are of relevance in the differential diagnosis of cerebellar infection are summarized in **Box 2**. The cerebellar and brainstem symptoms can postdate vesicular eruptions by several weeks and can develop while patients are receiving antiviral therapy.[21] Pure cerebellitis is uncommon but has been reported in immunocompetent adults.[22,23] All VZV syndromes can occur without a herpetic rash. Diagnosis is confirmed by detection of VZV DNA or anti-VZV immunoglobulin G in the CSF.

Box 2
Varicella-zoster

Epidemiology

Immunocompetent: usually older than 60 years

Immunocompromised: glucocorticoid use, natalizumab, fingolimod, calcineurin inhibitors, tumor necrosis factor-α inhibitors

Clinical presentations involving potential cerebellar signs

Vasculopathy: transient ischemic attack, ischemic or hemorrhagic stroke

Polyneuritis: Ramsay Hunt (V3 and VII)

  Vernet syndrome, lower cranial neuritis, glossopharyngeal, vagus, ataxia dysphagia

Segmental brainstem myelitis

Cerebellar ataxia

Diagnosis

Biopsy skin lesions, if present

CSF anti-VZV IgM, IgG or VZV DNA (pr)

Blood: Anti-VZV IgM

Anti-VZV IgG in CSF more often positive in chronic vasculopathy than is PCR

Treatment

Acyclovir 10 mg/kg IV every 8 hours × 2 weeks

Post-VZV encephalitis: check CD4+ count; if less than 500, consider valacyclovir 500 mg twice a day chronically

Abbreviations: IgG, immunoglobulin G; IV, intravenous; PCR, polymerase chain reaction.

Dengue

The territory of dengue fever, an arboviral infection, has expanded in many tropical countries and has been seen in the United States. An acute cerebellar syndrome has been reported as the presenting manifestation of dengue fever in Sri Lanka.[24] Another report also comes from Sri Lanka where more than 44,000 cases were seen in 2012, likely an underestimate as serologic tests were still not readily available in most hospitals.[25]

Influenza

Influenza viruses A and B can produce acute syndromes with hyperintensities in cerebellar hemispheres along with cytotoxic edema causing enough acute swelling to require decompressive craniotomy. H3N2 influenza and other influenza viruses, including H1N1, have been associated with brainstem/cerebellar encephalitis.[26]

Progressive Multifocal Leukoencephalopathy

Progressive multifocal leukoencephalopathy (PML) results from lytic infection of oligodendroglia by the JC polyomavirus. Most patients have human immunodeficiency virus (HIV) or lymphoreticular malignancy or are receiving drugs that alter T-cell function, though PML has been reported in patients with no apparent immune deficit.[27] Although most patients present with cognitive, visual, or motor impairment, the posterior fossa is also a favored site for PML. **Fig. 4** illustrates the rapid evolution of cerebellar PML in a patient with lymphoma. Cerebellar dysfunction can also dominate the clinical presentation when a mutated form of John Cunningham Virus (JCV) shifts the viral tropism from glial cells to cerebellar granule cells.[28,29] Most of these cases have been reported in patients who are HIV +, but recent reports detail JC virus granule cell neuronopathy in a patient treated with rituximab[30] and infection of neurons in cerebellar gray matter in JC virus infection associated with natalizumab.[31] Diagnosis is confirmed with the presence of JC virus in the CSF.[32] Apart from restoration of immune function, there is no established therapy for PML.

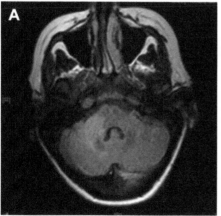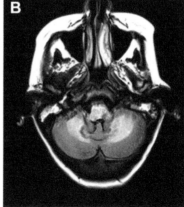

Fig. 4. Rapid progression of MRI fluid-attenuated inversion recovery (FLAIR) abnormality on this axial view of posterior fossa in HIV-negative patient with untreated small lymphocytic lymphoma. Patient became locked-in within 4 months of symptom onset. CSF was positive for JCV by polymerase chain reaction. Axial FLAIR images at presentation (*A*) and 4 months later (*B*).

Epstein-Barr Virus

In older children and young adults, infectious mononucleosis is the most commonly identified preceding infection causing APCA. The most common area of the brain affected is the cerebellum.[33] CSF may show lymphocytic pleocytosis or be normal; polymerase chain reaction (PCR) for Epstein-Barr virus (EBV) is often positive, though the presence of EBV in the CSF of normal hosts does not necessarily indicate a direct causal relationship to the clinical syndrome. EBV-associated APCA is distinguished by neurologic symptoms occurring 2 to 3 weeks after the mononucleosis symptoms, somewhat longer than in VZV-related APCA. MRIs are typically normal.[34]

The immunologic basis of EBV-associated postinfectious cerebellitis derives from reports of antibodies directed against Purkinje cells. Although most patients have a self-limited course with compete recovery, treatment directed at the immune response (plasmapheresis or intravenous immunoglobulin [IVIG]) can result in rapid improvement. If there is no improvement at the end of the first week of cerebellitis or if patients have cognitive or emotional symptoms, Schmahmann[35] recommend plasmapheresis or IVIG.

Enterovirus

In the past decade, it has been estimated that more than 6 million cases of enterovirus 71 have occurred worldwide, mostly in the Asia-Pacific region, with 2000 fatalities.[36] The virus presents with myoclonus, ataxia, nystagmus, tremor, or neurogenic pulmonary edema mimicking acute myocarditis. Opportunistic enteroviral meningoencephalitis has been reported in patients B-cell depleted from rituximab therapy.[37] Enterovirus is likely the second most common cause of rhombencephalitis, after *Listeria*, discussed later. Neurologic complications range from devastating brainstem encephalitis extending into the upper cervical cord to acute flaccid paralysis mimicking poliomyelitis to self-limited aseptic meningitis.

Respiratory Syncytial Virus

Cerebellar hemispheric cortical edema in the context of an acute respiratory illness has been reported in a young child with positive respiratory syncytial virus (RSV) negative for influenza A and B and enterovirus. Symptoms progressed rapidly to ataxia, hypotonia, and mutism. Symmetric DWI restriction was seen in the middle cerebellar peduncles and right dentate nucleus without contrast enhancement or supratentorial abnormalities. Five days of methylprednisolone led to complete MRI and clinical resolution.[38]

BACTERIAL INFECTIONS OF THE CEREBELLUM

Any bacterial infection that causes meningoencephalitis can produce cerebellar signs and symptoms. *Salmonella* species and other enteric fevers have been associated with a delayed cerebellar syndrome with mild CSF pleocytosis and good clinical outcomes.[39] *Mycoplasma pneumoniae* has also been associated with a cerebellar syndrome during or just after the acute phase of the illness.

LISTERIA MONOCYTOGENES AND RHOMBENCEPHALITIS

Of all the bacterial infections, this is the most important to recognize clinically and radiographically, as early treatment is lifesaving. Rhombencephalitis (RE) is a syndrome of multiple causes and disparate outcomes. Most clinicians use the terms *rhombencephalitis* and *brainstem encephalitis* interchangeably even though anatomically they connote slight differences. *Listeria* is the most common cause of infectious RE. *Listeria* RE occurs in healthy young adults, whereas immunocompromised patients have a less specific meningoencephalitic picture with or without multiple parenchymal abscesses. Food exposures include contaminated soft cheeses, delicatessen meats, and cantaloupe.

A biphasic clinical course with a flulike syndrome followed by brainstem dysfunction is typical; 75% of patients have CSF pleocytosis. Most patients have cranial neuropathies (VII and VI being the most common), and more than half have cerebellar signs. Almost 100% have an abnormal brain MRI scan that is very suggestive with fluid-attenuated inversion recovery (FLAIR) abnormalities in the dorsal pons and middle cerebellar peduncles as well as ring-enhancing abscesses in the posterior fossa (**Fig. 5**). Ampicillin is the treatment of choice.

After enteroviruses, herpes simplex virus (HSV) is the third most common infectious cause of RE (or brainstem encephalitis); about 80% of cases are caused by HSV1 and 20% by HSV2. About 50% only had involvement of the brainstem, whereas the other 50% also had supratentorial involvement of the temporal and frontal lobes. Other causes of similar brainstem syndromes are Behçet disease and MA2 paraneoplastic syndrome. Because *Listeria* and HSV are the most common treatable acute causes of RE, it is imperative to begin empiric therapy with ampicillin and acyclovir while cultures for *Listeria* and PCR for HSV are pending.[40]

FUNGAL INFECTIONS AFFECTING THE POSTERIOR FOSSA

Several fungi have a predilection for posterior fossa invasive parenchymal disease. In particular, angioinvasive *Aspergillus* species assume this pattern. Awareness of fungal infections was heightened in mid 2012 when cases of fungal-contaminated compounded methylprednisolone distributed by one New England facility were reported.

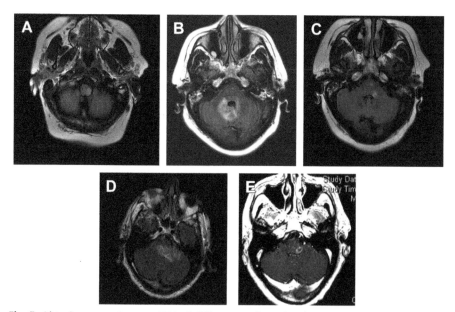

Fig. 5. *Listeria monocytogenes* RE in 2 different patients (*A–C*). FLAIR images showing scattered hyperintensities in pons and cerebellum (*D, E*). FLAIR image (*D*) and T1 with gadolinium enhancement (*E*) shows characteristic ring-enhancing pattern of an abscess.

As of mid 2013, more than 760 patients from 20 US states have developed meningitis or paraspinal infection with several dozen deaths.[41] Although the index case had *Aspergillus*, subsequent cases were caused by *Exserohilum rostratum*, a fungal pathogen not previously associated with human disease. Stroke caused by epidurally injected fungal pathogens usually involves the posterior circulation territory (**Fig. 6**).[42] Neutrophilic meningitis, vasculitis, and mycotic aneurysm formation characterize *Aspergillus* and other invasive fungal infections.

PRION-ASSOCIATED CEREBELLAR DISEASE
Creutzfeldt-Jakob Disease

Transmissible spongiform encephalopathies are invariably fatal illnesses that should be suspected in the setting of rapid cognitive decline often with gait and balance problems emerging early in the patients' course. However, about 38% of patients referred to one major center for prion disease testing had a nonprion-related condition.[43] In another center, treatable disorders misdiagnosed as Creutzfeldt-Jakob disease (CJD) amounted to nearly 7% of brain autopsies. Conversely, in a recent study of misdiagnosis of patients with sporadic CJD, diagnosis was quite delayed, with a mean time from onset to diagnosis of nearly 8 months.[44] Cerebellar symptoms were present in more than a quarter of the potentially treatable cases. Several recent cases of antivoltage gated potassium channel complex antibodies mimicking CJD have led

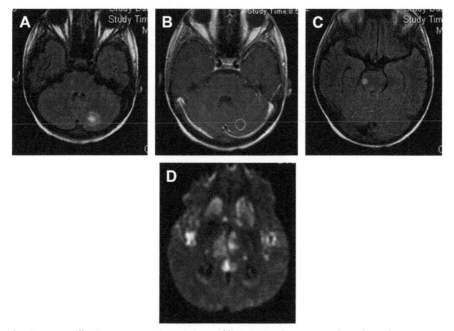

Fig. 6. *Aspergillus* in neutropenic recipient of liver transplant 1 month earlier. The posterior fossa is a favored site for this angioinvasive fungus that can cause hemorrhagic vasculitis and cerebral aneurysm. The image illustrates several features of this angioinvasive fungus: (*A*) Axial FLAIR shows hyperintensity in left cerebellum with ring enhances on gadolinium study. (*B, C*) FLAIR shows brainstem hyperintensity, likely another abscess, and also demonstrates sulcal hyperintensity in the posterior fossa suggestive of elevated protein, blood, or infection. (*D*) DWI MRI shows thalamic, basal ganglia, and corpus callosum areas of cytotoxic edema consistent with infarction.

to the recommendation that patients with suspected CJD be tested for these potentially suppressible autoantibodies.[45,46]

POSTINFECTIOUS SYNDROMES
Acute Postinfectious Cerebellar Ataxia

APCA is a sudden, pure cerebellar dysfunction that occurs mostly in children, typically some 10 to 15 days after a viral upper respiratory of gastrointestinal febrile illness.[47] Cerebellar ataxia of subacute onset with CSF pleocytosis is variously described as parainfectious, postinfectious, or postvaccinal. Fever and meningeal irritation may accompany nausea, headache, and acute onset of cerebellar symptoms. In young children, the most common preceding infection is varicella, whereas, in older children and young adults, infectious mononucleosis is the most commonly identified antecedent pathogen (see earlier EBV discussion).[48] Multiple other organisms have been implicated, including Mycoplasma, rotavirus, mumps, rubella, influenza, and VZV.[49] There is no clinical or radiographic evidence of demyelination or, if biopsy is obtained, of perivenular inflammatory changes, distinguishing the process from acute disseminated encephalomyelitis (ADEM). ADEM is typically more widespread, whereas, with acute peri-infectious cerebellar ataxia, the typical MRI appearance is confined to bilateral cerebellar hemispheric cortical edema and T2/FLAIR hyperintensity. Leptomeningeal enhancement along the cerebellar folia is often present. Involvement of the middle cerebellar peduncles and deep cerebellar nuclei has been reported with rotavirus encephalitis but is not etiologically specific.[50] At times, patients will have reversible splenial T2/FLAIR abnormalities.[51] In older patients, such a subacute cerebellar syndrome may suggest paraneoplastic process (see differential diagnosis section earlier in this article). New syndromes continue to be defined from cases previously thought to be idiopathic or postinfectious, and these should be recognized by neurologic consultants. Dalmau and colleagues recently have reported a series of teenagers and young adults with teratoma who are NMDAR antibody negative and have lower brainstem/cerebellar encephalitis with opsoclonus-myoclonus who respond to immunosuppressive therapies.[52]

REFERENCES

1. Sawaishi Y, Takada G. Acute cerebellitis. Cerebellum 2002;1:223–8.
2. Schmahmann JD, Weilburg JB, Sherman BC. The neuropsychiatry of the cerebellum- insights from the clinic. Cerebellum 2007;6:254–67.
3. Morales Odia Y, Minka M, Ziai WC. Severe leukoencephalopathy following acute oxycodone intoxication. Neurocrit Care 2010;13:93–7.
4. Jan W, Zimmerman RA, Wang ZJ, et al. MR diffusion imaging and MR spectroscopy of maple syrup urine disease during acute metabolic decompensation. Neuroradiology 2003;45:393–9.
5. Pittock SJ, Debruyne J, Krecke KN, et al. Chronic lymphocytic inflammation with pontine perivascular enhancement responsive to steroids (CLIPPERS). Brain 2010;133:2626–34.
6. Limousin N, Praline J, Motica O, et al. Brain biopsy is required in steroid-resistant patients with chronic lymphocytic inflammation with pontine perivascular enhancement responsive to steroids (CLIPPERS). J Neurooncol 2012;107:223–4.
7. Ortega MR, Usmani N, Parra-Herran C, et al. CLIPPERS complicating multiple sclerosis causing concerns of CNS lymphoma. Neurology 2012;79:715–6.

8. Marignier R, Chenevier Rf, Roegemond V, et al. Metabotropic glutamate receptor type 1 autoantibody-associated cerebellitis: a primary autoimmune disease? Arch Neurol 2010;67(5):627–30.
9. Becker EB, Zuliani L, Pettingill R, et al. Contactin-associated protein-2 antibodies in non-paraneoplastic cerebellar ataxia. J Neurol Neurosurg Psychiatry 2012;83(4):437–40.
10. Hoftberger R, Sabater L, Ortega A, et al. Patient with Homer-3 antibodies and cerebellitis. JAMA Neurol 2013;70(4):506–9.
11. Zuliani L, Sabater L, Saiz A, et al. Homer 3 autoimmunity in subacute idiopathic cerebellar ataxia. Neurology 2007;68(3):239–40.
12. Karmon Y, Inbar E, Cordoba M, et al. Paraneoplastic cerebellar degeneration mimicking acute post-infectious cerebellitis. Cerebellum 2009;8:441–4.
13. Gupta R, Maralani PJ, Chawla S, et al. Advanced neuroimaging findings of pseudotumoral hemicerebellitis in an elderly male required surgical decompression. J Neurosurg 2014;120:522–7.
14. Flanagan EP, Rabinstein AA, Kumar N, et al. Fulminant cerebellitis with radiological recurrence in an adult patient with Crohn's disease. J Neurol Sci 2014;336: 247–50.
15. Cho-Park YA, Perez DL, Milian TA, et al. Radiographic evolution of a rapidly reversible leukoencephalopathy due to metronidazole. Neurol Clin Pract 2013; 3:272–3.
16. Erdener SE, Kansu T, Arsava EM, et al. Brain MRI evolution of metronidazole intoxication. Neurology 2013;80:1816–7.
17. Hernandez Vega Y, Kaliakatsos M, U-King-Im JM, et al. Reversible vigabatrin-induced life-threatening encephalopathy. JAMA Neurol 2014;71:108–9.
18. Fushimi Y, Taki H, Kawai H, et al. Abnormal hyperintensity in cerebellar efferent pathways on diffusion-weighted imaging in a patient with heat stroke. Clin Radiol 2012;67:389–92.
19. Lee JS, Choi JC, Kang SY, et al. Heat stroke: increased signal intensity in the bilateral cerebellar dentate nuclei and splenium on diffusion-weighted MR imaging. AJNR Am J Neuroradiol 2009;30:E58.
20. Nagel MA, Gilden D. Complications of varicella zoster virus reactivation. Curr Treat Options Neurol 2013;15:439–53.
21. Calabria F, Zappini F, Vattemi G, et al. Pearls and Oy-sters: an unusual case of varicella-zoster virus cerebellitis and vasculopathy. Neurology 2014;82: e14–5.
22. Ratzka P, Schlachetzki JC, Bahr M, et al. Varicella zoster virus cerebellitis in a 66 year old patient without herpes zoster. Lancet 2006;367:182.
23. Moses H, Nagel MA, Gilden DH. Acute cerebellar ataxia in a 41 year old woman. Lancet Neurol 2006;5:984–8.
24. Withana M, Rodrigo C, Chang T, et al. Dengue fever presenting with acute cerebellitis: a case report. BMC Res Notes 2014;7:125–7.
25. Weeratunga PN, Caldera HP, Gooneratne IK, et al. Spontaneously resolving cerebellar syndrome as a sequela of dengue viral infection: a case series from Sri Lanka. Pract Neurol 2013;14(3):176–8.
26. De Santis P, Della Marca G, Di Lella G, et al. Subacute hydrocephalus in a patient with influenza A (H3N2) virus-related cerebellitis. J Neurol Neurosurg Psychiatry 2012;83:1091–2.
27. Gheuens S, Pierone G, Peeters P, et al. Progressive multifocal leukoencephalopathy in individuals with minimal or occult immunosuppression. J Neurol Neurosurg Psychiatry 2010;81:247–54.

28. Tan CS, Koralnik IJ. Progressive multifocal leukoencephalopathy and other disorders caused by JC virus: clinical features and pathogenesis. Lancet Neurol 2010;9:425–37.

29. Dang X, Vidal JE, Oliveria AC, et al. JC virus granule cell neuronopathy is associated with VP1 C terminus mutants. J Gen Virol 2012;93:175–83.

30. Dang L, Dang X, Koralnik I, et al. JC polyomavirus granule cell neuronopathy in a patient treated with rituximab. JAMA Neurol 2014;71(4):487–9.

31. Dang X, Koralnik IJ. Gone over to the dark side: natalizumab-associated JC virus infection of neurons in cerebellar gray matter. Ann Neurol 2014;4(4):503–5.

32. Berger JR, Aksamit AJ, Clifford DB, et al. PML diagnostic criteria: consensus statement from the AAN Neuroinfectious Disease Section. Neurology 2013;80: 1430–8.

33. Abul-Kasim K, Palm L, Maly P, et al. The neuroanatomic localization of Epstein-Barr virus encephalitis may be a predictive factor for its clinical outcome: a case report and review of 100 cases in 28 reports. J Child Neurol 2009;24:720–6.

34. Cho TA, Schmahmann JD, Cunnane ME. Case 30-2013: a 19 year old man with otalgia, slurred speech and ataxia. N Engl J Med 2013;369:1253–61.

35. Schmahmann JD. Plasmapheresis improves outcome in postinfectious cerebellitis induced by Epstein-Barr virus. Neurology 2004;62:443.

36. McMinn PC. Enterovirus vaccines for an emerging cause of brain-stem encephalitis. N Engl J Med 2014;370:792–3.

37. Ganjoo KN, Raman R, Sobel RA, et al. Opportunistic enteroviral meningoencephalitis: an unusual treatable complication of rituximab therapy. Leuk Lymphoma 2009;50:673–5.

38. Tang Y, Suddarth B, Du X, et al. Reversible diffusion restriction of the middle cerebellar peduncles and dentate nucleus in acute respiratory syncytial virus cerebellitis: a case report. Emerg Radiol 2014;21:89–92.

39. RIzek P, Morriello F, Sharma M, et al. Teaching NeuroImages: acute cerebellitis caused by Salmonella typhimurium. Neurology 2013;80:e118.

40. Jubelt B, Mihai C, Li TM, et al. Rhombencephalitis/brainstem encephalitis. Curr Neurol Neurosci Rep 2011;11:534–52.

41. Lahoti S, Berger JR. Iatrogenic fungal infections of the central nervous system. Curr Neurol Neurosci Rep 2013;13:399–408.

42. Kauffman CA, Pappas PG, Paterson TF. Fungal infections associated with contaminated methylprednisolone injections. N Engl J Med 2013;368(26): 2495–500.

43. Geschwind MD, Shu H, Haman A, et al. Rapidly progressive dementia. Ann Neurol 2008;64:97–108.

44. Patterson RW, Torres-Chac CC, Kuo AL, et al. Differential diagnosis of Jakob-Creutzfeldt disease. Arch Neurol 2012;69:1578–82.

45. Yoo JY, Hirsch LJ. Limbic encephalitis associated with anti voltage gated potassium channel complex antibodies mimicking Creutzfeldt-Jakob disease. JAMA Neurol 2014;71:79082.

46. Grau-Rivera O, Sanchez-Valle R, Saiz L, et al. Determination of neuronal antibodies in suspected and definite Creutzfeldt-Jakob disease. JAMA Neurol 2014;71:74–8.

47. Poretti A, Benson JE, Huisman TA, et al. Acute ataxia in children: approach to clinical presentation and role of additional investigations. Neuropediatrics 2012;44(3):127–41.

48. Klockgether T, Doller G, Wullner U, et al. Cerebellar encephalitis in adults. J Neurol 1993;240:17–20.

49. Desai J, Mitchell WG. Acute cerebellar ataxia, acute cerebellitis, and opsoclonus-myoclonus syndrome. J Child Neurol 2012;27:1482–8.
50. Takanashi J, Miyamoto T, Ando N, et al. Clinical and radiological features of rotavirus cerebellitis. AJNR Am J Neuroradiol 2010;3:1591–5.
51. Doherty MJ, Jayadev S, Watson NF, et al. Clinical implications of splenium magnetic resonance imaging signal changes. Arch Neurol 2005;62:433–7.
52. Armangue T, Titulaer MJ, Sabater L, et al. A novel treatment-responsive encephalitis with frequent opsoclonus and teratoma. Ann Neurol 2013;75(3):435–41.

Index

Note: Page numbers of article titles are in **boldface** type.

Neurol Clin 32 (2014) 1133–1148
http://dx.doi.org/10.1016/S0733-8619(14)00091-7
0733-8619/14/$ – see front matter © 2014 Elsevier Inc. All rights reserved.

neurologic.theclinics.com

United States Postal Service

Statement of Ownership, Management, and Circulation
(All Periodicals Publications Except Requestor Publications)

1. Publication Title	2. Publication Number	3. Filing Date
Neurologic Clinics	0 0 0 - 7 1 2	9/14/14

4. Issue Frequency	5. Number of Issues Published Annually	6. Annual Subscription Price
Feb, May, Aug, Nov	4	$300.00

7. Complete Mailing Address of Known Office of Publication (Not printer) (Street, city, county, state, and ZIP+4®)

Elsevier Inc.
360 Park Avenue South
New York, NY 10010-1710

Contact Person
Stephen R. Bushing

Telephone (Include area code)
215-239-3688

8. Complete Mailing Address of Headquarters or General Business Office of Publisher (Not printer)

Elsevier Inc., 360 Park Avenue South, New York, NY 10010-1710

9. Full Names and Complete Mailing Addresses of Publisher, Editor, and Managing Editor (Do not leave blank)

Publisher (Name and complete mailing address)

Linda Belfus, Elsevier Inc., 1600 John F. Kennedy Blvd., Suite 1800, Philadelphia, PA 19103-2899

Editor (Name and complete mailing address)

Joanne Husovski, Elsevier Inc., 1600 John F. Kennedy Blvd., Suite 1800, Philadelphia, PA 19103-2899

Managing Editor (Name and complete mailing address)

Adrianne Brigido, Elsevier Inc., 1600 John F. Kennedy Blvd., Suite 1800, Philadelphia, PA 19103-2899

10. Owner (Do not leave blank. If the publication is owned by a corporation, give the name and address of the corporation immediately followed by the names and addresses of all stockholders owning or holding 1 percent or more of the total amount of stock. If not owned by a corporation, give the names and addresses of the individual owners. If owned by a partnership or other unincorporated firm, give its name and address as well as those of each individual owner. If the publication is published by a nonprofit organization, give its name and address.)

Full Name	Complete Mailing Address
Wholly owned subsidiary of	1600 John F. Kennedy Blvd, Ste. 1800
Reed/Elsevier, US holdings	Philadelphia, PA 19103-2899

11. Known Bondholders, Mortgagees, and Other Security Holders Owning or Holding 1 Percent or More of Total Amount of Bonds, Mortgages, or Other Securities. If none, check box. ▶ ☐ None

Full Name	Complete Mailing Address
N/A	

12. Tax Status (For completion by nonprofit organizations authorized to mail at nonprofit rates) (Check one)
The purpose, function, and nonprofit status of this organization and the exempt status for federal income tax purposes:
☐ Has Not Changed During Preceding 12 Months
☐ Has Changed During Preceding 12 Months (Publisher must submit explanation of change with this statement)

PS Form 3526, August 2012 (Page 1 of 3 (Instructions Page 3)) PSN 7530-01-000-9931 PRIVACY NOTICE: See our Privacy policy in www.usps.com

13. Publication Title	14. Issue Date for Circulation Data Below
Neurologic Clinics	August 2014

15. Extent and Nature of Circulation		Average No. Copies Each Issue During Preceding 12 Months	No. Copies of Single Issue Published Nearest to Filing Date
a. Total Number of Copies (Net press run)		870	911
b. Paid Circulation (By Mail and Outside the Mail)	(1) Mailed Outside-County Paid Subscriptions Stated on PS Form 3541. (Include paid distribution above nominal rate, advertiser's proof copies, and exchange copies)	398	442
	(2) Mailed In-County Paid Subscriptions Stated on PS Form 3541 (Include paid distribution above nominal rate, advertiser's proof copies, and exchange copies)		
	(3) Paid Distribution Outside the Mails Including Sales Through Dealers and Carriers, Street Vendors, Counter Sales, and Other Paid Distribution Outside USPS®	155	167
	(4) Paid Distribution by Other Classes Mailed Through the USPS (e.g. First-Class Mail®)		
c. Total Paid Distribution (Sum of 15b (1), (2), (3), and (4))	▶	553	609
d. Free or Nominal Rate Distribution (By Mail and Outside the Mail)	(1) Free or Nominal Rate Outside-County Copies Included on PS Form 3541	106	88
	(2) Free or Nominal Rate In-County Copies Included on PS Form 3541		
	(3) Free or Nominal Rate Copies Mailed at Other Classes Through the USPS (e.g. First-Class Mail)		
	(4) Free or Nominal Rate Distribution Outside the Mail (Carriers or other means)		
e. Total Free or Nominal Rate Distribution (Sum of 15d (1), (2), (3) and (4))	▶	106	88
f. Total Distribution (Sum of 15c and 15e)	▶	659	697
g. Copies not Distributed (See instructions to publishers #4 (page #3))	▶	211	214
h. Total (Sum of 15f and g)	▶	870	911
i. Percent Paid (15c divided by 15f times 100)	▶	83.92%	87.37%

16. Total circulation includes electronic copies. Report circulation on PS Form 3526-X worksheet.

17. Publication of Statement of Ownership
If the publication is a general publication, publication of this statement is required. Will be printed in the November 2014 issue of this publication.

18. Signature and Title of Editor, Publisher, Business Manager, or Owner

Stephen R. Bushing

Stephen R. Bushing – Inventory Distribution Coordinator

Date
September 14, 2014

I certify that all information furnished on this form is true and complete. I understand that anyone who furnishes false or misleading information on this form or who omits material or information requested on the form may be subject to criminal sanctions (including fines and imprisonment) and/or civil sanctions (including civil penalties).

PS Form 3526, August 2012 (Page 2 of 3)

Moving?

Make sure your subscription moves with you!

To notify us of your new address, find your **Clinics Account Number** (located on your mailing label above your name), and contact customer service at:

Email: journalscustomerservice-usa@elsevier.com

800-654-2452 (subscribers in the U.S. & Canada)
314-447-8871 (subscribers outside of the U.S. & Canada)

Fax number: 314-447-8029

Elsevier Health Sciences Division
Subscription Customer Service
3251 Riverport Lane
Maryland Heights, MO 63043